THE CURRICULUM OF THE BODY AND THE SCHOOL AS CLINIC

This collection brings together cutting-edge research on the history of embodiment, health and schooling in an international context. The book distinguishes a set of educational technologies, schooling practices and school-based public health programmes that organise and influence the bodies of children and young people, defining the curriculum of the body.

Taking a historical approach, with a focus on the period in which mass schooling became an international phenomenon, the book is organised according to four major themes. The first positions the school as a modern clinical space, followed by the second that explores programmes and curricula which influence the discipline of and care for the body. The third section examines the role of the built environment on the organisation and experience of children's bodies, and the final section outlines the pedagogies, rules and routines that determine how the body is treated and experienced in school.

International and multidisciplinary in scope, this unique collection is of interest to postgraduate students and researchers in education and public health, as well as history, policy studies and sociology.

Kellie Burns is a historical sociologist at the University of Sydney interested in the intersections of gender, sexuality, health and schooling. Her research investigates the socio-historical role of schools as public health spaces across the late 19th and early 20th centuries, examining how ideas about childhood disease and health were constructed. She is also engaged in various projects about vaccination literacy and school-based vaccination clinics, historically and contemporaneously.

Helen Proctor is a professor of education at the University of Sydney, who uses historical methods and perspectives to examine the making of contemporary educational systems. She is interested in the history of how schools have shaped social and cultural life beyond the school gate, and how a range of relationships between schools, families and 'communities' have formed and changed from the late 19th to the early 21st centuries.

Critical Studies in Health and Education

Series Editors: Katie Fitzpatrick, Deana Leahy, Jan Wright, Jessica Fields, and Didier Jourdan

Critical Studies in Health and Education explores the sociological, critical and political approaches to health-related issues in education. The series underscores the discussions and debates surrounding the practice of health education and the development of solutions to the new ethical, practical, political and philosophical questions that are emerging within the field.

Creative Approaches to Health Education
New Ways of Thinking, Making, Doing, Teaching and Learning
Deborah Lupton and Deana Leahy

Teachers as Health Workers:
A Critical Understanding of the Health-Education Interface
Dr Louise McCuaig, Dr Eimear Enright, Professor Tony Rossi and Professor Doune Macdonald

School Food, Equity and Social Justice
Critical Reflections and Perspectives
Dorte Ruge, Irene Torres and Darren Powell

School Food Politics in Mexico
The Corporatization of Obesity and Healthy Eating Policies
José Tenorio

The Curriculum of the Body and the School as Clinic
Histories of Public Health and Schooling
Edited by Kellie Burns and Helen Proctor

THE CURRICULUM OF THE BODY AND THE SCHOOL AS CLINIC

Histories of Public Health and Schooling

Edited by Kellie Burns and Helen Proctor

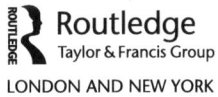
Routledge
Taylor & Francis Group

LONDON AND NEW YORK

Designed cover image: Lyle Fowler. (1936). Boys with polio taking lessons on outdoor verandah at Children's Orthopaedic Hospital, 33 Jacksons Road, Mt. Eliza. Harold Paynting collection, State Library Victoria.

First published 2024
by Routledge
4 Park Square, Milton Park, Abingdon, Oxon OX14 4RN

and by Routledge
605 Third Avenue, New York, NY 10158

Routledge is an imprint of the Taylor & Francis Group, an informa business

British Library Cataloguing-in-Publication Data
A catalogue record for this book is available from the British Library

ISBN: 978-1-032-26525-4 (hbk)
ISBN: 978-1-032-26523-0 (pbk)
ISBN: 978-1-003-28867-1 (ebk)

DOI: 10.4324/9781003288671

Typeset in Galliard
by MPS Limited, Dehradun

CONTENTS

CONTRIBUTORS

Karen E. Andreasen has a PhD in education and is an associate professor in education and pedagogical assessment in the Department of Culture and Learning at Aalborg University, Denmark.

Marta Brunelli is a professor in General and Social Education in the Department of Education, Cultural Heritage and Tourism Sciences at the University of Macerata, Italy.

Kellie Burns is a senior lecturer at the Sydney School of Education and Social Work at the University of Sydney, Australia.

Dale Allen Gyure is a professor of Architecture at Lawrence Technological University, USA.

Jim Harris is a senior lecturer in the Department of History at The Ohio State University, USA.

Felipe Hidalgo Kawada is a Chilean health sociologist currently working as a tutor and lecturer at the University of Sydney, Australia.

Frances Kelly is a senior lecturer in the School of Critical Studies in Education in the Faculty of Education and Social Work, Waipapa Taumata Rau/ University of Auckland, in Aotearoa New Zealand.

David Magro is a higher-degree research student in the Sydney School of Education and Social Work at the University of Sydney, Australia.

Jason L. Newton is an assistant teaching professor of American history at the University of North Carolina at Charlotte, USA.

Bethsaida Nieves is a visiting assistant professor of Latinx Studies at the University of Connecticut Storrs, USA.

Helen Proctor is a professor of Education History at the Sydney School of Education and Social Work at the University of Sydney, Australia.

Annette Rasmussen has a PhD in the sociology of education and is an associate professor at the Department of Culture and Learning at Aalborg University, Denmark.

Heloísa Helena Pimenta Rocha is a professor at the Faculty of Education, State University of Campinas (UNICAMP), Brazil and is a researcher at the Brazilian National Council for Scientific and Technological Development (CNPq).

Paolo Sanza is an assistant professor of architecture in the School of Architecture at Oklahoma State University, USA.

Henrique Mendonça da Silva is a professor at the Secretaria de Educação do Rio de Janeiro He holds a PhD in education from the State University of Campinas.

Ilektra Spandagou (She/her) (Gadigal land) is an associate professor of inclusive education at the Sydney School of Education and Social Work, University of Sydney, Australia.

Stella Meng Wang is a post-doctoral research fellow in the Department of Literature and Culture Studies at The Education University of Hong Kong, Hong Kong.

Heather Weaver is a cultural historian and research associate with the Sydney School of Education and Social Work at the University of Sydney, Australia.

ACKNOWLEDGEMENTS

We would first like to thank the Routledge Critical Studies in Health and Education Series Editors for their enthusiasm and encouragement around this project idea; mentioning in particular Deana Leahy for first suggesting we submit a proposal for their new series.

We are grateful to Vilija Stephens, Editor, Education and Behavioural Sciences, Routledge, Taylor & Francis Group for her support over the course of the book's writing and production, and to Georgia Oman, Editorial Assistant and Urvi Sharma, Project manager T & F Books Production.

We extend our heartfelt appreciation to the anonymous reviewers of our initial book proposal who provided good advice in going forward with the project.

Our colleague Heather Weaver edited this manuscript with tremendous care and commitment and worked with patience and expertise to advise and support chapter authors with their images.

We would like to acknowledge the University of Sydney and Australian Research Council funding awards that have supported our ongoing research and writing—both with separate projects and together. These include the University of Sydney Faculty of Education Program Grant (2013–15, Burns and Proctor), which initiated our decade-long collaboration on histories of health, bodies and schooling. Additionally, we mention here the University of Sydney's Faculty of Arts and Social Sciences Multidisciplinary Arts and Social Sciences Inaugural Fellowships (FASS MASSIF 2018, Burns); Sydney University Equity Prize (2023, Burns); Australian Research Council Future Fellowship (2015–2018, Proctor); and Australian Research Council Discovery Project award (2020–2024, Proctor—with co-investigators Jessica Gerrard and Susan Goodwin).

We are fortunate to have worked with supportive colleagues in a rich intellectual environment at the University of Sydney and for collegial conversations and responses to our papers at conferences such as the Australian Association for Research in Education, the Australian and New Zealand History of Education Society and the International Standing Committee for the History of Education.

We extend our gratitude to our wonderful array of authors—from five continents—who have shared their work in this collection, and also some two dozen colleagues around the world who reviewed the chapter drafts and offered brilliant feedback.

Kellie remains forever grateful for the love and support of her partner Kate Hansen and her two beautiful children Elliot and Jude.

Helen has benefited over many years from the boundless encouragement and good humour of Peter, Anna and Louisa.

INTRODUCTION

Bodies, health and schooling

Kellie Burns and Helen Proctor

In 1909, an eight-page article entitled 'Outline Scheme of Teaching Hygiene and Temperance' was featured in *The Public Instruction Gazette*, a monthly bulletin used to distribute circulars, instructions and departmental information to public school teachers across the Australian state of New South Wales. Published under the authority of the education minister, the piece provided detailed instructions around content and pedagogies to promote healthy conduct. The scheme of instruction listed a set of compartmentalised topics as related to 'the home', 'the person', 'eating and drinking' and 'illness', outlining the desired habits and rituals of personal and social conduct (p. 3). Hygiene was coupled with personal discipline, self-control and the observation of daily routines and rules. Students were to be taught punctuality and financial responsibility ('thrift') alongside keeping classrooms and homes clean and well ventilated. Likewise habits of personal cleanliness were coupled with a focus on maintaining good posture and the virtues of 'quiet speech, self-restraint and self-respect'. Detailed advice was given about how to appropriately teach hygiene and temperance to children at school according to age and stage. An overarching approach was that:

> hygiene should be so firmly pressed upon [children's] memories that they will never forget it. The rules of health impressed upon the children should therefore be few and direct, and as little as possible encumbered with technicalities or quasi-scientific expositions; indeed didactic teaching is necessary in this subject.
> (Minister for Public Instruction, 1909, p. 3)

This piece, one of many such materials in the historical records of public elementary schooling, offers a glimpse into the importance of the body in school pedagogies, routines and rituals at the turn of the 20th century and

DOI: 10.4324/9781003288671-1

highlights the role of the teacher in the management of potential contagions as well as the formation of healthy routines and habits. Moreover, it offers an illustration of how the expansive schools and school systems established by the state in 19th century Australia (and in many other places too) were intended neither merely to reflect current social values nor simply to teach reading, writing and arithmetic. Modern mass schooling was always a more ambitious project, aimed at shaping future citizens and their households—in mind and body (e.g. Campbell & Proctor, 2014, pp. iv–xvi; see also Kirk, 1998).

When the 1909 scheme of instruction for hygiene and temperance was circulated, public schooling was only a few decades old in Australia. Compulsory schooling had been promulgated in 1880 in the then colony of New South Wales and Australia had very recently become a Federation (this happened in 1901). Contemporary documents were full of essays and editorials about what this new Australian nationhood meant in terms of the purposes of mass schooling, even though public schools were governed by states rather than at the national level. Australia was often metaphorically depicted as a child in newspaper and magazine illustrations—full of promise, yet still vulnerable, and still learning. Both in Australia and internationally schools, in different ways in different historical periods and contexts, were key sites for the management of population health through hygiene curricula, school medical inspections and, from time to time, other programs such as mass vaccinations. Although schools were established to educate the masses, David Armstrong (1993) maintains, they 'also functioned as a laboratory in which the body of the child could be subjected to analysis, experimentation and transformation' (p. 402; see also Bakker, 2017; Gleason, 2005; Newman, 2022; Rocha & Silva, 2017). That these practices, in settler colonial Australia, produced, and upheld ideals of childhood health premised on White, western and middle-class models of Christian morality is both explicit and sub-textual in contemporary practices and documents (e.g. Browne, 1927; Horne & Sherington, 2013; Mackinnon & Proctor, 2013; Nakata, 2007; Sriprakash et al., 2022).

In the 1909 *Gazette's* syllabus, the teaching of temperance with hygiene is deemed more important for those children from 'poor homes', where it is assumed 'good habits' were not being taught or practised:

In the schools of prosperous neighbourhoods the parents will supply, or may be induced to supply, the practical training of good habits, for which the home is better equipped than the school. But in poor districts the school must endeavour in this particular, to supply the deficiencies of the home. Scholars who are not under good home influences must find at school the discipline of regular duties; without this it is almost hopeless to expect that children when they grow up will observe hygienic principles as part of the ordinary routine of life.

(Minister of Public Instruction, 1909, p. 3)

Parents, families and young people strategized around schools and schooling in complex ways and, as schooling credentials slowly became more important for employment and economic security, many found ways to navigate through the curriculum to find what was useful (e.g. Barron, 2022; Proctor & Weaver 2020). Nevertheless, whether viewed as official or unofficial curriculum, this example illustrates how the formulation of knowledge categories or curriculum subjectifies people—how it names, groups, separates, normalises and pathologizes the bodies and lives of schooling subjects—and how these are wedded to prevailing norms of class, gender, race, ability and locatedness. In the matter of schooling healthy child citizens, we are reminded of Alison Bashford's (2003) contention that lines of hygiene also produced boundaries of rule in many colonial and national contexts. Public health spaces, she argues, overlapped with other 'governmental line-making', including the making and maintaining of national borders, restricting immigration, and establishing and maintaining quarantine lines, 'racial cordons sanitaires and the segregative ambitions of a grafted eugenics and public health' (p. 1). All these, Bashford argues, 'produced identities of inclusion and exclusion, of belonging and citizenship, and of alien-ness' (p. 1).

In varied ways, the chapters assembled in this edited collection attend to the governmental line-making of schools and of school-based health interventions, asking what kinds of material and discursive effects these lines produce on the bodies of children, but also families and communities. The chapters represent original research from eighteen authors from five continents that in diverse though overlapping ways, promulgate the project of modern schooling as it was organised around the bodies of schoolchildren. The title of the collection, *The Curriculum of the Body and the School as Clinic*, extends our earlier thinking around two related concepts. First, 'the curriculum of the body'—a term we have used to encapsulate the multifarious educational technologies and discursive and material schooling practices that were enacted on or through the body (Burns et al., 2020; see also, Gleason, 2018; Rousmaniere & Sobe, 2018; Veiga, 2018). Second, the idea that schools can usefully be understood as 'clinical' spaces, in which health is addressed through teaching, through the management of bodies and spaces, and through health interventions such as publicly mandated screening and vaccination programs (Proctor & Burns, 2017; see also McCalman, 2009; Newman, 2022; Petrina, 2006).

The collection is organised into four thematic sections: (1) Clinical practices; (2) Programmes and policies; (3) Architecture and spatialities; and (4) Routines and disciplinary practices. The sections are not intended to demarcate distinct programs and practices and we acknowledge that the practices and effects of any kind of curriculum are always irregular, inconsistent and contested. The aim of grouping the chapters is to highlight common practices and overlapping discourses and, in some cases, to show the shared effects of schooling and public health interventions in seemingly divergent historical contexts, highlighting the role of key authorities, governmental norms and dominant bodies of knowledge in establishing normative ideas about both schooling and childhood health. The historical period in focus runs from the 19th to the 21st centuries, a time period when 'going to school' became the most common way of organising children's days and understanding their milestones—notwithstanding both formal and informal exclusions from these institutions on such grounds as race or disability. This era also marks a period of expansion in public health ideas and systems, and in the field of medicine, with infancy and childhood understood as important points of intervention in the making of healthy future populations. Schools, as the chapters in this collection show, were identified by governments and others as critical sites for shaping healthy attitudes and habits.

The three chapters in **Part 1**, **Clinical practices**, engage with the school as a temporary clinical space in which children's bodies were observed, diagnosed, categorised and pathologised from the 19th to mid-20th centuries in England, Brazil and Australia. They engage with the ways in which the projects of schooling and public health were associated with the modernisation of the state and its investments in the bodies of schoolchildren.

Jim Harris focuses on the provision of public health in English schools from 1875–1914, during the height of the British Empire, a time when the promotion of physical fitness and healthy development became important points of focus in public health. Children's bodies in schools were accessible to public scrutiny and could be subject to programmes enacted on their bodies in ways that were not possible via home and family. Harris considers how schools operated as sites for the collection of anthropometric data as a means of understanding British children's health and how school curricula and programmes were initially more narrowly focussed on disease control, before broadening out to aim at more ambitious goals of national population health.

Heloísa Helena Pimenta Rocha and **Henrique Mendonça da Silva** examine public debates about the creation of school hygiene clinics in the city of Rio de Janeiro in the first half of the 20th century. This chapter's authors focus on both the institutionalisation of this service and the practices for the treatment of detected diseases. Inspection work performed by physicians in schools reproduced the idea of schools as risky settings and produced new knowledge about children, their physical constitution, and childhood health and disease. Clinical practices in schools were legitimised through the publication of records and 'data' in public newspapers, government reports, and scientific journals.

Kellie Burns, Helen Proctor, Ilektra Spandagou and Heather Weaver explore the mediation of childhood polio in Australian media outlets in the 1920s–1950s. The authors locate the mid-20th century polio era within the broader context of an expanding welfare state, in which education, medicine and hospitals were positioned to manage the health of children with a combination of simple public health strategies (such as outdoor lessons), complex modern medical equipment (such as iron lungs) and, crucially, a positive attitudinal orientation to the future. Analysing a set of mass media images of cheerful children, with and without polio, the authors show how the bodily effects of the disease were often narrated as a deficit that could be overcome in order to achieve a 'promise of ablebodiedness'.

Part 2, Programmes and policies, collects four chapters which examine the design of syllabus and/or curriculum systems in the United States, newly US-annexed Puerto Rico, Denmark and Chile for various historical periods from the late 19th to the 21st centuries. In different ways, the chapters show how plans and proposals for system-level reform have responded to present concerns and anxieties—urban masculinity, race and colonialism, the role of women in a welfare state and childhood unfitness.

Jason L. Newtown examines the figure of 'physical culture' instructor and scientist Dudley Allen Sargent to explore how middle-class men in the late 19th- and early 20th-century US responded to anxieties about the emasculating effects of urbanisation by attempting to emulate an idealised version of the lifestyles and bodies of rural working-class men. Sargent's students literally copied the motions of workers in the gymnasium, performing exercises with names like 'Striking the Anvil', 'Driving Stakes' and 'Wood-Chopping' among others. As a teacher of physical educators, Sargent spread his ideas on the merits of the working class to teachers working in a range of educational institutions including schools across the United States.

Bethsaida Nieves addresses the connectedness of race, colonialism and schooling in Puerto Rico by describing how a normative Puerto Rican schoolchild was assembled as an object in need of reform through different kinds of authoritative public discourse during the first years of rule by the United States. The first part of Nieves' chapter explains how the assumption of a shared understanding of colonialist racial hierarchies was central to the questions asked and answered by informants during US Senate hearings on the administrative future of Puerto Rican institutions in 1900. The second part draws on a set of US-generated education documents which advocated the collection of racial data about schoolchildren and their teachers. As Nieves points out, reporting of this spurious quasi-scientific data opened a discursive space for correlating embodied race with educability, and the designing of education reforms based on that logic.

Annette Rasmussen and Karen E. Andreasen engage with home economics as a school subject in Denmark that was largely directed at girls and young women with the aim of contributing to family life. The home economics movement developed early in Denmark (1895 onwards) as both an educational subject and a professional field with its own curriculum, methods, textbooks and educational institutions. The authors read its broad and rapid expansion against the development of the Nordic welfare state, which, on the one hand, reduced the significance of the family and kinship relations in society, but on the other hand, promoted the nuclear family as a social norm, institutionalising patriarchal gender roles.

Felipe Hidalgo Kawada shifts the conversation to Chile, a nation recognised globally for pioneering neoliberal social and educational policies under the dictatorship of Augusto Pinochet (1973–1990). Hidalgo explores the introduction of a performative school market model comprising sophisticated control systems and accountability processes developed in the post-dictatorship period, analysing the deployment of a set of compulsory assessment tools for schools comprising comparative numerical ratings of health and wellness. He argues that tools of this kind represent a new phase in Chilean education and health policy where outcomes in both spheres are conjoined to produce population data that invisibilises social inequalities in both national health outcomes and schools.

In **Part 3, Architecture and spatialities,** four chapters examine how the built environment of schools was intended to, or operated to, influence or mandate certain kinds of movements and arrangements of bodies across space. The chapters, looking at cases from the 19th- to 20th-century US, Fascist Italy, early to mid-20th-century Hong Kong and 1940s New Zealand, respectively, offer a variety of perspectives on the relationships between bodies and rooms, rooms and buildings and the indoor and outdoor worlds of schooling and childhood.

Dale Allen Gyure examines architectural innovations to introduce more light and air into American classrooms in the early 20th century. The 'pavilion' classroom was envisioned with the aim of making students' bodies healthier and overcoming the health risks posed by the traditional 'closed box' classroom. The adoption of this design precipitated changes to internal classroom organisation, furniture design and novel approaches to teaching and learning. Gyure argues that while the non-directionality and flexibility available in pavilion classrooms constituted a generative environment for modern 'progressive' pedagogies, its roots were firmly planted in early-century health movements aimed at protecting young students' bodies from infectious diseases.

Paolo Sanza addresses the built environment of *colonie* summer camps for children, which were popular in Italy from the 1930s to the 1960s. The chapter examines the metamorphosis of the children's camps during the Fascist period, highlighting the regime's curriculum for sports, leisure and fascist indoctrination, while analysing some of the edifices that were specifically designed for this purpose by architects favoured and sponsored by the regime, and still survive. These structures, argues Sanza, are interesting for how they responded to the brief of fashioning spaces that could simultaneously educate, heal, facilitate play, foster friendship and conform to the regime's ideals. Such buildings, Sanza proposes, can be understood to exemplify architecture as a pedagogical machine.

Stella Meng Wang maps a detailed landscape of buildings, outdoor spaces and school timetables in Hong Kong during the early decades of the 20th century, considering how travelling colonial sanitary, medical and educational experts influenced the development of new health infrastructure for schoolchildren. She argues that architectural reform, hygiene education and medical inspection were most rigorously carried out in the state-sponsored English schools (English medium) that educated a multiracial, but predominantly Chinese middle-class cohort, while the poorer but much more populous vernacular Chinese schools were neglected despite being criticised by European inspectors for their unsanitary conditions.

Frances Kelly shifts the focus to late 1940s Aotearoa New Zealand when modernist design and social democratic town planning were heralded as means to ensure all members of society had access to well-designed housing, schools, recreation areas and opportunities for purposeful sociability. Kelly considers how core precepts of post-war town planning—which emphasised the distribution of spaces for active and virtuous forms of leisure—were taught to young New Zealanders through state-sponsored school publications which encouraged pupils to take responsibility for actively shaping the towns and communities they live in.

Part 4, Routines and disciplinary practices, focusses on classroom routines, learning practices, school regulations and the materials of instruction. It deals with the everyday noise of schooling. The three chapters, two from Australia and one from Italy, offer quite divergent examples, describing, respectively, a method for teaching gymnastics without special equipment, debates over proposals to ban corporal punishment, and the forms and purposes of school uniforms.

Marta Brunelli offers a fascinating example of the so-called 'gymnastics among the school desks', a means of increasing Italian schoolchildren's fitness in Italy by conducting physical fitness lessons in ordinary classrooms. She analyses how, despite hygienic and pedagogical criticisms by educators and hygienists, this practice existed in Italian schools for over a century, consolidating during the Fascist period (1922–1943), continuing in the post-war period and surviving until the 1960s. With its authoritarian approach, this practice helped to keep alive a traditional pedagogical vision of the pupil's body as an object of discipline. The practice also shaped the school experience and influenced the school culture of the time through a heavy, reciprocal conditioning between spaces, bodies and pedagogies.

Helen Proctor, Kellie Burns and David Magro describe how corporal punishment—the disciplining of unruly, mainly male, school students by hitting them with a cane or strap—became a hot topic of public debate in Australia during the 1980s, the last decade in which the practice was not only legal but apparently widespread. The chapter documents some of the activities of a nascent grassroots community group called Parents and Teachers Against Violence in Education (PTAVE) and considers how this longstanding, violent practice could, at this historical moment, animate public interest in how schools operated, and challenge the idea that schools were little worlds, sealed off from the outside.

In the final chapter of the collection, **Heather Weaver** examines mass-market texts and images of Australian children in school uniforms. Weaver uses the gendered and classed school uniform as a springboard for examining public responses and interpretations of attempts to 'modernise' school uniforms from the latter half of the century to the present. Newer looks such as sweatshirts, polo shirts and sunhats—worn by both boys and girls in public primary schools and comprehensive high schools—were often characterised by the media as 'modernising' older styles, conveying the suggestion that traditional single-sex school wear, still prevalent, was elitist and outmoded. The chapter also engages with representations of 'unisex' schooled bodies, including schoolgirls wearing trousers and schoolboys wearing skirts and dresses.

References

Armstrong, D. (1993). Public health spaces and the fabrication of identity. *Sociology*, *27*(3), 393–410.

Bakker, N. (2017). School medical inspection and the 'healthy' child in the Netherlands, 1904–1970. *History of Education Review*, *46*(2), 164–177.

Barron, H. (2022). *The social world of the school.* Manchester University Press.

Bashford, A. (2003). *Imperial hygiene: A critical history of colonialism, nationalism and public health.* Palgrave Macmillan. 10.1057/9780230508187

Browne, G. (1927). Introduction. In G.S. Browne (Ed.), *Education in Australia* (pp. vxii–xxi). Macmillan & Co.

Burns, K., Proctor, H., & Weaver, H. (2020). Modern schooling and the curriculum of the body. In T. Fitzgerald (Ed.), *Handbook of historical studies in education* (pp. 1–21). Springer. 10.1007/978-981-10-0942-6_34-1

Campbell, C., & Proctor, H. (2014). *A history of Australian schooling.* Allen & Unwin.

Gleason, M. (2005). Race, class, and health: School medical inspection and 'healthy' children in British Columbia, 1890–1930. In C.K. Warsh, & V. Strong-Boag (Eds.), *Children's health issues in historical perspective* (pp. 287–304). Wilfried Laurier University Press.

Gleason, M. (2018). Metaphor, materiality and method: The central role of embodiment in the history of education. *Paedagogica Historica*, *54*(1–2), 4–19. 10.1080/00309230.2017.1355328

Horne, J., & Sherington, G. (2013). Education. In A. Bashford & S. Macintyre (Eds.), *The Cambridge history of Australia: Volume 1: Indigenous and colonial Australia* (pp. 367–390). Cambridge University Press.

Kirk, D. (1998). *Schooling bodies: School practice and public discourse, 1880–1950.* Leicester University Press.

Mackinnon, A., & Proctor, H. (2013). Education. In A. Bashford, & S. Macintyre (Eds.), *The Cambridge history of Australia: Volume 2: The Commonwealth of Australia* (pp. 429–451). Cambridge University Press.

McCalman, J. (2009). Silent witnesses: Child health and well-being in England and Australia and the health transition, 1870–1940. *Health Sociology Review, 18*(1), 25–35. 10.5172/hesr.18.1.25

Nakata, M.N. (2007). *Disciplining the savages, savaging the disciplines.* Aboriginal Studies Press.

Newman, L. (2022). Bodies of knowledge: Historians, health and education, *History of Education.* 10.1080/0046760X.2022.2112767

NSW Minister of Public Instruction. (1909, January 30). Outline scheme for teaching hygiene and temperance. *The Public Instruction Gazette, 3*(1), 2–10.

Petrina, S. (2006). The medicalisation of education: A historiographic synthesis. *History of Education Quarterly, 46*(4), 503–531.

Proctor, H., & Burns, K. (2017). The connected histories of mass schooling and public health. *History of Education Review, 46*(2), 118–124.

Proctor, H., & Weaver, H. (2020). Family, community and sociability: 1920–present. In J. Harford & T. O'Donoghue (Eds.), *A cultural history of education in the modern age* (pp. 81–98). Bloomsbury Academic.

Rocha, H.H.P., & Silva, H.M. (2017). The dangers of infection: School medical inspection in Brazil (the 1910s). *History of Education Review, 46*(2), 150–163. 10.1108/HER-02-2016-0015

Rousmaniere, K., & Sobe, N.W. (2018). Education and the body: Introduction. *Paedagogica Historica, 54*(1–2), 1–3.

Sriprakash, A., Rudolph, S., & Gerrard, J. (2022). *Learning whiteness: Education and the settler colonial state.* Pluto Press.

Veiga, C. (2018). The body's civilisation/decivilisation: Emotional, social, and historical tensions. *Paedagogica Historica, 54*(1–2), 20–31. 10.1080/00309230.2017.1358290

PART 1
Clinical practices

1

RAISING A HEALTHY NATION

Provisioning public health in English schools, c. 1875–1914

Jim Harris

Williams and Mooney (1994) calculate that 78% of the English population lived in cities by the year 1901, up from roughly 50% in the middle of the 19th century. With this rise in urbanisation, the deleterious impacts of city life on the health of English citizens became an important matter for public health. Municipal sanitary reforms, whose origins Hardy (1993), Hamlin (1998) and Porter (1999) trace at least to the mid-19th century, sought to mitigate some of the 'damage' wrought by city life and were particularly effective at reducing the spread of infectious diseases. However, sanitary reforms alone were insufficient to improve the physical health of the many 'puny and ill-developed' English children, as the Scottish physician James Cantlie (1885) described them (p. 33), whose productive role in military and the political economy of the nation and empire had become a major focus of contemporary public health administrators' attention. Cantlie's language was extreme but still representative of upper- and middle-class nationalist fears about 'national efficiency' and the possibility of imperial decline vis-à-vis the other 'Great Powers' that in turn influenced efforts to 'improve' the lives of the working classes.

Protecting children's health required carefully managed public health interventions early on in life, but public health administrators often faced resistance to what Mooney (2015) has described as 'intrusive interventions' into the intimate aspects of English daily life, such as public health inspections and regulations inside the privacy of the home, which were frequently perceived as the act of an overreaching state apparatus. One way in which public health sought to bypass this resistance involved targeting children outside the home. As children grew into early childhood and left home for primary school education, they became more accessible to public health administrators. In turn, this allowed for more opportunities for medical interventions intended

DOI: 10.4324/9781003288671-3

to promote their healthy development without creating the perception of the state invading the privacy and intimacy of the house and home.

To demonstrate how English schools became increasingly embedded in expanding systems of public health, this chapter traces the history of public health in English schools from the mid-1870s, at which time public health efforts were still largely focused on disease control, through the first decades of the 20th century, when the role of public health became embroiled in the nationalist 'child saving' mission during the age of high imperialism. By the first decade of the 20th century, public health efforts in schools became increasingly proactive to ensure children were not only free from disease, but also properly nourished, growing up healthy and in a physical condition to benefit from their education, as contemporaries increasingly believed that the future of the nation and the empire hinged on their physical and bodily well-being. To borrow Armstrong's (1993) language, schools became a sort of 'laboratory' in which children were subject to 'analysis, experimentation and transformation' (p. 402). In schools, children were observed for signs of disease, and their health was *analysed* as they were routinely measured to ensure that neither disease, malnourishment, nor environmental hazards were adversely affecting their physical development into adolescence. In cases where children were found suffering, schools began to provide a space for *experimentation* with treatments ranging from the provision of free meals to simple clinical practices that would, in theory, *transform* them into a healthier future generation. All the while, because the children were under the public supervision of the Board of Education and Local Education Authorities while at school, this was believed to be less 'intrusive' than other aspects of public health.

Origins in infection control

The practice of promoting public health in English schools predates the 20th century, of course, and the origins of public health in schools were narrower in scope and focused on issues of contagion and disease control. As Burns et al. (2019) note, during the 19th century, the rise in mass schooling created new health risks as crowded public schools often became sites for the opportunistic spread of infectious diseases. Hirst (1991) adds that between 1848 and 1872, 'infectious diseases were the main cause of death among the school age population' averaging 412.8 deaths per 100,000 living (p. 108). Thus, beginning in 1851 Medical Officers of Health were permitted to enter and observe schools, at least for cases of smallpox, though they rarely did (Woodward, 1995).

By the 1870s, doctors increasingly adopted the (correct) conclusion that overcrowded, unventilated schools, often with defective plumbing, were prime sites for infectious diseases to spread. In 1875, *The Lancet* established a

Commission on the Sanitary Condition of Public Schools that forcefully argued for the importance of sanitary reforms in schools. It offered suggestions with regards to hygiene, temperature, ventilation and waste removal from classrooms (and dormitories) to reduce students' exposure to infectious diseases (Report of the Lancet Sanitary Commission, 1875). Hirst (1991) adds that beginning in 1876, Medical Officers of Health called for legislation that barred infected children from attending schools to avoid an outbreak of common childhood diseases (like diphtheria, measles and scarlet fever). However, the implementation of many of these reforms proved too costly for many local education authorities to bear. By the year 1880, when Parliament enacted free and compulsory primary education nationwide, medical authorities largely accepted that schools created a high-risk site for exposure to infectious diseases, while still debating the best course of action to prevent outbreaks in schools.

Building a coordinated system in which schools became connected with larger municipal public health efforts remained difficult for several reasons. First, even though the 1875 Public Health Act obligated teachers to notify the health department of suspected cases of infectious diseases among their students, individual cases often went unnoticed, especially as class sizes grew. Second, medically untrained teachers often made 'diagnostic' mistakes. Third, school boards often impeded rather than aided municipal Medical Officers of Health from working with teachers to identify infections within schools, issuing their own regulations to teachers on health matters (Mooney, 2015).

Once a system was established to identify cases of children with disease, medical authorities sought to establish a means of mitigating an outbreak within schools. Developing such a process also proved difficult, and, initially, put school officials at odds with municipal public health administrators. Under Local Government Board policy, a student who was diagnosed with an infectious disease could be barred from school until cleared by medical examination. This was highly contentious. In small, poorly ventilated, working-class homes, it was nearly impossible to isolate a sick child, meaning that if one child contracted a disease, then the entire family likely needed to be barred from attendance at school until the course of infection passed. In the event of a larger outbreak within a school, a common practice was to simply close the entire school. But this practice was rarely effective in stopping a highly transmissible disease like measles, which became infectious among close contacts before cases became visibly identifiable by the tell-tale rash, and thus could easily spread throughout a school before the first cases were even clearly identified. Thus, school closures were largely ineffectual at best in stopping disease outbreaks. In addition, school closures had serious financial consequences, as schools' funding (and teachers' salaries) were partially determined by attendance (Mooney, 2015). Educators often concealed outbreaks rather than reporting them to the municipal health authorities, which, according to

Hirst (1991) created no shortage of animosity between educational and sanitary authorities. Municipal Medical Officers of Health understood these difficulties associated with school closures, but nevertheless generally supported the practice.

The city of Manchester provides a useful case study. During an 1898 outbreak of measles, Medical Officer of Health James Niven (1899, pp. 88–89) praised the School Board for providing his office with a daily list of cases, which allowed for 'prompter action' to ensure isolation of the patients and better charting of the course of the outbreak. At the same time, Niven was aware of the 'heavy responsibility' upon his office, and the difficult choice he had to make in ordering the closure of schools. Niven concluded that the benefits of delaying and slowing the course of an outbreak of measles by closing schools outweighed the costs. The School Board disagreed, strenuously, when Manchester faced another epidemic of measles that was 'more violent than ever' (killing 699 and infecting 13,980 children) the following year, which forced many children's services to close, including schools. Niven (1900, pp. 78–83) insisted that 'prompt action' must be taken when the presence of measles became apparent in schools. Teachers were asked to report cases directly to the Health Authorities. But this often happened too late, as measles is most infectious in its pre-symptomatic stage, making detection difficult. Thus, even when cases were reported diligently by teachers, reports often came too late to stop an outbreak within a school, and so school closures seemed necessary.

This animosity between school and municipal public health authorities was not relieved until a reform to the Education Code (Article 101) in 1892 created an important exception to the reduction in schools' funding due to low attendance if reduced attendance resulted from an order from the Sanitary Authorities. This made school officials much more amenable to cooperation. However, when Article 101 was revoked in 1903, this financial uncertainty briefly reemerged, until the practice of whole-school closures began to fall out of favour during the first decade of the 20th century, such that Kerr (1916) declared school closures 'as obsolete as quarantine'. He argued that their effect on stopping the spread of measles 'was quite illusory' because a student became infectious days before the rash appeared (pp. 248–249). Instead, he encouraged the more targeted practice of individual pupil exclusion, measured by immune status (since second cases of measles were rare). The Board of Education agreed that 'the prompt exclusion of individual children' was a better course of action in disease prevention and would cause the 'least amount of interference with the education of the majority of the children in a school' (Mooney, 2015, p. 112).

So, to summarise, divisions and tensions characterised the relationship between school authorities and municipal public health administrators until the 1890s when, Hirst (1991) reports, a 'more co-operative, even collaborative approach began to emerge' in many municipalities as both understandings of disease aetiology and educational and public health policy changed (p. 113). I would suggest that this softening resulted from a growing acceptance of a contagionist theory that 'placed less emphasis on the need to control the school, and more on the need to isolate individual cases' (Hirst, 1991, p. 114). This emphasis on the individual also increased working-class willingness to accept more public health interventions, though access to the home was still met with a high degree of resistance. As school administrators became more willing to work with municipal public health administrators towards the common goal of preventing a disease outbreak in schools, we then see the first layers of a foundation for raising a healthy nation being laid in English schools by the 1890s.

In addition, in 1890 W.R. Smith was appointed as the first School Medical Officer, in London. His position was only part-time, and his primary responsibility was to provide medical guidance on the ventilation and sanitation of the school. Other towns followed suit. Bradford was the first town to appoint a full-time School Medical Officer, James Kerr, in 1893. Unlike Smith, Kerr was responsible for examining students, looking for signs of infection (Newman, 1939; Woodward, 1995). Also beginning in the 1890s, doctors urged school officials to be methodical in their record-keeping of case histories, absences and presence of diseased children, as well as greater cooperation between school medical authorities and parents (Mooney, 2015, pp. 96–98). At roughly the same time, growing sales of medical textbooks like Arthur Newsholme's *School Hygiene* (first published in 1887) further illustrated a growing belief that schools must be healthy environments for students.

In some ways, as the Scottish physicians and medical examiners Mackenzie and Matthew (1904) argued in their popular textbook *The Medical Inspection of School Children*, concerns about infectious diseases 'played an enormous, perhaps an exaggerated part' in shaping medical examination in schools, but it is indisputable that concerns about diseases in schools established a relationship between municipal public health and educational authorities (p. 2). As this relationship developed, school-aged children were subjected to other types of medical examinations and interventions. However, the process of integrating public health into schools in a regular and systematic manner remained a slow and gradual process that would not be fully formalised until the establishment of the School Medical Service in 1907, which we will return to at the end of this chapter.

Expansion: Monitoring for malnutrition and school meals for public health

As English medical personnel began working with and directly in schools in the last decade of the 19th century, they began to not only monitor for infectious diseases but other indicators of poor health as well. Doctors encouraged careful monitoring of the height, weight, teeth, eyesight, hearing and skin of schoolchildren as metrics for physical and mental well-being (Woodward, 1995, p. 132). In 1904, the Inter-departmental Committee on Physical Deterioration (1904), which was tasked with surveying the physical condition of the population at large, asserted that 'a systematized medical inspection should be imposed as a public duty on every school authority' (p. 65). By 1907, as Dwork (1987) makes clear, inspections had become commonplace in English schools. These inspections were not merely attempts to tabulate statistics on average heights and weights but to identify the nearly one-fifth of schoolchildren in need of intervention to ensure their healthy development.

Like concerns about infectious diseases spreading in schools, concerns about the condition of children's physical and bodily health also emerged in public health discourse during the last decades of the 19th century. *The British Medical Journal* warned that if a child was 'pale and feeble and depressed, badly fed and clothed and housed, and surrounded by all the most depressing influences of sanitary neglect', extended school days would do more harm than good to their 'badly nourished brains' (Educational Pressure, 1880, p. 892). J. Milner Forthergill (1889) lamented that driving 'children like a flock of sheep, through a certain series of examinations' while they were in poor health and malnourished did more harm than good and feared that 'a system of education, which kills off the weak children, is [of] doubtful advantage' (pp. 92–93).

Concerns about malnutrition garnered special attention in these discussions. An 1889 study conducted by the British Medical Association found that 43,000 children in London board schools were 'inadequately fed', and this was stunting growth and inhibiting mental capacity for education (Feeding the Hungry Children, 1889). According to Frances Warner (1892) of the London Hospital, malnourished children were visibly 'thin, pale or delicate-looking' (p. 538). Warner suggested that determining the severity of a child's malnourishment required physical examination of the limbs and torso as well as the face. Abnormalities in cranial development (21 inches in circumference at age seven was considered average), spinal development (measured by the curvature of the spine and symmetry of the head balance) or nervous defect (such as eye twitches or hand imbalance) all potentially indicated malnourishment. Yet, despite vivid reports of sickly, malnourished children, many contemporaries believed that providing meals to these starving children was 'an unnecessary intrusion on the responsibilities of parents' (Welshman, 1997, p. 7).

By the first decade of the 20th century, concerns about the physical condition of school-age children became more pronounced amid growing fears of national and imperial 'degeneration'. One commentator wrote in *The British Medical Journal* that there 'can be little doubt that one of the chief causes of this degeneracy in young people is to be found in the insufficient food on which it seems to be expected that the hard work of school life should be performed'. They insisted that schools should provide a diet that was 'good for boys' so that they might 'reach the highest possible physical and mental development' (The Food Factor in Education, 1903, p. 424). James Kerr (1916), the first full-time school medical officer, went even further, arguing that 'if the food supply is scanty ... growth will be impeded, and children will be stunted specimens of humanity' (p. 195). Under these circumstances, it appeared as though the importance of feeding these necessitous children began to outweigh concerns about 'intrusion' into the responsibilities of parents.

Malnourished children were easily identifiable in schools where they were subject to regular observation, and this further reinforced the role schools could play in raising a healthy nation. Contemporaries generally agreed that schools could also be sites for direct interventions, including providing nourishing meals to children. One commentator in *The British Medical Journal* believed 'when those in control of the school are directly responsible for the feeding of the children ... there is no excuse for the diet being other than sufficient in quantity and suitable in quality' (The Food Factor in Education, 1903). In 1904, the *Report of the Inter-departmental Committee on Physical Deterioration* (1904) made clear that a substantial population of school-aged children were malnourished, and the committee urged schools to serve reduced-cost meals in a systematic way so that the diets of malnourished children could carefully regulated, unlike in meals taken at home (Davin, 1996). That same year, James Kerr, along with school board member Margaret McMillan and city councillor Fred Jowett, introduced the first municipally funded programme for school meals in Bradford (Vernon, 2007).

A year later, the *Report of the Inter-departmental Committee on Medical Inspection and Feeding of Children Attending Public Elementary Schools* (1905) expanded on the need for systematic feeding of school-aged children. Tasked with determining which children should receive subsidised or free meals, the manner of serving them and what foodstuffs they should provide, the committee advised that a relief committee rather than teachers should select the children to receive meals; that permanent and regular feeding of those children most in need would do much greater good than feeding a larger number of children irregularly; that meals should be provided every school day and throughout the year; and meals should be properly served to train in both manners and suitably prepared food.

In 1906, W.T. Wilson and Thomas Macnamara introduced the 1906 Education (Provision of Meals) Act into Parliament, which allowed public elementary schools to provision meals to the pupils—and either recover the costs by billing the parents or with public funds from the Board of Education. According to Vernon (2007), the voluntary nature of the Act made it attractive across political lines. To appease conservative dissenters, Chief Medical Officer of the Board of Education George Newman (1939) explained in his memoirs that the Board of Education programme for feeding schoolchildren aimed only to supplement at-home feeding of the children, but above all else to ensure that the child received 'sufficient and stable food'. To Newman, the provision of school meals was not an act of an overreaching state, but a supplement to home feeding to prevent 'disability, defect or weakness, physical or mental—threatening or actual—of the child's body' (pp. 332–333).

The school meals programme was not simply a new form of poor relief (although malnutrition was often the function of poverty); it was another major example of how schools became important sites of public health reform in the early 20th century as the provision of school meals to necessitous children did aid in their healthy development. However, the permissive nature of the Act made its adoption uneven across Great Britain before 1907. Thus, this important Act was not a permanent or absolute solution to the problem of malnutrition in English children. Rather, as Welshman (1997) notes, the 1906 Education (Provision of Meals) Act laid the foundation for further legislation later in the century, beginning with the expanded Education (Provision of Meals) Act of 1914, which expanded state funding for school meals, and even more far-reaching legislation in the 1940s that made the earlier permissive Acts compulsory.

Consolidation: The School Medical Service

Monitoring for infectious diseases linked schools with broader municipal public health efforts administered by the Medical Officers of Health. The provision of nourishing meals in schools further emphasised the importance of work schools could do to promote and improve children's health. But the irregularity of public health interventions in schools across English cities made further codification necessary. To this end, on 28 August 1907, Parliament passed the Education (Administrative Provisions) Act (1907), which empowered Local Education Authorities 'to provide for the medical inspection of children immediately before or at any time of, or as soon as possible after, their admission to public elementary school'. In addition, the Board of Education was obligated to 'make arrangements … for attending to the health and physical condition of the children educated in public elementary schools' for the duration of their education. According to Harris (2003), even conservative Members of Parliament like Sir William Anson supported this bill, because the physical condition of the schoolchild had been established as a matter of 'national importance' (p. 96). The following year, the School Medical Service was established to serve as an administrative centre for the medical inspection of school-aged Britons, and according to Mooney (2015) marked 'an important milestone in social welfare in Britain' (p. 114).

Passing this Act was another foundational moment in shaping the role the schools would play in a provisioning public health to English children in the early 20th century, but many problems remained unresolved with regards to the implementation and funding of school medical inspection. As Harris (1995) has argued, many questions arose about the process and scope of medical examinations: for example, should only sick children be inspected or should all children be inspected? Where would the inspections take place? Eventually, the Board of Education concluded that 'all children must periodically come into the hands of the doctor ... to enable every school child to take full advantage of the education provided for it by the State' (Newman, 1913, p. 194). The Board of Education directed school medical examiners to inspect children a minimum of three times: at the age of five, seven or eight, and ten. Doctors were also encouraged to provide a fourth examination at age 13 or 14 as the child was leaving primary school. Newman (1913) recalled that this was an enormous task, requiring the inspection of approximately two million children per year. Inspectors were required to address a list of eight questions, and to determine if the child was suffering from any type of physical deficiency that might inhibit his healthy development into adolescence and adulthood (pp. 199–200):

1 Has the child had any illness in the past which would be likely to affect his physical future?
2 What is the present condition of his body as regards cleanliness and nutrition?
3 Are his senses normal?
4 Has he sound or decayed teeth?
5 Are the throat and tonsils normal and healthy?
6 Is he normal and sound in mind?
7 Does he show any signs of disease or deformity (rickets, tubercle, rheumatism, rupture, glandular disease, ringworm, anaemia, epilepsy, psychoneurosis, etc.)?
8 Has he any weakness or defect unfitting him for ordinary life and physical exercise, or requiring any exemption from any branch or form of instruction?

The first few years of school inspections revealed that much work still had to be done to improve the health of English children. Despite improvements in hygiene and prevention of infectious diseases since the 1890s, Newman (1913) reported that three 'morbid conditions' still afflicted enormous numbers of children: upwards of 70% of children suffered some form of dental decay; at least 120,000 children needed 'prompt treatment annually' for defects of vision and diseases of the eye; and another 95,000 cases of diseases of the ear, nose and throat that required annual attention (p. 203). Other conditions afflicting the school child included skin diseases, tuberculosis, rickets, nervous maladies, malnutrition, rheumatic fever and common infectious diseases (measles, whooping cough, scarlet fever and diphtheria). The outcome of these early inspections conducted by the School Medical Service provided doctors with a more thorough 'knowledge of the physical and mental condition of the school-child population of Britain' (Newman, 1913, pp. 208–209), which in turn helped bring about more careful attention to the threats to the health of children and further efforts to provide individualised treatments to necessitous children.

The formation of the School Medical Service not only established a clear responsibility for schools within growing networks of public health, but also gradually gave rise to the formation of the school as a clinical space. Under the new 1907 Education (Administrative Provisions) Act, medical inspections were mandatory, but the Act also granted permissive powers to schools to provide treatment for childhood ailments or physical defects. Some Local Education Authorities exercised this optional power, developing quite elaborate school clinics. In 1908, there were just seven school clinics across England and Wales, but by the outbreak of the First World War, this number had risen to 179 (Hirst, 1989).

School Medical Officers justified the need to offer treatment in schools lamenting the high rates of 'defects' among students and even greater concern about parents' inability to act upon the child's condition, which often resulted from unavailability or inaccessibility of necessary remedies or access to hospitals. With low treatment rates outside of schools, reformers ranging from socialists to trade unionists also urged the Local Education Authorities to provide treatments inside the school for diseased and disabled children. Bradford schools established a model for other municipalities to follow in expanding the services provided by the School Medical Service: from solely a site for observation and diagnosis, into a clinical space that offered basic treatments for ear and skin diseases, defective eyes and teeth, and cases of ringworm, all of which Hendrick (1994) notes, were not mandatory but permissive under the 1907 Act. As Hirst (1989) further notes, providing treatment also benefited the schools themselves, as absences continued to cost schools funding after the repeal of Article 101. As a result of this pressure, a handful of local education authorities saw value in providing treatments in schools (including the provision of glasses, dental care, adenoid and tonsil removal and the use of X-rays to eliminate ringworm) and began to establish clinics for treatment directly in schools, rather than solely collecting diagnosis and then referring students to a hospital that they often did not attend.

In offering these simple treatments, and by blurring 'the boundaries between preventative and curative medicine' (Mooney, 2015, p. 215), School

Medical Services was generally effective in providing affordable and accessible treatments to children and became a significant partner in promoting public health in early 20th-century England. But, in establishing sites for treatment, school medical officials temporarily once again put themselves at odds with other systems of public health. Newman (1908, as cited in Hirst, 1989), initially argued that schools should 'point out defects and disease and ... leave treatment as far as possible to the ordinary channels' (p. 326). But when the position of the School Medical Officer was frequently a duty assigned to the municipal Medical Officer of Health (or one of their deputies), this tension between municipal and school-sponsored public health often subsided.

Conclusions and legacies

According to George Newman (1926), who served as the Chief Medical Officer for the Board of Education from 1907 to 1919 and then Chief Medical Officer to the Ministry of Health from 1919 to 1935, 'the health of the child is the foundation of the national health' (p. 70). This commonly held belief shaped the ways schools became an important partner in public health. Schools offered public health officials a physical environment in which they could monitor children's health to ensure that they were growing up healthy and fit amid fears of national 'degeneration' around the turn of the 20th century, while avoiding concerns about public health becoming overly 'intrusive'. But this was only possible if school officials were willing to partner with municipal public health authorities.

This chapter has sought to lay out some of the ways that a partnership between school authorities and municipal public health authorities emerged in England from the late Victorian and early Edwardian years as schools became important places for provisioning public health. Both school and public health authorities were both keenly aware of the importance of children's health, but forming a public health partnership was not without its hurdles. Much like the broader history of public health, the origins of this partnership were rooted in efforts to protect children from dangerous infectious diseases that often spread inside schools, but the financial consequences of school closures due to disease outbreaks created tensions that inhibited an early partnership. By the early 20th century, though, as public health efforts became increasingly proactive and especially focused on children as this 'foundation of the national health', the relationship between schools and municipal public health began to grow closer. As public health officials became increasingly focused on proactive measures aimed at raising a healthy nation, partnering with schools as important sites for interventions became increasingly important. Providing nutritious meals, a potentially 'intrusive' act, became possible in schools and expanded the ways public health could improve the healthy development of the 'puny' children that Cantlie and others feared. This expansion gave way to further roles for schools to play after the passage of the 1907 Education Act. The data collected by periodic monitoring of children in schools equipped public health officials with more precise knowledge of the conditions and ailments of English children, and in turn created the opportunities for more targeted treatments at a critical developmental juncture in the child's life. Thus, by 1914, English schools had become an important partner in public health campaigns.

As a final thought, it should also be noted that the formation of the School Medical Service and its growth before the First World War is not an endpoint but rather an origin story. The role of schools as sites of public health would continue to grow and expand throughout the first half of the 20th century. By the mid-century, for example, the Education Act (1944) would greatly expand state authority over education by reconstituting the Board of Education as the Ministry of Education, mandating that local education authorities must provide school meals and milk in the case of hardship, provide compulsory medical inspection for all children ages two to 15 (a much-widened age range), and also greatly expand the free medical and dental treatments that Local Education Authorities were expected to provide through the School Medical Service (Hendrick, 1994).

References

Armstrong, D. (1993). Public health spaces and the fabrication of identity. *Sociology*, *27*(3), 393–410.

Burns, K., Proctor H., & Weaver, H. (2019). Modern schooling and the curriculum of the body. In T. Fitzgerald (Ed.), *Handbook of historical studies in education* (pp. 1–21). Springer. 10.1007/978-981-10-0942-6_34-1

Cantlie, J. (1885). *Degeneration amongst Londoners: A lecture delivered at the Parkes Museum of Hygiene, January 27, 1885.* Field & Tuer.

Davin, A. (1996). *Growing up poor: Home, school and street in London, 1870–1914.* Rivers Oram Press.

Dwork, D. (1987). *War is good for babies and other young children: A history of the infant and child welfare movement in England, 1898–1918.* Tavistock Publications.

Educational Pressure (1880) *The British Medical Journal*, *1*(1015), 892–893.

Feeding the Hungry Children (1889). *The British Medical Journal*, *2*(1510), 1295.

Fothergill, J. (1889). *The town dweller: His needs and his wants.* H.K. Lewis.

Hamlin, C. (1998). *Public health and social justice in the age of Chadwick, 1800–1854.* Cambridge University Press.

Hardy, A. (1993). *The epidemic streets: Infectious disease and the rise of preventative medicine, 1856–1900.* Clarendon Press.

Harris, B. (1995). *The health of the schoolchild: A history of the School Medical Service in England and Wales.* Open University Press.

Harris, B. (2003). Educational reform, citizenship and the origin of the School Medical Service. In M. Gijswijt-Hofstr & H. Marland (Eds.), *Cultures of child health in Britain and the Netherlands in the twentieth century* (pp. 85–101). Rodopi.

Hendrick, H. (1994). *Child welfare: England, 1872–1989.* Routledge.

Hirst, J.D. (1989). The growth of treatment through the School Medical Service, 1908–18. *Medical History, 33*(3), 318–342.

Hirst, J.D. (1991). Public health and the public elementary schools, 1870–1907. *History of Education, 20*(2), 107–118.

Inter-departmental Committee on Physical Deterioration (1904). *Report of the Inter-departmental Committee on Physical Deterioration.*

Kerr, J. (1916). *Newsholme's school hygiene: The laws of health in relation to school life* (14th ed.). George Allen & Unwin.

Mackenzie, W.L., & Matthew, E. (1904). *The medical inspection of school children: A textbook for medical officers of schools, medical officers of health, school managers and teachers.* William Hodge.

Mooney, G. (2015). *Intrusive interventions: Public health, domestic space, and infectious disease surveillance in England, 1840–1914.* University of Rochester Press.

Newman, G. (1913). *The health of the state* (3rd ed.). Headley Brothers.

Newman, G. (1926). *An outline of the practice of preventive medicine: A memorandum addressed to the Minister of Health.* His Majesty's Stationery Office.

Newman, G. (1939). *The building of a nation's health.* Macmillan.

Newsholme, A. (1887). *School hygiene: The laws of health in relation to school life.* Swan Sonnenscheine, Lowrey, & Co.

Niven, J. (1899). *Report on the health of the City of Manchester, 1898.* Henry Blacklock.

Niven, J. (1900). *Report on the health of the City of Manchester, 1899.* Henry Blacklock.

Porter, D. (1999). *Health, civilization and the state: A history of public health from ancient to modern times.* Routledge.

Report of the Inter-departmental Committee on Medical Inspection and Feeding of Children Attending Public Elementary Schools. (1905). Wyman & Sons.

Report of the Inter-departmental Committee on Physical Deterioration. (1904). Darling & Son.

Report of the Lancet Sanitary Commission on the sanitary condition of public schools. (1875). *The Lancet, 105*(2703), 859–861.

The Food Factor in Education (1903). *The British Medical Journal, 2*(2225), 424–425.

Vernon, J. (2007). *Hunger: A modern history.* Harvard University Press.

Warner, F. (1892). Abstracts of the Milroy lectures on an inquiry as to the physical and mental condition of school children. *The British Medical Journal, 1*(1628), 538.

Welshman, J. (1997). School meals and milk in England and Wales, 1906–45. *Medical History, 41*(1), 6–29.

Williams, N., & Mooney, G. (1994). Infant mortality in an 'age of great cities': London and the English provincial cities compared, 1840–1910. *Continuity and Change, 9*(2), 185–212.

Woodward, J. (1995). The school medical officer before the School Medical Service: England and Wales, 1850–1908. In J. Woodward, & R. Jütte (Eds.), *Coping with sickness: Historical aspects of healthcare in a European perspective* (pp. 121–146). European Association for the History of Medicine and Health Publications.

2

SCHOOLING AND MEDICAL ASSISTANCE

The school clinics in Rio de Janeiro[1]

Heloísa Helena Pimenta Rocha and
Henrique Mendonça da Silva

The importance of health issues, in the institutionalisation of the modern school, materialised in a varied set of initiatives between the end of the 19th century and the beginning of the 20th century. These initiatives, set up in distinct centres of power, were guided by the recurring claim of the need for hygiene inspection of schools and students, as a requirement that should accompany compulsory schooling established in different countries. These guidelines were referred to in various international congresses, such as the International Congress of Schooling (Brussels, 1880), II Latin-American Scientific Congress (Montevidéu, 1901), School Hygiene Congress (Paris, 1904, 1910) and II School Hygiene and Physiological Education Congress (Paris, 1905). One of the aims of these events was to intervene in the structure of these educational systems (Moreno, 2006, 2009; Rocha, 2009; Rocha & Silva, 2017; Terrón, 2000; Viñao, 2000; Viñao & Moreno, 2000).

The concern with aspects linked to health comprised the risk of transmission of diseases arising from the clustering of children in the same space; abnormal spine curvature due to body posture during school activities; as well as the problems caused by lighting problems, airing and hygiene in the school buildings. These themes were also registered in the School Hygiene Treaties produced in different countries, many of which crossed frontiers, becoming a reference in the qualification of doctors and teachers, for example, those of Burgenstein (1934), Méry and Génévrier (1914) and Riant (1884).

In a similar vein, the Brazilian doctor Clemente Ferreira, very much in line with these discussions and aware of the implementation of medical inspection services in various countries, stated at the beginning of the 20th century: 'In every country where schooling is compulsory, the logical corollary should be compulsory medical inspection' (1909, p. 305).

DOI: 10.4324/9781003288671-4

The results of the inspection work carried out by doctors, some with the support of teachers, gradually reinforced the thesis of the dangers of schooling and of the need for interventions on the bodies of the students. An example of this can be found in the diagnosis given by a health inspector in the city of Rio de Janeiro, the then capital of Brazil: 'Observed as a whole, the school population's state of health, merely by its aspect, was not recognized as the best in all schools' (Moncorvo Filho, 1913, p. 20). The same diagnosis was repeated in other regions of the country. One health inspector, on a visit to a school in the state of São Paulo, was shocked at the 'physical deficiency that was obvious in the students, as a consequence of malaria and jaundice', to the point that he could imagine he was looking at the courtyard in a children's hospital, as the children's appearance was so unhealthy (Neiva, 1918, p. 710).

Focussing on the setting up and practice of the school clinics in Rio de Janeiro, as one of the developments of medical school inspections, this chapter intends to contribute a reflection on the 'curriculum of the body' (Burns et al., 2020, p. 4), a concept that seeks to distinguish 'a set of educational technologies, schooling practices and school-based public health programmes that have been enacted on or through the body'. As proposed by the authors, the concept is not limited to the formal contents of schooling but includes 'texts', 'discourse', 'practices' and 'institutions', allowing the questioning of various dimensions of what is taught and learned at school, in line with representations of childhood and convictions in relation to the ways in which school can intervene in the lives of children and their families.

This chapter therefore seeks to examine the discourse in defence of the creation of school clinics in the city of Rio de Janeiro in the first half of the 20th century, in addition to the process of institutionalisation of this service and the practices established for the treatment of conditions detected, in their links with the wider ongoing movement beyond national frontiers (Bakker, 2017; Pozo Andrés, 2000; Rodríguez-Ocaña, 2003). Working together with the schools of this city between the 1930s and 1950s, the clinics, created for the purpose of treating the medical conditions that affected students, boasted x-ray services, clinical analysis laboratories, as well as dental, ophthalmological, ear-nose-and-throat and dermatological departments.

The analysis of these discourses and initiatives allows one to observe the forms of intervention on school health issues. Based on theoretical reflections of contagion expressed in the previous century, medical attention viewed the school, at first sight, as one of the places that could put children's health at risk, due to the insalubrity of the areas and of the handling of the contaminated objects among other factors. Developments in microbiology and knowledge regarding viruses and their transmission resulted in an emphasis on individual relationship with disease and states of health and were responsible for the shift of focus of the interventions from buildings to students' bodies themselves. This shift took place in a set of practices of individual hygiene and infantile body investigation.

Thus, in the second decade of the 20th century, apart from the initiatives geared towards the installations, the carrying out of exams and registers of physical and intellectual development, together with the output of indices of normal and abnormal standards could already be seen. The physiological studies of scholars offered the assumptions on which the anthropometric, clinical and laboratorial procedures were based and that were emphasised during this time. The school clinic was inserted into this growth knowledge movement of social medicine, which intended to arrest the health risks that stem from school attendance.

Linked to public education administration, the clinics participated in the production of knowledge about children, their physical constitutions and the diseases they suffered from and their way of life, with repercussions on their daily practices. The records of the clinics' performance were published in newspapers geared towards the general public, such as *O Paiz, A Rua* and *O Comércio*. The doctors involved in this project released the results of their research in scientific journals (*Brazil Médico* and *Folha Médica*) and public education administrative reports. These documents make up the empirical basis of this chapter.

The initiative to create clinics reveals the production of clinical and thera-peutic knowledge inside the city's public education system, representing a shift in the then-adopted model, which reverted mainly to the identification of health risks, with the aim of preventing sickness. Analysing the disputes that surrounded the institutionalisation of this service, the aim of this chapter is to capture indications of discursive and institutional investments regarding the body of the children who attended the schools. In other words, we intend to examine the ways the body of the student became the object of a range of discourse and practices focussed not only on the prevention of diseases and the preservation of health, but also on the treatment of the infirmities detected, in a period during which school began to be represented as a key element in the interventions organised by doctors (Viñao, 2000). From this perspective, the reflections by Rodríguez-Ocaña highlight that 'the issue of the health, disease and care of children provides paradigmatic case studies within modern history' (2003, p. 17).

To explore these inquiries, this chapter is divided into three sections. In the first part, we examine two initiatives that aimed to establish institutions attending to the needs of schoolchildren in Rio de Janeiro, based on the model that tried to move away from simple inspection, towards also offering medical treatment for identified diseases. In the second part, we highlight the arguments used to justify these initiatives, focussing on the importance placed on data regarding the state of health of the school population and the eco-nomic impacts of infantile illness on the schooling project. Lastly, we observe some practices carried out in the school clinics and the role of this new modality of school health practices in the expansion of medical action.

A time of inaugurations and disputes

April 1930 saw the inauguration of the first clinic for the medical treatment of children who attended public schools in the city of Rio de Janeiro (Clínica Escolar Oscar Clark). Reporting on the event, the city's newspapers observed that the initiative was in line with the adoption of a new action model that did not restrict itself to conventional practices for the detection of diseases.

> Until quite recently, our preventive medicine services for schoolchildren were limited to their inspection and diagnosis of morbid states. Not one step was taken towards the organic recovery of these sick youngsters, the majority of whom were deprived of resources for adequate effective treatment.
>
> (A Clínica Escolar, 1930)

The event brought together medical intellectuals, political authorities and members of high society, apart from a group of scouts outside the building. The institution's patron, Dr Oscar Clark, gave a speech in which he invited participants to foresee a new action model that moved away from existing practices by medical school inspectors that 'naively dreamed of the possibility of the existence of a school population free of diseases and physical deficiencies by the simple creation of an official medical inspection service in municipal schools' (Clark, 1930). As part of the ceremony, the group toured consulting, measurement checking and sterilisation rooms, along with laboratories and specialist clinic offices.

Ten years later, in 1940, another medical space, the PMC (the Osvaldo Cruz Pedagogical Medical Centre), would emerge to attend to school-children. At the inauguration, the director of instruction gathered the press to present the new institution and give the reasons that justified its creation: 'the alarming health condition of the population attending schools in Rio de Janeiro', caused both by diseases and insufficient food (Centro Médico Pedagógico, 1940).

Those present at the ceremony listened to speeches by medical and peda-gogical authorities that addressed the social and financial damage to school and society brought on by lack of health, the strategies to combat the problem of children's health, and the place of the initiative in this fight (Centro Médico Pedagógico, 1940):

> The inauguration of the Pedagogical Medical Centre's main services by the Federal District City Hall is principally aimed at **early diagnosis**, the ultimate objective of individual medicine which is obliged to avoid physical and anatomopathological modifications through specific and opportune treatment.

> Public education statistics tell us that in 1938, in elementary day schools, 100,948 children were registered, with only 67,821, in other words 67.18%, passing to the next year. The average pass rate corresponds to 33,127 failing the year.
>
> The averages furnished do not determine the limit of responsibility of the medical service, making it obligatory to globally consider the **percentage of students redoing the year as a functional pedagogical medical anomaly**.
> (Emphasis in original)

A decade separated the inauguration of these two spaces dedicated to the clinical treatment of the city's school population. On both occasions, the newspapers reported the justifications of the public authorities, emphasising the advantages and advances that the creation of these services represented. The list of arguments cited the 'alarming' proportion of sick children, physical precariousness as a limiting educational factor and the inadequate use of public resources given the number of students failing the year. The justifications were based on medical and pedagogical arguments, mediated by concepts, statistical data, innovations and the updating of scientific paradigms. Possibilities for improving the physical state of children and their school performance through adequate treatment and the expansion of medical practices in school health were pronounced as necessary and in keeping with the new advances in medicine. While analysing these arguments, we will examine some of the grounds on which they were based, including schoolchildren's state of health, the funds invested in education (correlated to attendance and failure rates and the expansion of school attendance) and openness to scientific innovations. Administrative reports from the Department of Education produced during the 1920s had introduced questions about this type of problem, as the statistics showed that in the first half of the decade, out of a total of more than 52,000 students enrolled, a third failed the school year (Leão, 1926).

The intention of endowing the city of Rio de Janeiro with services geared towards student health was nothing new. Yet although the school clinic was hardly the first initiative in this direction, its establishment represented an important shift, especially if one considers that the functions of these services, albeit registered in the City's legislation and expressed as opinions by some members of the body of inspectors, were not therapeutic.

Concerns regarding the inspection of the sanitary conditions of the buildings and students date back to the 19th century, as can be seen by the recommendations approved in international congresses carried out at the time. In the case of Rio de Janeiro, these discussions resulted in regulations never leaving the drawing board. Two further attempts, in 1910 and 1916, had similar results. The 1910 experiment lasted a mere few months, abandoned due to poor support from politicians and a lack of resources. However, it did produce an encouraging report on the sanitary conditions of the buildings and school materials, and the problems related to student health (Moncorvo Filho, 1913).

School medical inspection was effectively implemented in 1916, following a model that guided work for decades, which established the diseases that should be the target, along with preventive measures and control methods. The services consisted merely of inspection, with a marked tone of medical policing, in which the practice of isolation from school was predominant, in addition to a push for the acquisition of individual rules concerning hygiene. According to the law, it was not the place of the inspection team to treat diseases found in schoolchildren; their activities were to focus on controls against the risks of contagion. It thus fell to the medical inspector 'to detect and prevent transmittable diseases and stop propagation in the environment; to remove the danger of contagion as soon as possible'. Once the problem was identified, the doctor 'will communicate it to the services administration, who will inform those responsible so that they will be alerted and take adequate measures for treatment' (Estado do Rio de Janeiro, 1916).

The prevalence of disease among schoolchildren in the city was easily observed. The first moments of inspection activities revealed the need for medical-scientific knowledge to deal with the cases of sickness, as shown by the articles and reports published in the press, which dealt with the aetiology, prevention and treatment of these diseases.[2] The newspapers scathingly exposed the limits of inspection, in the ways in which it was implemented: 'The programme did not consider preventable diseases, it only dealt with contagious diseases, as if there were no preventable non-contagious diseases whose prophylaxis is of clear value' (Inspeção Médica Escolar, 1916). The reports regarding the inadequacy of the services gave rise from the very beginning to questions regarding the inspection model, accompanied by suggestions for new practices, which in fact came from members of the body of the medical inspectors themselves.

The connections between the sick state of schoolchildren and their modest or even negative educational results, expressed in numbers that apparently spoke for themselves, went against the flow of the modern Brazil project, defended by intellectuals at the time (Herschmann, 1996; Herschmann & Pereira, 1994). Along the same lines, the education administration inquired: what can be done to deter school abandonment? More than 31,000 children registered in first grade; 15,000 in second; a little over 9,000 in third; in the last grade (seventh year) there was an impressive number of 955 (Leão, 1926, p. 9). The measures taken to contain school abandonment included promotions and an increase in salary for teachers, as well as health assistance action based on attention to food. According to Paulilo (2011, 2020), facing the impossibility of a reform according to the law, and due to the low budget for public teaching, the option taken was the organisation of new programmes establishing actions in the field of hygiene, school sanitation and assistance for schoolchildren.

The sick state of schoolchildren in Rio de Janeiro as observable data

The census regarding the health of schoolchildren and the data collected on medical records, set up in the 1920s, resulted in the production of more accurate knowledge about the health condition of those who attended the city of Rio de Janeiro's schools. The data allowed for statistical analyses that represented an important strategy in the articulation and legitimacy of a model based on the prevention of cases of illness. The 'physical format of a child from Rio de Janeiro', established from 6,500 medical records, served as a basis for the production of a 'monthly weight and height graph in the classroom' (Leão, 1926, p. 56).

Between 1924 and 1925, actions aimed at improving the state of school-children's health were implemented, with the goal of changing the character of inspection services. These efforts ranged from providing milk and a bowl of soup to those deemed below-average in development to offering outreach to the 'school for feeble children', created in 1926, on the outskirts of the city, in an experimental, improvised way (Dalben & Silva, 2020).

As per the evaluation of some inspectors, however, some schoolchildren presented such a fragile state of health that the strategies adopted were ineffective, requiring specific, lengthier clinical care, which was not always possible. In addition to the costs, the municipal teaching structure itself was an obstacle: there were no funds for treatment and the creation of medical infrastructure; the number of inspectors was insufficient, making the adequate monitoring of children's medical history unfeasible. Apart from this, there was not only a lack of assistants and specialist doctors, but also the facilities and conditions needed for precise diagnosis (laboratories, dental and ophthal-mology offices and clinics for more specific investigations). All of this led to a halt of therapeutic activities of the school health services.

During the 1920s, there were constant discussions about the need for innovation and expansion. The cases compiled between 1928 and 1930 (Clark, 1930, pp. 361–367) revealed the high proportion of morbid states. In 1929, for example, there were 5,748 school visits, with 22,166 children examined out of the 70,000 who attended school (Veloso, 1929, p. 4). The incidence of disease, in both variety and degree, was expressed in the examination results: 18,000 presented some type of illness. The cases were characterised as 'diseases, illnesses, physical defects and malnutrition', with the predominating conditions being: 'Anaemia—2,796; Malnutrition—2,212; Acute infectious diseases—176; Tuberculosis—218; Syphilis—1,187; Intestinal worms—1,129; Hookworm—699; Leprosy—6; Malaria—75; Mental disability—295; Physical deficiencies—213' (Clark, 1930, p. 64).

When publications such as the *Jornal do Comércio* and *O Globo* made the statistical data widely available, they heightened public awareness, while at the same time mitigating internal disputes between the inspection service doctors, and between these doctors and the education authorities. Targets of criticism included the identification of contagious cases, their isolation and 'hygiene education' in the methods established (Lima, 1985). The medical inspectors were divided when facing questions as to the most efficient model (Rocha & Silva, 2017): vigilance against the dangers of contagion or treatment of the sick schoolchildren? Prophylaxis or assistance?

In the model adopted by school medical inspection, the discovery of a disease among schoolchildren did not guarantee access to medical care. According to legislation, it fell to the parents, many of whom had no available resources, to seek help. More accurate knowledge about the general state of schoolchildren exposed the size of the problem. In the first half of the 20th century, the city of Rio de Janeiro was precariously assisted in terms of the clinics, hospitals and dispensaries that were geared towards children's health: just four institutions offered child health care. In addition to this, services were badly distributed, leaving many peripheral and rural regions uncovered (Silva, 2017). The numbers and analyses published in newspapers with wide circulation and educational journals offer indications of discursive and institutional investments regarding the bodies of the children who attended the city's schools, revealing the disputes between initiatives focussed on prevention, and those geared towards the treatment of illnesses.

According to some medical inspectors and doctors, the data showed that health initiatives in schools faced the challenge of guaranteeing the continuity of learning. To this end, they argued that it was fundamental to ensure the treatment of morbid conditions that children presented. They drew attention to the specialists and spaces needed for the implementation of a wider public health programme, which included the carrying out of more complex diagnoses and clinical treatment. Thus, the creation of a school clinic, with professionals such as school nurses, became more evident in the discourses. The clinics were an innovation that came from developments regarding school health in England, pointing to an international circulation of intervention models in children's health, and indicating ways in which Brazilian doctors took on issues debated internationally. As Bakker (2017, p. 165) points out, whereas in England and Wales school doctors treated children's diseases, in other countries like Holland, their activities were strictly limited to prevention, with the treatment of children and the creation of clinics not being within their scope.

In Rio de Janeiro, this proposal was initially defended by doctor Luiz Barbosa (1916). While criticising the results obtained from the inspection services and compulsory isolation from school, the doctor proposed that 'the essential thing will not exactly be to relate physical disabilities, pathological traits, the presence of ailments or infections that debilitate the body, but to follow this testing with the treatment of young sufferers' (Barbosa, 1916). Thus, as per Armstrong (1993), more than a teaching and learning space, the school offers the opportunity to analyse, experiment and transform.

The economic impacts of ill health in schoolchildren

The issue of the 'healthy child' changed classrooms into spaces for the preventive management of children's health in the 20th century in Brazil and various other parts of the world, in line with investments and projects of modernity (Bakker, 2017; Gleason, 2013). As Rodríguez-Ocaña (2003, p. 17) highlights, 'child history reveals the strategic character of health in modern industrial world, and accordingly, the relevant role of medicine as a cultural agency, insofar that medical care of children is one of the elements defining the status of children in our days'.

The expansion of school attendance and educational achievements in Rio de Janeiro was notable throughout the first half of the 20th century, making issues related to children's health a subject for discussion. The report by the city's Public Education Board relayed the existence of 300 schools in 1924/ 1925, with 68,000 and 70,000 students, respectively, registered, and 53,831 attending school on average (Leão, 1926, p. 23). A decade later, in 1935, school attendance reached on average two out of three children between the ages of 7 and 12, which made the city's school system the largest in the country: 'the closest to a universal public school that Brazil possesses', according to Dávila (2006, p. 125).

The expansion of initiatives in school health in Rio de Janeiro was preceded by economic reflections on the costs of school failure. Since the 1910s, when medical inspection was formally established, questions related to attendance, repeating a year and dropping out of school, in their correlations with the amounts spent, began to weigh heavily in the discussions of legislators, doctors and educational authorities. Between 1919 and 1924, school attendance reached 60%, and the costs continued to rise steadily (Leão, 1926). According to one of the Instruction directors, 'There is no region where a student costs more public money than in the Federal District' (Azevedo, 1932, p. 60). Even so, the number of children failing per year remained high, even as 50,000 students were waiting for school places. This situation led education authorities to review their position.

School health measures, which were limited to actions related to body hygiene, physical education and food education, were then seen by the doctors themselves as insufficient. They determined that a dual objective should guide these actions: ensuring that students followed their course of schooling, and treating the pathologies that hindered this course. It was necessary to establish some agreement on ideas and actions. Thus, in a speech in 1932, the director of public instruction asserted:

> Although the medical inspector has to be above all a health educator, a propagator of social hygiene … recourse to school Clinics or school outpatient services is an imperative, in which treatment is given by contracted specialists and pathologists, under the direction and vigilance of school doctors. …
>
> The personal, direct observation convinced me of the need to organize the service of treatment for poor students in school clinics distributed throughout the diverse districts and equipped with laboratories for research and biological tests, and specialist clinical offices.
>
> (Azevedo, 1932, p. 78)

Once again, at the time of the setting up of the PMC Oswaldo Cruz, in 1940, arguments surrounding the structural problems of student failure resulting from health conditions were raised:

> In general, the children in the Federal District are malnourished and sick … . The distribution of school meals was intensified last year, with wonderful results. Seeing that 50% of schoolchildren repeating the first year according to statistics were malnourished minors, underfed and sick, not having, therefore, the natural elements of physical and intellectual defence.
>
> (Assistência Médica, 1940)

As can be seen, between 1930 and 1940, spaces for more integrated action in public health in Rio de Janeiro's city schools were set up, focussed not only on the detection of diseases, the dissemination of knowledge on cleanliness and inculcation of individual hygiene habits, but also on analysis, experimentation and treatment. Some doctors involved in this discussion were evidently attentive to the opportunity to widen the social medicine field of action, incorporating new scientific paradigms, which entailed more individualised action, mediated through diagnosis and more specific treatments, combining investigative, scientific knowledge production and treatment actions.

Renovations in social medicine and the spreading of scientific action range

In the midst of disputes involving school doctors and educational authorities, the inauguration of the Clínica Escolar (School Clinic) Oscar Clark in 1930 and the PMC Oswaldo Cruz in 1940 came about as a medical-scientific determination, and from the production of clinical and therapeutic knowledge inside the public education system in Rio de Janeiro. These initiatives brought about a new proposition for the medical-social action proposal. Regarding the relevance of this 'new frontier', which corresponded to advances in disease knowledge, its agents, its causes and forms of dissemination, as well as the updating of action models, it is worth paying attention to reflections by Rodríguez-Ocaña (2003, p. 35), whose research entails 'institutionalization in a transnational space of tasks concerning vigilance and the defence of health', which was expressed in a circulation network of sanitary ideas.

In the scope of these discussions on new scientific certainties, the term 'active medicine', used frequently by those involved in the Clínica Escolar and the PMC project, bore the fundamental concerns of social medicine at the time: prevent disease and treat its manifestations (Baldwin, 1999; Rosen, 1994). The intended form consisted of the individualisation of health procedures, by means of 'the imperative need for preventive medicine tests on all students' (Clark, 1930, p. 36) and for treatment based on the results obtained. To this end, the clinic was to carry out laboratory, radiological and eye exams, also paying attention to respiratory, hearing and skin problems.

Once the disease was detected, a new set of interventions on the child's body was carried out. Thus, the school clinics took advantage of the opportunity to produce medical-social strategies, through a shift in methods and objectives: diagnostic evaluation, therapeutic prescription and its application. School clinics were also used as a place for the production of science, in which research, scientific dissemination and medical training were interlinked.

The analysis of these practices offers indications of the changes in the profile of school medical activity that the clinics represented in Brazil and, more specifically, in Rio de Janeiro, from the 1930s onwards. These practices are different from the model adopted in the initial decades of the 20th century, when the first experiments were implemented in the city with the main objective of deterring the transmission of contagious diseases among schoolchildren through the detection of cases and isolation of those contaminated according to the model adopted in several countries at the time, as shown by the communications presented in many international congresses. One of the precursory studies on school health in Brazil points out the following forms of action and the pillars that sustained the great part of these practices:

School health or, more precisely, school hygiene at the time, occurred at the intersection of three doctrines: that of medical policing, through the inspection of health conditions of those involved in teaching; that of sanitation by prescription and respect for the salubrity of the teaching areas; and that of puericulture, by the dissemination of rules of living for teachers and students and intervention in favour of a more 'physiological' pedagogy, that is, more adequate for the schoolchildren's bodies to which it applies.

(Lima, 1985, p. 85)

The adoption of individualised medical assistance (therapeutic and rehabilitative) in the city's school clinics led to the writing of dozens of texts, published in major Brazilian scientific journals such as *Brazil Médico* and *Folha Médica*, and became a recurring theme at education and hygiene congresses from the 1920s onwards. Two pathological conditions gained distinction in the medical production: tuberculosis and cases of anaemia caused by malnutrition. Tuberculosis was a disease seen as emblematic of the school health problems in Rio de Janeiro (Rocha & Silva, 2017) and was the object of painstaking investigations, such as the study published in *Brazil Médico* by doctor Martins Pereira, director of the CE Oscar Clark and of the PMC. Practices of radiological exams were adopted as standard procedures for the formulation of student medical records, with the identification of tuberculosis in mind. The experience described in the article, 'A Tuberculose Entre os Escolares do Rio de Janeiro' (Tuberculosis Among Students in Rio de Janeiro), which combined thorax measurements and research on the bacillus in the sputum of children seen at the CE, offered more precision to the treatment, as well as to the organisation of the statistics (Pereira, 1932, 33–34).

The systematic testing of students was aimed at the formulation of plans for the prevention and treatment of children who were pre-tubercular, extremely weak or with the disease in a consumptive state. Confronting this infirmity, for the best part of the first half of the 20th century, included a wide variety of procedures, among which was the regeneration and strengthening of the body by nature, represented as one of the most accepted therapeutic repertoires, as shown by ongoing experiments at the time in various countries (Freire & Leony, 2011). Dr Martins Pereira did not deviate from these practices. After diagnosis, according to him, 'there would be the absolute necessity for sanatoriums at the beach or in the mountains for preventive treatment … in the sea or mountain air, with full-time physical education and food' (Pereira, 1932, p. 12). The individualisation of knowledge, through clinical and laboratory analyses, would promote actions such as the distribution of medication: worm medicine against intestinal parasites; quinine for malaria; and iron sulphate, salvarsan and tonics (cod liver oil) for cases of anaemia and other formulas manipulated by the institution's pharmacy.

According to the doctor, with regards to the children who presented advanced cases of 'fever, weight loss, expectorated bacilli', adenopathies or pulmonary lesions, 170 were treated with experimental medication from a combination of cod liver oil and copper salts. In total, 4,000 injections were applied, with no verified intolerance, local or general reaction, as stated by the doctor who led the experiment. His notes on prophylaxis and treatment registered three cases, with information on anamnesis, treatment, quantity, periods and medication dosage, as well as evolution and results of new laboratory tests and radioscopy (Pereira, 1932). One of them refers to a nine-year-old child described as malnourished, anaemic and with signs of adenopathy. This child weighed 20 kg and remained under treatment for three months, receiving 20 injections of 1 mL of the medication, with a weight gain of 1.8 kg, described as progressive improvement, verified in the radiology tests.

Using the resources available in the clinics, the results of student blood tests were also investigated in order to create clinical standards. Haematological research on the haemo-sedimentation of blood was carried out in 1940 by two doctors, Manoel Roiter and Aloysio de Paula, aiming at establishing the use of the test on all those examined at the school clinics. The doctors sought to define an average reaction time, with a view to discovering standards for the city's public-school students that could indicate some disease.

The experiment for testing the standards, the possibilities of medications and the treatment brought together 33 children sent to the CE Oscar Clark. Three groups were set up: children considered normal, which included those with worms, colds, hypertension, adenoids and tonsilitis. The second group included children with signs of more serious pathologies, who underwent more sophisticated (radiological) clinical exams and a more detailed anamnesis. Some were reallocated to the first group after tests, others went to a third group, which consisted of children whose tests pointed towards inflammation with causes not yet clarified and who had to be submitted to new tests, with a view to discovering the disease.

Another front of medical-scientific action was the investigation of cases of anaemia among schoolchildren, which allowed for the establishment of a geography of spaces in the city where factors that presupposed this condition were presented. To the medical eye guided by investigations carried out in the clinics, some children attending public schools in Rio de Janeiro lived in outlying poorer zones, some significantly rural, apart from others who lived in urban zones marked by the city's topography, with its hills and favelas—communities characterised as improvised, densely populated, precariously served by public authorities regarding sanitation and living conditions. This situation could also be found in the poor areas on the city's outskirts.

According to doctors who were linked to the school clinic projects, the sanitary conditions to which the children were exposed were responsible for the results obtained: 80% of the students had worms, which produced anaemic states, aggravated by malnutrition.

Our schools in Rio de Janeiro are attended by an army of profoundly anaemic children. What are the causes? In the first place, deficient diet, both in quantity and quality. Great numbers of children have just one meal a day. This meal is always the same: rice and beans and coffee with bread. Many according to our enquiries rarely eat even a little meat, eggs or vegetables. The most affordable foodstuffs for the poor are starchy foods and milk.

Animal-based foods (meat, fish, eggs, liver, kidneys etc.) that are rich in these factors are more expensive, rarely accessible to the multitude of impoverished children who attend municipal schools.

(Pereira, 1942, pp. 303–304)

As noted above, there was an attempt to resolve the dietary shortages suffered by children in public schools with measures attentive to diet through programmes for the distribution of milk and more nourishing meals in school spaces (Paulilo, 2019, 2020). The data gleaned by these clinics, based upon scientific studies different from those behind the creation of school inspection services, allowed for the consumption of certain foods to be considered as part of school health actions. The doctors recognised that the habit of eating food rich in nutrients was not enough to prevent certain illnesses. Intense anaemic states, verified by haematological studies, pointed to a precarious diet caused by poverty and the need for treatment with the use of drugs.

Final considerations

Proctor and Burns defend the need for a 'more engaged, empirical investigation of the interconnected histories of mass schooling and public health' (2017, p. 118). Drawing attention to investments by national states in mass schooling and public health projects between the 19th and 20th centuries, these researchers highlight the centrality of health in school diffusion processes. They thus advise that the investigation of the connections between education and health includes, among other aspects, questions about professional groups and the fields of knowledge that are involved in the proposal of measures geared towards ensuring the salubrity of school, preserving the health of students and their families and teaching them new ways of life. These measures—which focussed on spaces, teaching materials and their uses, and the daily practice of reading, writing and physical exercise—focussed largely on the bodies of students, participating in the constitution of a set of representations on childhood and its education.

This chapter intends to contribute towards reflection on the 'curriculum of the body' (Burns et al., 2020) and, more particularly, on 'clinical practices'. Investigating historical aspects of the institutionalisation of school health services in the city of Rio de Janeiro in the first half of the 20th century, it seeks to consider the definitions and practices that gained priority, in tune with models in circulation internationally. The study allowed for the observation of a movement of redefinition based on a willingness to transcend the disease and offer a response to the diffusion of schooling, the modernisation of the country and the updating of social medicine.

Advances in surgical techniques, clinical practices and laboratory analyses, the development of drugs, as well as investments geared towards the inculcation of hygienic habits, caused a shift in the focus of actions regarding school conditions—with a view to containing the risks of contagion—and concerns about cleanliness and body posture, towards new practices that include individual examination, recording and direct treatment of pathologies. This shift represented a redirection in investments in schoolchildren's bodies.

Notes

1 This chapter in part derives from research carried out with funds from the CNPq (Brazilian National Council for Scientific Technological Development)—Process 312088/2021-3 and FAPESP (The São Paulo Research Foundation)/Thematic Project *Saberes e práticas em fronteiras* (Knowledge and practices in borders project—Process 2018/26699-4) coordinated by Diana Vidal, in which Heloísa Helena Pimenta Rocha acts as an associate researcher.
2 The newspaper *A Rua*, in a series of articles published in 1916, entitled 'A Inspeção Médica Escolar' (Medical School Inspection) was the precursor for a deeper analysis of the questions related to school health, launching medical terms and debates to a wider audience while at the same time promoting greater visibility related to these questions. From 1920 to 1930, the newspaper *Correio da Manhã* also dealt with the theme, highlighting vast subject matter on prophylaxis and assistance on what was considered the main diseases, showing which trends were visibly under dispute. The article 'Pela Saúde da Infância Escolar' (For Infant School Health), published in 1930 by the newspaper *Jornal do Comércio*, and an article printed by the newspaper *O Globo* followed by official reports entitled 'Os Serviços Médicos Escolares' (School Medical Services) (1928) are also worthy of note.

References

A clínica escolar. (1930, April 30). *O Paiz*, 2.
Armstrong, D. (1993). Public health spaces and the fabrication of identity. *Sociology*, *27*(3), 393–410.
Assistência médica. (1940, January 30). *Jornal do Comércio*, 4.
Azevedo, F. (1932). *Novos caminhos e novos fins: A nova política da educação no Brasil*. Companhia Editora Nacional.
Bakker, N. (2017). School medical inspection and the 'healthy' child in the Netherlands, 1904–1970. *History of Education Review*, *46*(2), 164–177.
Baldwin, P. (1999). *Contagion and the state in Europe, 1830–1930*. Cambridge University Press.
Barbosa, L. (1916, July 24). Clínica escolar. *O Paiz*, 1–2.
Burgenstein, L. (1934). *Higiene escolar* (L. Davidovich, Trans.; 3rd ed.). Atlantida.
Burns, K., Proctor, H., & Weaver, H. (2020). Modern schooling and the curriculum of the body. In T. Fitzgerald (Ed.), *Handbook of historical studies in education* (pp. 1–21). Springer. 10.1007/978-981-10-0942-6_34-1
Centro Médico Pedagógico. (1940, January 27). *Jornal do Comércio*, 4.
Clark, O. (1930). Higiene escolar. *Folha Médica*, 61–69.
Dalben, A., & Silva, H. (2020). Sol e ar fresco no combate à tuberculose: Experiências de educação ao livre no Rio de Janeiro (1910–1920). *Cadernos CEDES*, *40*(112), 218–232. 10.1590/CC232227

Dávila, J. (2006). *Diploma de brancura: Política social e racial no Brasil, 1917–1945.* Editora da UNESP.

Estado do Rio de Janeiro. (1916). *Regulação do serviço de inspeção médica escolar* (Decreto 1.580). Tipografia do Jornal do Comércio.

Ferreira, C. (1909). A inspeção médica dos colegiais. *Imprensa Médica, 17*(20), 305–312.

Freire, M., & Leony, V. (2011). A caridade científica: Moncorvo Filho e o Instituto de Proteção e Assistência à Infância do Rio de Janeiro (1899–1930). *História, Ciências, Saúde-Manguinhos, 18,* 199–225. 10.1590/S0104-59702011000500011

Gleason, M. (2013). *Small matters: Canadian children in sickness and health.* McGill-Queen's University Press.

Herschmann, M. (1996). Entre a insalubridade e a ignorância: A construção do campo médico e do ideário moderno no Brasil. In M. Herschmann, S. Kropf, & C. Nunes (Eds.), *Missionários do progresso: Médicos, engenheiros e educadores no Rio de Janeiro* (pp. 11–67). Diadorim.

Herschmann, M., & Pereira, C.A.M. (1994). O imaginário moderno no Brasil. In M. Herschmann, & C.A.M. Pereira (Ed.), *A invenção do Brasil moderno: Medicina, educação e engenharia nos anos 20–30* (pp. 9–42). Rocco.

Inspeção Médica Escolar. (1916, April 4). *A Rua,* 4.

Leão, A. (1926). *O ensino na capital do Brasil.* Tipografia do Jornal do Comércio.

Lima, G. (1985). *Saúde escolar e educação.* Cortez.

Méry, H., & Génévrier, J. (1914). *Hygiène scolaire.* J.B. Baillière et Fils.

Moncorvo Filho, A. (1913). *Guia do médico escolar.* Typ. Baptista de Souza.

Moreno, P.L. (2006). The hygienist movement and the modernization of education in Spain. *Paedagogica Historica, 42*(16), 793–815.

Moreno, P.L. (2009). Cuerpo, higiene, educación e historia. *Historia de la educación, 28,* 23–36.

Neiva, A. (1918). Relatório sobre as escolas de Iguape, Cananéia e Ararapira, apresentado pelo Dr. Arthur Neiva. *Anuário do Ensino do Estado de São Paulo,* pp. 708–714.

Os serviços médicos escolares. (1928, May 29). *O Globo,* 2.

Paulilo, A. (2011). *A Reforma Carneiro Leão no Distrito Federal (1922–1926).* Autores Associados.

Paulilo A. (2019). Inventivas administrativas nas reformas da instrução pública (Distrito Federal 1922–35). *Cadernos de História da Educação, 18*(1), 191–207. 10.14393/che-v18n1-2019-11

Paulilo, A. (2020). Casos e histórias da profissionalização docente no Instituto de Educação do Distrito Federal (1928–1935). *História da Educação, 24,* e87354. 10.1590/2236-3459/87354

Pela saúde da infância escolar. (1930, May 1). *Jornal do Comércio,* 4–5.

Pereira. A. (1932). *A tuberculose na idade escolar.* Clinica Escolar Oscar Clark.

Pereira. A. (1942). A anemia na idade escolar. In O. Clark (Ed.), *Hematologia* (pp. 301–310). Calvino e Mello.

Pozo Andrés, M. (2000). Salud, hygiene y educación: Origen y desarrollo de Inspección Médico-Escolar en Madrid (1900–1931). *Areas: Revista de Ciencias Sociales, 20,* 95–119.

Proctor, H., & Burns, K. (2017). The connected histories of mass schooling and public health. *History of Education Review, 46*(2), 118–124.

Riant, A. (1884). *Hygiene scolaire: Influence de l'ecole sur la sante des enfants.* Hachette.

Rocha, H.P. (2009). Education, health and production of knowledge about the childhood in Brazil. *History of Education & Children's Literature, 4*(1), 199–216.

Rocha, H.P., & Silva, H.M. (2017). The dangers of infection: School medical inspection in Brazil (the 1910s). *History of Education Review, 46*(2), 150–163. 10.1108/HER-02-2016-0015.

Rodríguez-Ocaña, E. (2003). La salud infantile, asunto ejemplar en la historiografía contemporánea. Dynamis, *23*, 27–36.

Rosen, G. (1994). *Uma história da saúde pública.* Hucitec.

Silva, H. (2017). *A higiene escolar além das palavras: Oscar Clark e o tratamento médico escolar* (Doctoral thesis), Universidade Estadual de Campinas, Brasil.

Terrón, A. (2000). La higiene escolar: un campo de conocimiento disputado. *Areas: Revista de Ciencias Sociales, 20*, 73–94.

Veloso, A. (1929, May 15). Profilaxia ou assistência? *Correio da Manhã,* 4

Viñao, A. (2000). Higiene, salud y educación en su perspectiva histórica. *Areas: Revista de Ciencias Sociales, 20*, 9–24.

Viñao, A., & Moreno, P. (2000). Introdución. *Areas: Revista de Ciencias Sociales, 20*, 7.

3

THE MEDIATION OF CHILDHOOD HEALTH DURING THE POLIO ERA IN AUSTRALIA

Kellie Burns, Helen Proctor, Ilektra Spandagou, and Heather Weaver

From the 1930s to the 1950s, Australians endured various outbreaks of polio-myelitis, with rates of infection initially highest amongst young children. Polio generated widespread public fear as the means of transmission was not fully understood for some time, there were no cures or treatments until the intro-duction of vaccinations in 1956, and infection with the polio virus could be fatal, or could result in paralysis of the limbs or muscles controlling the lungs, requiring immobilisation in cumbersome casts or braces, or assistance with breathing in iron lung machines. Patients able to leave the hospital sometimes remained disabled for life. Although the fear and risk management of polio were significant features of social life, histories of Australia during this period pay relatively little attention to the disease (e.g. Smith, 1997). Likewise, in the small number of historical studies about polio in Australia, the ways in which the disease both shaped and was shaped by broader understandings of childhood health and disability are underrepresented. The most comprehensive engage-ments with polio histories in Australia are two doctoral theses, the first, John H. Smith's (1997) social history of polio in Western Australia, and the second, Kerry Ann Highley's (2009) rich medical history of polio, which informs her subse-quent book *Dancing in my Dreams* (Highley, 2014). Both authors prioritise the experiences of polio patients and acknowledge the significant place of polio in the public imagination. Also seminal is Anne Killalea's (1995) *The Great Scourge: The Tasmanian Infantile Paralysis Epidemic, 1937–8.* Joan London's (2014) closely researched novel, *The Golden Age,* albeit fictional, offers rich insights into the daily lives of children and young people with polio living in a convalescent hospital in the Western Australian city of Perth in the 1950s.

Despite this relatively limited engagement with the disease's significance in shaping understandings of 'the child', the place of the polio in the public

DOI: 10.4324/9781003288671-5

imagination is evidenced by Alan Marshall's *I Can Jump Puddles* (1956), an autobiographical novel about growing up in rural Victoria with the effects of polio. A common text in Australian primary schools, Marshall depicts an exciting and happy 'post-polio' childhood in which his days are defined by friendship and play. Australian boyhood is constructed through traditional tropes of masculinity, celebrating mateship, outdoor play and testing the limits of the physical body in the context of rural living. The original cover for the edition used in schools features two boys, one on crutches, with their dogs racing down a hill through eucalyptus trees. As Dora Vargha (2018) argues, pictures of children displaying bravery in the face of polio were prominent around the world in the 1950s, used to heighten awareness and appeal to people's emotions to promote vaccination and raise funds for patient care.

In his critical reading of *I Can Jump Puddles*, Dylan Holdsworth (2017) considers how Marshall engages the relationships between disability, masculinity and Australian national identity. He argues that naturalised masculine ideals centred on the body are reproduced through rituals of risk-taking and physical challenges. Alan recalls his countless attempts to keep up with the other boys by pushing his body to the point of physical exhaustion or harm (e.g. riding horses, climbing and descending a mountain), reinscribing 'hegemonic masculine conceptions of what the body *should* do' (p. 115) and highlighting the significance of able-bodiedness to hegemonic masculine norms. Marshall's canonical text proposes that overcoming the limits disability places on childhood is a noble project of the self and one that is characteristically Australian.

This chapter examines other representations of children living with polio in Australia from the 1930s to the 1950s. Drawing on images from the print and screen news sources dominant in Australian mass culture at that time—newspapers, magazines and newsreels—consideration is given to how the public representation of bodies of school-aged children living with polio reflected and contributed to dominant ideas about disability, childhood health and in relation to conventional contemporary tropes of 'good' or 'normal' Australian childhoods in this period. Historians of health and medicine have established that public health's management of disease has always been a political exercise, rather than a merely neutral response to external conditions, raising questions of governance, authority and sovereignty (e.g. Anderson, 2005). Furthermore, health care and interventions focussed on school-aged children shaped racialised, gendered and disabled norms and experiences (e.g. Armstrong, 1993; Gleason, 2013; Proctor & Burns, 2017). Polio is no exception, and our focus is on what the mediation of polio tells us about the norms that organised childhood and childhood health. We begin by theorising the use of news media images in historical research about childhood health and schooling.

The 'turn to images' in historiography

How and when to use visual forms of data such as photographs, documentaries and film in historiography has been widely debated (e.g. Allender et al., 2021). Using visual texts as historical materials challenges the methodological traditions of reconstructionists who regard validated sources as evidence of a recovered past and view empirical methods as transparent and objective (Booth, 2005). This traditional approach to history deems photographs and films to be visual illustrations of the past that support 'the facts' gathered from other validated sources (Burke, 2001). Ian Grosvenor (1999) notes that the photographic image 'had truth-value, it was self-evident and evidence of the "real"; it was a witness and had documentary status' (p. 84); it therefore defied comment or analysis.

Over the past 50 years, however, a growing number of historians have argued that visual texts can promote deep criticality in the way historical sources are understood and used. This is often referred to as the 'pictorial turn' and describes the use by historians of visual texts to enact a reckoning with 'the constructed nature of what constitutes historical evidence' (Tucker, 2009, p. 3). Photography and film-making have been recognised as active in meaning-making and situated within a broader set of knowledge regimes, institutional practices and historical relations. The idea that historical photographs or other visual texts are prediscursive or atheoretical has also been challenged, and the theoretical writings of philosophers, cultural and media theorists, anthropologists and critical historians have developed critical historiographies that prioritise visual texts (e.g. Booth, 2005; Grosvenor, 1999). Those working on marginalised histories have further suggested that photographs are critical to telling stories that have otherwise been overlooked or erased from written historical documents and archives. Focus is thus paid not only to what is *in* the images, but also what is absent or elided.

Attention to historical images has been particularly valuable in offering new perspectives on embodied histories of schooling (Allender et al., 2021; Newman, 2022). The use of photographs and other visual sources to understand the historical intersections between public health and schooling is salient given that from the turn of the 20th century photographs were used by school medical inspectors to record the conditions of both school facilities and children's health. American medical historian Bert Hansen (2009) maintains that the dissemination of medical imagery in the public domain strengthened popular faith in the social utility of science and generated widespread public enthusiasm for scientific knowledge and a view of medicine as fundamentally humane and democratic. Additionally, medical photography has long been an important part of clinical care in some areas of medicine to document patients' care and progress, and also has captured life and community in hospitals. Recent engagements with the traditional conception of photographs as entirely objective forms of fact gathering have called into question objectivity and subjectivity as historical values and how 'particular ideals surrounding visual representation in science and medicine emerged and developed within a longer, complex series of changing epistemic values and concepts of truth' (Tucker, 2009, p. 4).

The term *mediation* has emerged in analyses of visual texts, signalling a shift away from the idea that images are mere representations of the real and/or that there is a simple or singular reading that can be made of an image (e.g. Brady et al., 2018). Mediation encapsulates the multiple and contested ways in which photographs and other visual and media texts are made meaningful within and through the broader material and discursive contexts in which they are produced, disseminated and viewed.

Childhood polio at the intersections of medical and educational discourses

Within the broader context of an expanding welfare state in Australia, discourses surrounding children's bodies living with polio afforded new authority to social institutions such as schools, hospitals, prisons and so on, and to the professionals who ran them—teachers, doctors, nurses and social workers. Individually and collectively, these institutions and professionals were invested in understandings of childhood as a distinct period of development separate from adulthood, defined by innocence, naivety, vulnerability and dependence (Burns & Proctor, 2022). The expansion of mandatory schooling in the 19th and 20th centuries was significant in establishing a set of priorities for childhood; how, where and with whom children should spend the bulk of their days, but also what appropriate tasks were or were not for young bodies.

With schooling compulsory in many parts of the world, the everyday rituals and practices of schooling served to organise, categorise and separate bodies at school (e.g. Burns et al., 2020; Proctor & Burns, 2017). Canadian historian Mona Gleason (2013) explains that the growing emphasis on childhood health at the dawn of the 20th century led to the development of formal health curricula in schools, as well as the expansion of resources and medical services directed at improving children's health. Medical knowledge about childhood and healthy development was given foremost authority and was significant in defining social attitudes about children—and normative childhoods. It also strongly informed how teachers understood and approached children's learning, discipline and socialisation in early classrooms. As such, understanding the curriculum of the body as it operated in and through a particular context or moment in time entails the close critical reading of knowledge practices about children's health, produced in and through the medical and public health discourse. School-based approaches to health and hygiene, but also frameworks used to define a 'normal' or 'healthy' child or childhood, were strongly informed by dominant framings in medicine and other scientific domains and deemed credible and unbiased.

Polio offers a useful case for understanding the connected domains of medicine and schooling in ordering children's bodies and lives. The polio crisis of the mid-20th century occurred at a moment when both schools and childhood medicine were highly invested in the making of 'healthy' future citizens (Gleason, 2013). The efforts to manage polio therefore utilised the knowledge, expertise and resources of medicine, public health, hospitals and schools. Schools were widely implicated in national efforts to control the spread of the polio virus. Newspapers during this period featured headlines—such as 'Infantile Paralysis: Many Districts Isolated, More Schools to be Closed' (1937), 'Polio Scare Hits Back-to-School' (1949), and 'Polio Fear Keeps Pupils from School' (1953)—that reflected and reinforced public perceptions of risk and mounting concern amongst parents and authorities about schools as sites for the spread of the polio virus. Along with schools, public pools, theatres and events with large gatherings were considered risky for children (e.g. Need for Precaution on Polio, 1950). Concern about the unsanitary conditions of schools because of overcrowding, poor lighting and ventilation and inadequate sewerage systems was longstanding, however, during periods of disease outbreak or epidemics the management of school environments became a strong focus (e.g. Gard & Pluim, 2014; Pineau & Frechtel, 2022). Compulsory schooling brought children together from across populations, making schools a locus for anxiety about contagious disease. Routines that fostered personal and social hygiene proliferated, and attention was paid to the spaces around and between the bodies of children in an effort to minimise the spread of infectious diseases. Concern was not only merely focussed on dirty or unhygienic school settings, but also on the body and bodily habits of the child, and by extension their family (e.g. Armstrong, 1993; Kirk, 1998). Headlines that reported risk, case numbers and schools or communities with known infections served to generate fear, but also to re-victimise and stigmatise those affected by polio (Pineau & Frechtel, 2022).

School authorities and teachers scrambled to modify physical and material elements of classrooms and schools that might facilitate the spread of disease. These were coupled with somewhat unconventional pedagogies such as moving children outside for lessons, where the exposure to fresh air and sunshine was thought to provide benefit, but also where the limitations of poor indoor ventilation were overcome. Figure 3.1 shows a public-school lesson in the city of Melbourne, Victoria in 1949 ('Out to Beat Polio'). Featured in the *Sun* (a newspaper from Sydney, New South Wales, Victoria's neighbouring state), the accompanying text notes that while classrooms at the school had recently been renovated, 'no risks were being taken' and this school was 'out to beat polio'. Both the text and image composition promote public reassurance in the hyphenated to decision-making of teachers and school

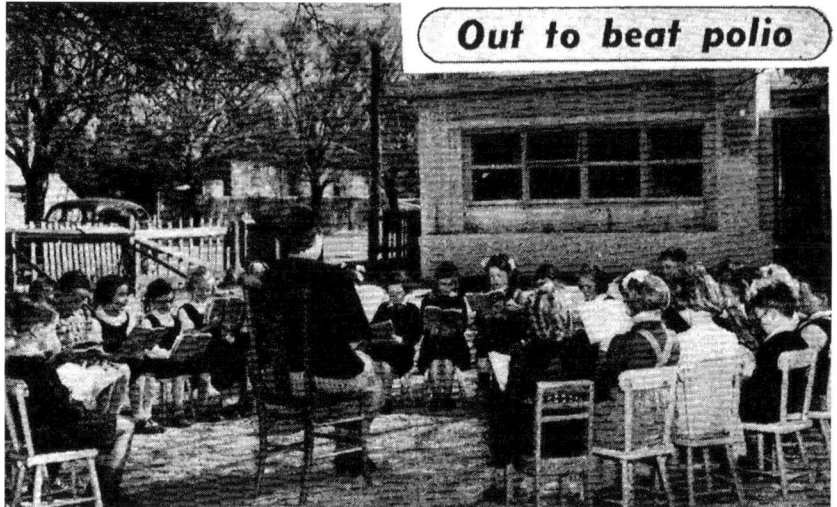

FIGURE 3.1   Outdoor learning to 'beat polio' at a Victorian school, 1949.

Source: Out to Beat Polio. (1949, September 9), *The Sun*, 5.

administrators as frontline professionals in combatting polio. Moreover, the message is that school learning and the routines of the classroom remain consistent regardless of broader social challenges. The children are sitting in an orderly and well-managed arrangement despite the shift to the outdoors—learning and the routines of school must endure in the face of health crises.

In the efforts to maintain hygiene standards in schools, newspapers also assigned roles to parents, specifically mothers, and their children. The Melbourne *Herald* encouraged mothers to send children to school with 'their own hand towels and drinking vessels for the water fountain'—this advice appeared below a photograph of two schoolgirls dutifully and smilingly using cups brought from home to 'show what all schoolchildren should be doing during the epidemic' (Here's a Tip for Mothers, 1949). The *Herald* reinforced this message the following week with a photograph of a three-year-old pre-school boy in suburban Melbourne filling his personal cup with water—in this instance, the newspaper explained, the water was delivered from communal taps that had been carefully modified with chicken wire to prevent mouths from touching shared surfaces (Taps Wired at School, 1949). Contracted from water, food or objects that had been contaminated by the faeces or mucous of an infected person, polio was shrouded in shame and associated with poverty and dirty living conditions in the early 20th century (National Museum Australia, n.d.). However, the more advanced a country in public health standards of hygiene, the more likely it was to experience epidemics of polio. To this end, polio was often referred to as the 'disease of public progress' (Highley, 2009). Like the students sitting outside in Figure 3.1, with their prettily arranged hair and neat clothing, those depicted bringing their cups from home convey both conscientiousness and cleanliness. Such images offered a double message—that it was possible for 'ordinary' children to catch polio—and that taking care of the environment could help to make such children safe.

The concern of parents, schools and authorities was understandable given the statistics; polio notifications in Australia peaked between 1936 and 1940, with over 2,500 cases annually, and then again between 1944 and 1956 with slightly lower annual totals (Australian Institute of Health and Welfare (AIHW), 2018). As the century progressed, the intervals between epidemics in Australia became shorter, suggesting the disease was becoming endemic (Highley, 2009). Deaths from polio peaked in 1951 at 357 nationally (AIHW, 2018), and the epidemics from 1951 to 1953 saw the median incidence of polio double that of the 1937–1938 epidemic (Highley, 2009). There were an estimated 20,000–40,000 Australians who were diagnosed with paralytic childhood polio between the 1930s and 1960s, resulting in acute disability, extended hospital stays and some experiencing the effects decades later of having had polio (Highley, 2009).

Educational and medical discourses also intersected in what Yoshida and colleagues (2017) refer to as the 'education of difference' provided to children living with a polio disability. Their work gathers the schooling experiences of English-speaking Canadian children in the 1940s and 1950s affected by polio. They argue that meanings about polio and disability were learned both at school and through the medical interventions (e.g. surgeries and physiotherapy) children underwent. This 'education' was framed by ableist ideas of disability as deficit, and the aim was to mend and correct 'crippled' bodies in order to 'normalise' the lives of children affected by polio to make them 'less disabled' or 'normal'. Historian Daniel J. Wilson (2005) notes during outbreaks in the 1940s and 1950s in the United States, the fear of becoming crippled or immobilised was pervasive, and this fear was reinforced by the myriad images of children with infantile paralysis used by organisations such as the March of Dimes trying to raise funds for polio care. Drawing on Paul Longmore (1997), Wilson (2005) argues that infantile paralysis—being confined or losing autonomy and control—was antithetical to American aspirations for childhood and citizenship. In Australia, similar tropes were wedded to ideas about childhood development and children as future citizens. Disability operated as an interruption to normal, healthy childhood development. Intellectual disability was viewed as a complete interruption of normative development as children with an intellectual disability were thought to not be able to achieve the maturity, independence and rationality characterising adulthood (Earl, 2017; Gleason, 2013). Physical disability on the other hand was perceived as something that could be fixed, with the impact on a normal, productive future minimised (Gleason, 2013).

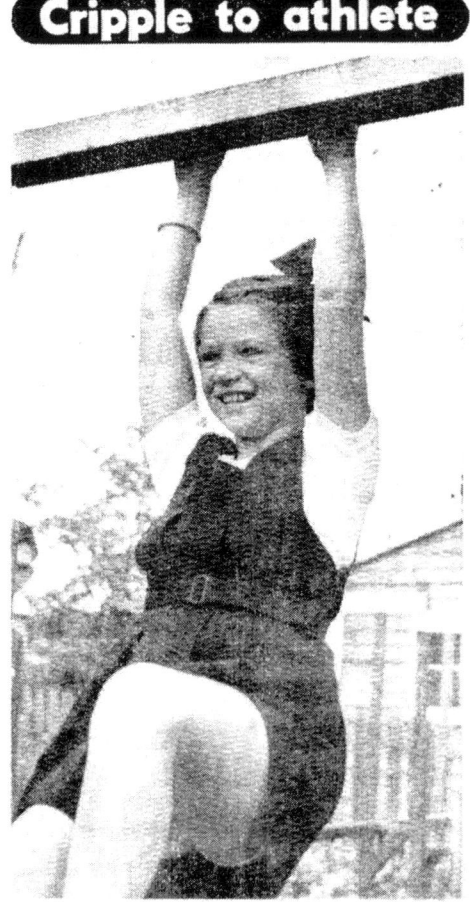

FIGURE 3.2   Barbara McGregor, from Cripple to Athlete (1950).

Source: Cripple to Athlete. (1950, October 18), *The Sun*, 5.

Figure 3.2 is a 1950 photograph featured in the Sydney *Sun* newspaper. Young Barbara McGregor of Punchbowl, an outer suburb of Sydney, is pictured playing exuberantly in her school uniform, having made a 'full recovery' from polio. The accompanying text explains that in eight short months, with the aid of physical exercise, Barbara, who had been 'paralysed down one side' and needed to be 'wheeled to school', was now a member of a church physical culture team (Cripple to Athlete, 1950). Given that one is disabled because of the structural and attitudinal barriers that organise meanings and representations of disability, images of this kind were significant in producing and upholding simple dichotomies between disabled and non-disabled, where the former is pejoratively framed as something to be avoided or conquered.

The promise of able-bodiedness through treatment, rehabilitation and ultimately recovery provided strong justification for internalised acceptance of the disability status as a deficit to overcome. The British sociologist and disability activist, Paul Abberley (1987) opens his seminal analysis of disability oppression with autographical information. He contracted polio when he was five and 'spent six weeks in an iron lung, eight months in a hospital bed, and by the age of seven had regained sufficient mobility to attend a state primary school' (p. 5). Later in his life, he felt 'annoyance and resentment' for the requests to talk about disability as part of his academic work as he 'had spent most of [his] life, as many "successful" disabled people do, attempting as far as possible to deny and ignore what is in fact a very obvious collection of impairments' (p. 5). The necessity for material, physical and emotional investment in regaining and maintaining the non-disabled status is established through the medical responses to disability and has long-term implications.

The assumed threat to normalcy led some practitioners to pay close attention to the well-being of hospitalised children (Gleason, 2013). Significantly, in the 20th century, illness caused by an infectious disease was increasingly treated and managed in institutional settings rather than within the confines of the family home, dramatically changing the experiences of patients. Many patients with infantile paralysis in Australia were treated in an infectious disease ward and subsequently in a convalescent hospital (Highley, 2009, 2014). Gleason (2013) describes the important place of health and bodies in memories of childhood—injured bodies, burdensome bodies, fevered bodies and sick and healing bodies. These memories reflect dominant social discourses about childhood, childhood health and the child/adult relationship. This is perhaps most acutely illustrated in the memories of those children who spent months, sometimes years, in hospitals without their parents and with visiting hours greatly restricted. Apart from wanting to minimise the spread of infectious disease brought into hospitals from visitors, it was also thought to be in the best interest of children to be left in the hands of medical staff who could focus intensely on the child without the distractions of the parents or the child–parent dynamics (Gleason, 2013).

During periods of isolation in the infectious disease ward, children with polio had no access to their parents, often for weeks or months. Kerry Highley (2009) documents the memories of children with polio in Australian hospitals away from their parents and siblings. She notes that often children misunderstood why they had contracted polio or why they were enduring painful hospital stays, with some survivors believing they had caught the polio virus because of their bad behaviour at home or at school. The early stages of polio, in which many were isolated, were extremely painful, and painkillers were not administered as there was concern they could exacerbate the severity of the disease (Highley, 2009). Even when patients were deemed safe to interact with their families, they often endured long periods of immobilisation and/or painful rehabilitation. Highley notes that unlike patients who suffered spinal cord injuries, polio patients retained full sensory awareness during the early acute phase of the disease. The pain suffered by patients was fraught with misunderstanding and misinterpretation. For example, a dominant school of thought was that pain was linked to movement, and as such patients endured long periods of prescribed immobilisation, thought to reduce the pain. The therapeutic methods pioneered by Australian bush nurse Sister Elizabeth Kenny challenged traditional clinical approaches that relied on immobilisation. Kenny acknowledged the significant pain experienced by polio patients and prescribed hot compresses in the acute phases of the disease, and passive movement exercises once patients could withstand it (Highley, 2009; also see Rogers, 2021).

The polio virus could also paralyse the intercostal muscles, compromising the ability to breathe, and patients would be put into iron lung machines which accommodated the patient's body up to their neck. While respirators saved children's lives, being restricted and isolated in them was often traumatising (Highley, 2009; Wilson, 2005). Living in these enormous respirators was a terrible ordeal, involving long periods of restriction and isolation (Highley, 2009; Wilson, 2005). Despite this, news media depicted children in iron lungs as being resolute, happy and cared for. For example, Figure 3.3, a photograph from the tabloid magazine *Pix* (Plucky Child Fights Disability, 1941), shows a young girl with a carefully arranged ribbon in her hair smiling while undergoing hours-long treatment in a mechanical respirator; the accompanying text reads, 'She used to spend eight hours a day in the respirator, but this has now been reduced to six. Even boredom … does not subdue her high spirits. Nurses say she is always happy and bright' (see also Paralysed Boy Learned to Breathe, 1943). Newsreels spread similar images. Cinesound Productions filmed news footage at the Austin Hospital, in Melbourne, released in numerous reels, showing 'children crippled by infantile paralysis [undergoing] treatment in iron lungs and [attending] physiotherapy'—this included multiple shots of children in respirators smiling at the camera (*Science Guides Child Welfare*, 1941). The images of these children worked to counter terrifying ideas of life with polio and construct the polio child as possessing a certain strength and durability and promise for rehabilitation, with the right care in a gleamingly clean, modern hospital. Shifting public perceptions of iron lungs would not have been an easy task, given that in his study of the medical technology and its use, David Rothman (1997) notes that often there was a delay in placing children in iron lungs, thus worsening the effects of the paralysis because of perceptions of the apparatus as 'coffin life' and its association with severe disability.

The pictures of children in iron lungs also posit that life in hospital is as close to normal as it possibly can be. Towards this end, news outlets depicted children with polio playing cricket (*Science Guides Child Welfare*, 1941),

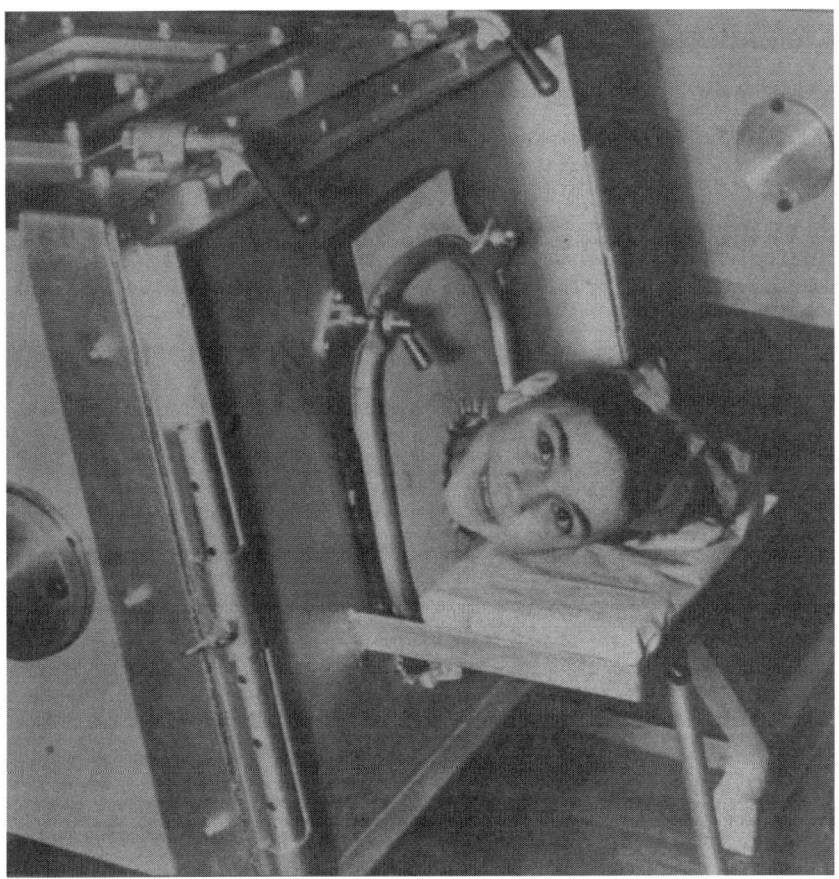

FIGURE 3.3 'Plucky' child in an iron lung, 1941.

Source: Plucky Child Fights Disability. (1941, February 15), *Pix*, 13.

creating artworks (e.g. Plucky Child Fights Disability, 1941; Paralysed Boy Learned to Breathe, 1943), and celebrating their birthday, as in Figure 3.4, a photograph featured in a 1937 issue of the South Australian *Chronicle* showing young Barbara Hindley 'recovering from infantile paralysis' and celebrating her seventh birthday at the Children's Hospital in Frankston, Victoria (Cheery Victims of Paralysis, 1937). Figure 3.4 captures the girl's apparently high spirits despite significant immobilisation. Normal childhoods were constructed through events like birthdays and also through the routine of schooling in hospital.

The education of children living in hospital served to ensure they did not fall behind in their normal pathway of development despite their circumstances. Print media captured school life in hospital settings, often

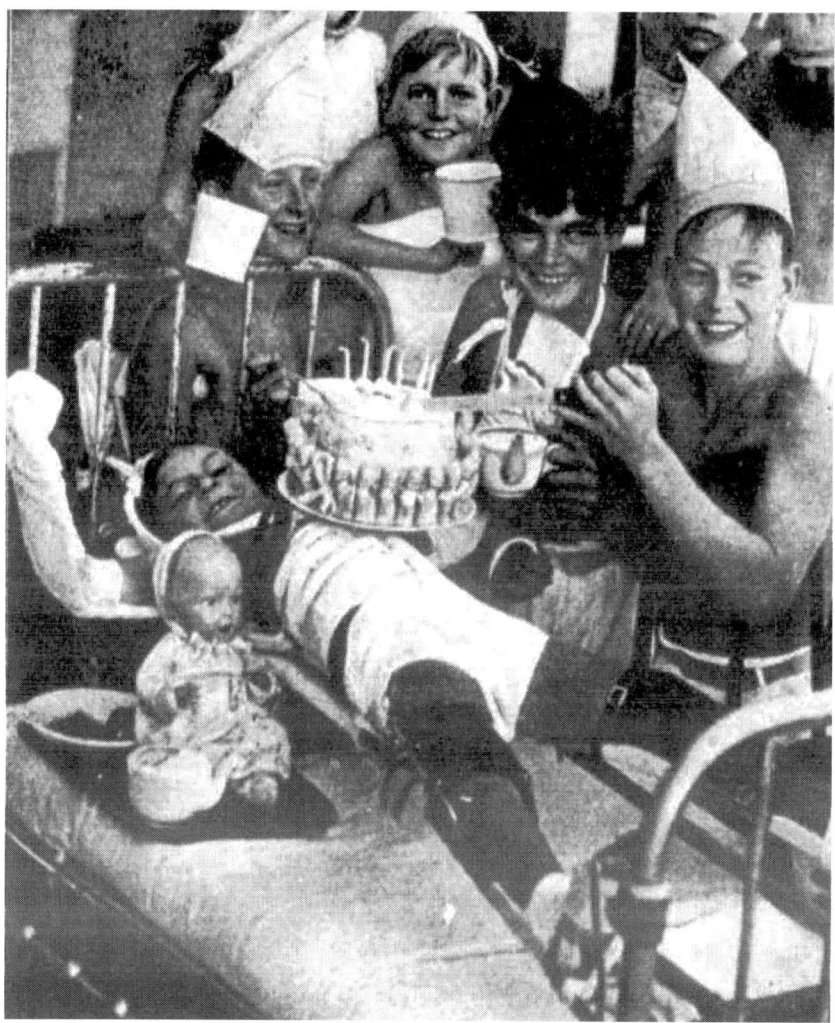

FIGURE 3.4 'Cheery victims' celebrate a birthday, 1937.

Source: Cheery Victims of Paralysis. (1937, December 2), *The Chronicle*, 37.

highlighting the attention paid to children by visiting dignitaries. The magazine *Pix* ran a photograph of a teenager 'stricken with infantile paralysis' being visited and taught by Clive Evatt, the New South Wales Minister for Education (Paralysed Boy Learned to Breathe, 1943). The *Sun*, a Sydney newspaper, published an image of an eight-year-old 'being instructed by Mrs. A. Higgins, of the Education Department at Prince Henry Hospital' (Hospital School Popular, 1946). The new schools established in hospitals are particularly visible in news articles like A School of a Different Kind (1950) in the

Sydney Morning Herald and Unusual School (1950) in the *Sunday Herald* about the Fred Birk's Activity School annexed to the Royal Alexandra Hospital for Children in Sydney. The special nature of these schools is presented as the means for future inclusion in society by providing educational and vocational opportunities.

As some hospital schools became hybrid schools, educating not only children in their wards but also those from the community, some students did not experience the transient nature of attending a hospital school. What is missing from the discourse is a public discussion of the schools that the students returned to and how they adapted or not to their needs. Highley (2009) notes that persistent misunderstandings about how polio was contracted and spread meant that some schools destroyed children's possessions, burning books and other items and fumigating their lockers. Likewise, as late as the 1950s, many Australians believed that children who had contracted polio remained contagious even after rehabilitation. Altenbaugh (2006) discusses how exclusion and segregation were the responses that students experienced when they returned to school in the United States. When students were allowed back in their schools, they experienced at best casual integration, which was dependent on students' ability to compensate for their impairments. The schism between the adapted, specialised environment of the hospital and rehabilitation setting and the 'normal' school environment constitutes also a schism in the reporting and representations around polio. While the detailed empirical work has not been done for Australia, there is no reason to imagine that reintegration was systematically supported by schools, or that significant structural adjustments were made to buildings or furniture (e.g. Campbell & Proctor, 2014; Slee, 1993).

Conclusion

Understandings of childhood polio and disability in Australia reflect broader social norms and approaches to childhood health and development promoted by medical and public health authorities. The case study of polio demonstrates how the curriculum of the body intersects with education and medical/public health discourses and experiences. It also highlights how 'schooling' children and managing (un)healthy bodies has long extended beyond the traditional brick and mortar school, suggesting that schooling in hospital and formal hospital schools represents a relatively unexplored area of research.

There is still work to be done in understanding the historical relationships between polio, childhood health and the place of schooling in the lives of Australian children living with infantile paralysis. There is a dearth of work asking how different children and different bodies were impacted by periods of hospitalisation and treatment. Take, for example, the polio outbreaks in the late 1930s and early 1940s in migrant camps in NSW and Tasmania, where children from these camps were brought to public hospital for care. Newspapers warned of childhood infections, blaming 'insanitary conditions of the migrants' who were said to be 'not using modern lavatories provided for them' and 'swimming in [the local creek] ... which has been polluted by sewage' (Migrant Camp Menace, 1950; also e.g. Polio Hits Migrants, 1951). These infected and contagious bodies are mediated differently from the bodies explored in this paper. Future research should attend to the ways in which the care of children with polio was underscored by assumptions about race, class and gender. Canadian childhood historian Mary-Ellen Kelm (1998) stresses that the bodies of Indigenous children have always been more vulnerable in institutional settings, including schools and hospitals, experiencing physical, emotional and sexual abuse. It is critical for new work to consider how to prioritise the oft invisibilised experiences of First Nations people and their racialised experiences at the intersections of medical care and education. The representations gathered for this research illustrate the overinvestment in the white child as the image of polio survival and recovery.

Finally, a growing body of historical research focuses on the materialities of schooling (e.g. Brunelli & Meda, 2017; Lawn & Grosvenor, 2005). The artefacts associated with infantile paralysis and polio care, including casts, splints, crutches, large crane-like devices that lifted and moved patients, and iron lungs, reflect cultural values around science, childhood and disability and shape the experiences and memories of people affected by polio and therefore point towards an important area of investigation in the field.

References

A School of a Different Kind. (1950, April 6). *Sydney Morning Herald*, 2.

Abberley, P. (1987). The concept of oppression and the development of a social theory of disability. *Disability, Handicap & Society*, 2(1), 5–19.

Allender, T., Dussel, I., Grosvenor, I., & Priem, K. (2021). *Appearances matter: The visual in educational history*. De Gruyter Oldenbourg.

Altenbaugh, R.J. (2006). Where are the disabled in the history of education? The impact of polio on sites of learning. *History of Education*, 35(6), 705–730.

Anderson, W. (2005). *The cultivation of whiteness: Science, health and racial destiny in Australia* (New ed.). Melbourne University Press.

Armstrong, D. (1993). Public health spaces and the fabrication of identity. *Sociology*, 27(3), 393–410.

Australian Institute of Health and Welfare (AIHW). (2018). Polio in Australia.

Booth, D. (2005). Evidence revisited: Interpreting historical materials in sport history. *Rethinking History*, 9(4), 459–483. 10.1080/13642520500307990

Brady, A., Burns, K., & Davies, C. (2018). *Mediating sexual citizenship: Neoliberal subjectivities in television culture*. Routledge.

Brunelli, M., & Meda, J. (2017). Gymnastics between school desks: An educational practice between hygiene requirements, healthcare and logistic inadequacies in Italian primary schools (1870–1970). *History of Education Review*, 46(2), 178–193.

Burke, C., Cunningham, P., & Grosvenor, I. (2010). Putting education in its place: Space, place and materialities in the history of education. *History of Education*, *39*(6), 677–680.

Burke, P. (2001). *Eyewitnessing: The uses of images as historical evidence*. Reaktion Books.

Burns, K., Proctor, H., & Weaver, H. (2020). Modern schooling and the curriculum of the body. In T. Fitzgerald (Ed.), *Handbook of historical studies in education* (pp. 1–21). Springer. 10.1007/978-981-10-0942-6_34-1

Burns, K., & Proctor, H. (2022). *Growing up. Education, change and society* (5th edition), (pp. 25–47). Oxford University Press.

Campbell, C., & Proctor, H. (2014). *A history of Australian schooling*. Allen & Unwin.

Cheery Victims of Paralysis. (1937, December 2). *The Chronicle*, 37.

Cripple to Athlete. (1950, October 18). *The Sun*, 5.

Earl, D. (2017). Australian histories of intellectual disabilities 1. In *The Routledge history of disability* (pp. 308–319). Routledge.

Gard, M., & Pluim, C. (2014). *Schools and public health: Past, present, future*. Lexington Books.

Gleason, M. (2013). *Small matters: Canadian children in sickness and health, 1900–1940*. McGill-Queen's University Press.

Grosvenor, I., Lawn, M., & Rousmaniere, K. (Eds.). (1999). *Silences and images: The social history of the classroom*. Peter Lang.

Hansen, B. (2009). *Picturing medical progress from Pasteur to polio: A history of mass media images and popular attitudes in America*. Rutgers University Press.

Here's a Tip for Mothers. (1949, September 8). *The Herald*, 5.

Highley, K. (2014). *Dancing in my dreams: Confronting the spectre of polio*. Monash University Publishing.

Highley, K. A. (2009). *Mending bodies: Polio treatment in Australia*. [Doctoral dissertation, Australian National University]. ANU Open Access Theses. 10.25911/5 d51575e8340a

Holdsworth, D. (2017). More than puddles: Disability and Masculinity in Alan Marshall's *I can jump puddles*. In C. Loeser, V. Crowley, B. Pini (Eds.), *Disability and masculinities* (pp. 105–123). Palgrave Macmillan UK. 10.1057/978-1-137-53477-4_5

Hospital School Popular. (1946, October 3). *The Sun*, 5.

Infantile Paralysis: Many Districts Isolated, More Schools to be Closed. (1937, July 24). *The Age*, 25.

Jordanova, L. (2010). [Review of the book *Picturing medical progress from Pasteur to polio: A history of mass media images and popular attitudes in America*, by B. Hansen]. *Isis*, *101*(4), 896–897. 10.1086/659701

Kelm, M.-E. (1998). *Colonizing bodies: Aboriginal health and healing in British Columbia, 1900–50*. UBC Press.

Killalea, A. (1995). *The great scourge: The Tasmanian infantile paralysis epidemic, 1937–1938*. Tasmanian Historical Research Association.

Kirk, D. (1998). *Schooling bodies: School practice and public discourse, 1880–1950*. Leicester University Press.

Lawn, M., & Grosvenor, I. (Eds.). (2005). *Materialities of schooling: Design, technology, objects, routines*. Symposium.

London, J. (2014). *The golden age*. Random House.

Longmore, P.K. (1997). Conspicuous contribution and American cultural dilemmas: Telethon rituals of cleansing and renewal. In D.T. Mitchell, & S.L. Snyder (Eds.), *The body and physical difference: Discourses of disability* (pp. 134–160). University of Michigan Press.

Marshall, A. (1956). *I can jump puddles* (School ed.). F.W. Cheshire.

Migrant Camp Menace. (1950, January 8). *The Sun*, 40.

National Museum Australia. (n.d.). *Defining moments: Polio vaccine introduced in Australia*. Retrieved 19 June 2023 from: https://www.nma.gov.au/defining-moments/resources/polio-vaccine-introduced-in-australia

Need for Precaution on Polio. (1950, December 12). *The Townsville Daily Bulletin*, 1.

Newman, L. (2022). Bodies of knowledge: Historians, health and education. *History of Education*, (ahead of print), 1–16. 10.1080/0046760X.2022.2112767

Out to Beat Polio. (1949, September 9). *The Sun*, 5.

Paralysed Boy Learned to Breathe. (1943, October 9). *Pix*, 18–19.

Pineau, P., & Frechtel, I. (2022). Health, illness, and schools in Argentina: Marks of epidemics in the history of a changing relation. *Paedagogica Historica*, *58*(5), 676–690. 10.1080/00309230.2022.2077119

Plucky Child Fights Disability. (1941, February 15). *Pix*, 12–13.

Polio Fear Keeps Pupils From School. (1953, August 1). *The Daily Telegraph*, 8.

Polio Hits Migrants. (1951, April 2). *The Mercury*, 3.

Polio Scare Hits Back-to-School. (1949, September 6). *The Herald*, 3.

Proctor, H., & Burns, K. (2017). The connected histories of mass schooling and public health. *History of Education Review*, *46*(2), 118–124.

Rogers, N. (2021). Polio and its role in shaping American physical therapy. *Physical Therapy*, *101*(6), pzab181. 10.1093/ptj/pzab126

Rothman, D.J. (1997). Beginnings count: The technological imperative in American health care (pp. 42–66). Oxford University Press.

Science guides child welfare [Newsreel]. (1941, September 26). Cinesound Productions. Title 73121, National Film and Sound Archive.

Slee, R. (Ed.). (1993). *Is there a desk with my name on it? The politics of integration*. Routledge.

Smith, J.H. (1997). Fear, frustration and the will to overcome: A social history of poliomyelitis in Western Australia. [Doctoral dissertation, Edith Cowan University]. Edith Cowan University Research Online. https://ro.ecu.edu.au/theses/921

Taps Wired at School. (1949, September 16). *The Herald*, 1.

Tucker, J. (2008). Objectivity, collective sight, and scientific personae. [Review of the book *Objectivity*, by L. Daston, & P. Galison]. *Victorian Studies*, *50*(4), 648–657. 10.2979/VIC.2008.50.4.648

Tucker, J. (2009). Entwined practices: Engagements with photography in historical inquiry. *History and Theory: Studies in the Philosophy of History*, *48*(4), 1–8. 10.1111/j.1468-2303.2009.00513.x

Unusual School. (1950, May 14). *Sunday Herald*, 1.

Vargha, D. (2018). Polio and disability in Cold War Hungary. In M. Rembis, C. Kudlick, & K.E. Nielsen (Eds.), *The Oxford handbook of disability history* (pp. 369–384). Oxford University Press. 10.1093/oxfordhb/9780190234959.013.22

Wilson, D.J. (2005). Braces, wheelchairs, and iron lungs: The paralyzed body and the machinery of rehabilitation in the polio epidemics. *The Journal of Medical Humanities*, *26*(2–3), 173–190. 10.1007/s10912-005-2917-z

Yoshida, K., Ferguson, S., & Shanouda, F. (2017). Breaking the rules: Summer camping experiences and the lives of Ontario children growing up with polio in the 1940s and 1950s. In R. Hanes, I. Brown, & N.E. Hansen (Eds.), *The Routledge history of disability* (pp. 455–484). Routlege. 10.1201/9781315198781-31

PART 2

Programmes and policies

4

EDUCATING THE UNDERWORKED

Dudley Allen Sargent and the influence of the rural worker on American physical culture, 1875–1919

Jason L. Newton

In 1875, at the age of 12, the stout and strong Louis Cyr started working in the lumber camps of Québec, Canada. By his 20s, he became the self-declared strongest man in the world, travelling Europe and North America in strongman shows. Cyr's powerful body drew the attention of Dr Dudley Allen Sargent, the influential American physical culture instructor. Using measuring tapes, callipers and resistance machines Sargent deduced that Cyr was, in fact, one of the strongest people alive (Beiderhase, 1906; Thomas de la Peña, 2003). Sargent's testimony was important. He was an expert in anthropometry and measured hundreds of students and famous examples of masculine power in order to create his physical culture curriculum and improve the health of young people. To Sargent, rural workers like Cyr demonstrated how middle-class men could fight the degrading effects of urban industrialism.

As a teacher at Bowdoin, Yale, Harvard and his own private schools, Sargent spread his ideas to 3,000 physical educators, one-third of all the teachers trained in this area in the United States by 1920. Though Sargent had conceptions of both the powerful manual labourer's body and ill-formed middle-class bodies, both conceptions were weakly connected to contemporaneous realities. Nevertheless, Sargent's students spread what they learned about workers' physicality across the country, having a great effect on the physical education part of the mass schooling movement in its formative years (Bennett, 1999; Sargent & Sargent, 1927).

This chapter explores Sargent's life and career to demonstrate how universities in the United States incorporated an idealised manual-worker bodily image into their physical culture curriculum. Sargent's curriculum demonstrates the reactionary sentiment at the foundation of physical culture. According to Sargent, as the propagators of urban corporate capitalism became more sedentary, and as hyper-specialisation of work became a driving feature of the economy, the bodies of

DOI: 10.4324/9781003288671-7

American men became unbalanced and effeminate. Sargent's curriculum, which was designed to correct these problems, reflected what later historians of gender called a 'crisis in masculinity/manhood' (Bederman, 1995; Douglas, 1977). He thought that the world that students would enter after graduation was poisonous to proper masculine health. Sargent and his contemporaries in physical culture and higher education nostalgically considered how the environments and work of early American 'pioneers'—loggers, farmers and Indian fighters—had positively affected the health and character of the nation (Turner, 1920). Natural masculinity could only be found outside the industrial city among people doing antiquated types of work which bestowed them with naturally masculine and healthy physiques (Baron, 2006; Bederman, 1995; Devlin, 2005; Jordan, 2016; Kidd, 2004; Kimmel, 2005; Macleod, 2004; Newton, 2017; Park, 2007a; Putney, 2001; Rotundo, 1993; Slavishak, 2008; Winter, 2002).

Importantly, Sargent's understanding of the healthy masculine body reflected his nationalistic and racist preconceptions which excluded black and brown people as well as the new immigrant class from eastern Europe and Asia. Moreover, it was devoid of overt class politics. As opposed to being a champion of the working class, Sargent's curriculum was inspired by and created by an idealised American worker that was mostly depoliticised. Working-class muscularity had a separate significance for socialists, syndicalists and unionist audiences. For these reasons, this chapter does not use the term working class to refer to Sargent's understanding of the healthy male body.

Still, Sargent was looking down the social and economic hierarchy for examples to help form his physical culture curriculum. Curriculum studies have often focussed on the way that curricula imposed western elite standards onto colonial subjects, immigrants or slum dwellers (Proctor, 2020). The narrative of lower-class disempowerment is firmly entrenched in the history of the American 'Progressive Era', a period named after elite reformers. Sargent's curricula are a helpful about-face, wherein the elite body is the subject of reform and the subaltern body the ideal. Cyr and other specific kinds of manual labourers influenced the curricula instituted in the most prestigious universities in the United States, affecting the most powerful people in the country, including future American presidents, as we will see below.

Curricula like Sargent's were, according to Helen Proctor, 'organized exhibition[s] of connected knowledge for the purpose of educating people', typically to prepare them for the future they will grow into (2020). Sargent and many other physical culture teachers were attempting to use curricula to resurrect aspects of an ideal past. In *No Place of Grace* (1981), historian T.J. Jackson Lears called those Americans who began to celebrate the past in this way *antimodernists*. Shannon L. Walsh's recent book sees Sargent as ahead of his time in forming the self-centred and isolated neoliberal subject. By not placing Sargent into the context of a larger antimodernist movement, Walsh fails to see that Sargent's curriculum was, in fact critiquing the direction of modern society, not foreshadowing it (Walsh, 2020). In doing this, Sargent's curriculum implicitly dictated what type of work, environments and bodily forms were properly masculine, and which were effeminate, and embedded these standards into mass schooling.

To better understand the reactionary roots of modern physical education, the first section of this chapter explores real models of masculinity that Sargent studied. The second explains the problems that antimodernists like Sargent sought to fix: unhealthy cities and the bodies they created. The idealised lives of rural workers as interpreted by Sargent is the subject of the third section as is the practical solutions to these problems. Sargent wrote extensively about how his teaching was inspired by his own life experiences and observations of 'real men' with whom he came into contact. These topics are explored in section four. One student who was affected by Sargent's lessons was American President Theodore Roosevelt, and aspects of his education are discussed in section five. This section shows Sargent's curriculum involved more than mimicry of working-class bodies. Antimodernist curricula encouraged students to go outside of the classroom to seek out rural workers and their environments in order to improve their own health.

How workers' bodies were built

Sargent drew inspiration from real working people, though these were most often famous people and people from his past (Black, 2013). Louis Cyr was clearly important for Sargent. Cyr professed that he built his strength by working on farms and in forests, but even when not working, Cyr pushed stones, rolled tree trunks, climbed trees, carried sacks of grain and lifted animals for exercise (Norwood, 1982). The Cyr family moved to America in 1878, one of the millions who made the trip to America to work in its factories. Cyr found factory work restrictive, so he took up farm work. By 1881, he was again working in logging camps, but crowds came to watch him. Thereafter Cyr performed as a strongman full-time, travelling the United States, Canada and England, challenging others to lift competitions that drew large crowds and were reported on widely (Weider, 1976).

Cyr's famous body was built by manual labour as was the body of one of his close friends John L. Sullivan, heavyweight boxing champion and one of the most famous men in America. Like Cyr, Sullivan came from a working-class background. When Sargent measured Sullivan, he declared the boxer one of the most powerful and 'girthy' men ever recorded. Sargent formed a close relationship with the pugilist, even helping him write his autobiography (Gorn, 2010; Kasson, 2001; Kimmel, 2005; Sullivan & Sargent, 1892). To Sargent, Cyr and Sullivan were representative of a white American working-class body, even though clearly these were extraordinary examples.

Unhealthy cities, unhealthy capitalism

Sargent's analysis of Cyr and Sullivan took place in the context of changes in American demographics and work. The number of American cities with

100,000 residents rose from 15 to 68 between 1870 and 1920. Production in these new urban spaces was powered by water, coal and eventually electricity, seemingly making human muscles obsolete. Between 1870 and 1940, the old middle class of farmers, businessmen and free professionals dropped from 85% of the working population to 44%. The percentage of Americans producing goods dropped from 77% to 46%. Between 1870 and 1910, the number of clerical workers—so-called 'brain workers'—in the country quadrupled (Lears, 1981; Lebergott, 1966; Mills, 1951). Authors like Jacob Riis, Upton Sinclair, Robert Woods and Josiah Strong convinced thousands of readers that industrialised cities, and the new types of work found in them, would negatively affect American health (Lears, 1981; Mills, 1951; Prescott, 2007; Strong, 1907). Nevertheless, this was the environment that many teachers imagined children and young adults would likely grow into.

Reactionary antimodernist argued that brain work stripped men of the authority and authentic masculinity of previous generations. Brain workers were entrenched in corporate structures where abstract forces like economic recessions could quickly change their fates and destroy them. Moreover, male brain workers were increasingly working alongside women in the office as equals (DeVault, 1995; Prescott, 2007; Srole, 2012). The rural life that antimodernists imagined gave men independent control over land, children, women, servants and animals. Farmers, farm labourers, lumbermen, small craftsmen and other rural workers toiled in homosocial groups, dictated the terms of their own lives, and at the same time pursued health-building activities.

The physical manifestations of urban industrialisation were obvious to Sargent. 'It is not only possible in many cases to distinguish individuals by their calling', Sargent found, 'but the particular branch of work in which they are engaged can be easily determined by its influence upon their physical structure' (Sargent, 1912). Sedentary occupations required the 'use of only small parts of the body, such as the fingers and hands', and this led to 'various kinds of local palsies, deformities, and nervous collapses' (Sargent, 1914a). Brain workers disproportionately suffered from 'neurasthenia', a disease with symptoms like headaches, tiredness and possibly even death (Beard, 1881; Rotundo, 1993). In *Gunn's New Family Physician*, James Gunn argued that:

> The active countryman, the farmer, the hunter, the common labourer, and those who take much exercise in the open air, do not suffer from this nervous debility and weakness. It is usually those of sedentary habits, who are confined to the house and the office.
>
> (Gunn et al., 1868)

Dyspepsia was a nonspecific stomach or bowel problem that, like neurasthenia, was found most often among the urban middle class. Dr Dio Lewis, the author of *Our Digestion: Or, My Jolly Friend's Secret*, argued that previous generations had more hardy stomachs because '[o]ur grand- fathers lived and worked in the open air. We live and work in stove heat. They worked hard— chopping and digging. We sit and move our fingers' (1872).

Alongside brain workers, the health of the urban working class was also supposedly in danger. According to one report from 1909, in the steel mills of Pittsburgh, men, women and children faced 'damaging noise parching heat … irritating dust that breeds throat and lung trouble … the vital wear and tear is tremendous: the hair of the steel worker grows grey at thirty-five'. When workers returned home 'under the shadow of the smoke-breathing mills', they dealt with overcrowded and unsanitary conditions (Bjorkman, 1909). Famous American author Jack London wrote that a child worker resembled a 'sickly ape, arms loose-hanging, stoop-shouldered, narrow chested, grotesque and terrible' (1911). Antimodernists juxtaposed the brain worker and the sickly factory hand with the robust and healthy rural worker.

Besides the obvious harms of the city, scientists and academics argued that modern production methods caused maladies indirectly. Experts like Sargent argued that people had a quantifiable amount of 'nervous' or 'vital' energy. In his *The Law of Civilization and Decay* (1895), historian Brooks Adams explained vital energy was analogous to all other energy: 'Whenever a race was so richly endowed with the energetic material that it does not expend all its energy in the daily struggle for life' Adams wrote, 'the surplus may be stored in the shape of wealth'. Industrial wealth was the apex of this crisis. According to Adams, 'the steam-engine [was] the most perfect of all vents of centralizing energy'. Widespread use of the steam engine meant that 'the economic, and, perhaps, the scientific intellect is propagated, while the imagination fades, and the emotional, the martial, and the artistic types of manhood decay' (Adams, 1903).

Labour's gender power

Brooks Adams argued social decay could be halted by 'the infusion of bar- barian blood' and many young men found this barbarous influence partici- pating in football, wrestling and boxing (Gorn, 2010; Lears, 1981; Mrozek, 1989; Park, 2012; Townsend, 1996). Others looked to rural workers. To antimodernists, rural work and environments were more authentic and more 'natural' (Wood, 1880). According to physician and social worker Richard Clarke Cabot, outdoor work recovered men's 'pioneer instinct … [that] ancient hunger to subdue the challenges which we meet, to tame what is wild' (Cabot, 1914). H.W. Foster wrote in the *Independent* magazine in 1900, '[i]t is generally conceded that the country-bred boy has made for himself a strong record. Necessity, difficulties, effort, struggle, are essential factors in main- taining a vigorous stock'. Through his struggle with nature the 'country-bred boy' gained 'fearlessness, pluck, self-reliance, activity, responsibility, patience, endurance [and] judgment. … For his labor he is rewarded with strength of body' (Foster, 2000). Civil War veteran Henry C. Merwin (2000, p. 317) urged urban Americans to:

> [l]eave the office … Consult the teamster, the farmer, the woodchopper, the shepherd, or the drover. You will find him … healthy in mind … free from fads, [and] strong in natural impulses … From his loins, and not from those of the dilettante, will spring the man of the future.

Geology teacher, native of the rural US state of Kentucky, and Sargent's colleague, professor Nathaniel Shaler, was sceptical of the 'tenderfoot' mannerisms of most students and professors at Harvard and believed that the loggers, miners and other rural workers of his native state provided examples of how the student body could be improved. 'This type of strong uneducated man, while he had little learning often had more life than those bred in academic places', Shaler wrote (Townsend, 1996).

On farms, quarries, railroads, lumber camps and other work sites across the country wage labourers were competing with one another in staged trade-based competitions that were as popular as many professional sporting events. These competitions, which Frank Zarnowski called 'work-sports', highlighted rural men's near super-human strength, agility and health (Zarnowski, 2013).

Unwell urbanites sought rural workers' environments to improve their health (Lansing, 2009). In his *American Nervousness* (1881), Charles Beard advised sufferers of neurasthenia to participate in 'camp cures' in the country or forest. Cabot extended the idea of the camp cure into a 'work cure'. Speaking to both the male and female patient, Cabot wrote that '[t]he patient's "rest cure" may not rest her at all. She may find that nothing rests her but work'. Cabot continued, arguing the patient should learn '*how* to work—a lesson which he usually needs very sorely' (Cabot, 1914). Sargent also had a camp in a forested part of the rural American state of New Hampshire where his students could connect directly with the outdoors (Hutchinson, 2015; Sargent, 1906).

Educating the underworked

Sargent learned from famous male figures, the problems of the city, but also his own life experiences. Born in 1849, Sargent spent his youth in the seaside towns of Hingham, Massachusetts and Belfast, Maine. Sargent admired his father's 'good physique', built through ship carpentry. He also admired the 'great seafaring men' of his communities (Sargent & Sargent, 1927). After his father died, Sargent began balancing school with manual labour jobs. His first experience of 'man's work' was helping construct a military battery. He also worked as a seaman, lumberjack and farm labourer.

Young Sargent was interested in the 'laws of health' but had few opportunities to exercise systematically. He decided to make his paid labour build his physique: 'Ploughing, mowing, tacking, pitching, hoeing, chopping, digging, hoisting, and all diversified forms of labour that fall to the lot of the country boy, were classified according to their specific effect in developing certain muscles of the body'. He wrote that this manual labour, alongside practicing gymnastics in a barn, built his body. He joined a circus as a strongman in 1867 and in 1869, at the age of 18, was hired to run the gymnasium at Bowdoin College in the American state of Maine (Cottrell, 1994; Leonard, 1915; Sargent & Sargent, 1927). Early physical educators like Sargent had few domestic examples to draw on to form a physical culture curriculum. The discipline had been developing since the 1830s, but the Association for the Advancement of Physical Education was not founded until 1885 (Leonard, 1915; Park, 2007a, 2007c; Sargent & Sargent, 1927).

The idea that work built strong bodies was common knowledge, however. Since the American Revolution in 1775, teachers advised students to do manual labour as part of normal curricula because of a belief in the health-building effects of hard work (Leonard, 1906). Cornell University's founder Ezra Cornell (1807–1874) argued for 10–20 hours of manual labour for students per week (Bishop, 1962; Wright, 1953). At the People's College in Havana, New York students were required to do 'bona fide labor in some branch of productive industry'. New York Central College, Connecticut Agricultural College, the New York State College of Forestry and Michigan Agricultural College all adopted labour requirements (Faculty Minutes, 1916; Park, 1987; Rudolph, 1962).

At Bowdoin, Sargent looked to the hinterland for inspiration. Maine was a very rural state with only 19 people per square mile on average in 1870. Sargent saw that 'it was customary for many students to work about farms, or in shops and mills or at some kind of physical labor … in order to … pay their college expenses'. The 'boys who came from farms, mills, and lumber camps' exhibited 'sheer strength, if little grace or agility' and 'generally showed a superior physique' compared to those who did not work', Sargent wrote. He sometimes compared college athletes to college workers. Oarsmen developed legs and backs but their 'shoulders and chests did not compare with those of the lumberman'. Sargent observed that 'some of the most prominent athletes … laid the foundation for their strength and agility while doing farm work or … some form of manual labor that gave them all-round exercise' (Sargent, 1889, 1914a; Sargent & Sargent, 1927).

This idea of all-around exercise or work was important because it countered the effects of the modern division of labour. 'Agricultural pursuits have always been among the hardiest and healthiest' Sargent wrote, 'as were the primitive trades of the carpenter, the blacksmith, the wheelwright, the gunsmith, etc. … these trades … furnished a man with a great deal of all-round activity' (Sargent, 1889, 1914a).

As is clear from the above quote, Sargent's understanding of history also shaped his methods. He wrote (1914a, pp. 5–6):

the life of primitive man implies a constant struggle with natural forces. … the progress of civilization has always depended upon the overcoming of material obstacles. Force has met force, and the energy and strength required in clearing forest, breaking up ground, laying out roads, and in building towns and cities with their numerous trades and industries, have given energy and strength to the masses.

Human muscles and health were built through working in nature: 'In the early history of American settlement we find no necessity for physical training … a frontier life kept our … ancestors free from nervous debility and muscular feebleness' (Sargent, 1914a, 1914b; Sargent & Sargent, 1927). In forming his curriculum, he posited that (1889, p. 63):

[i]f actual labor will produce such good physical results in certain directions, why will not a system of exercises in the gymnasium, resembling actual labor, accomplish the same result in opposite directions, and in this way be made to supplement the deficiencies of one's occupation, and to develop him where he is weak.

Realising that not all students could adventure outdoors regularly he also designed exercise apparatus that mimicked the 'work of natural labor' (Sargent, 1889, 1906; Sargent & Sargent, 1927). In her *The Body Electric* (2003), historian Carolyn Thomas de la Peña argued that Sargent saw machines as key to sculpting healthy bodies, but this chapter shows that Sargent's exercise machines were only designed to reproduce the effect that rural work had on the body.

While employed at Bowdoin, Sargent earned a BA, gave an award-winning oration titled 'Does Civilization Endanger Character?' and then went to Yale School of Medicine. There he taught gymnastics and, after graduating, ran a private gym. In 1879, he took a post as director of Harvard's Hemenway Gymnasium, which he held until 1919. He also continued operating private gyms (Sargent & Sargent, 1927).

At Harvard, Sargent observed weak students who had 'never made a fire, chopped a stick of wood, driven a nail, or actually worked'. By work, Sargent was clearly referring to his personal conception of proper masculine work, the type that he had done as a child, and the type that workers like Cyr and Sullivan had engaged in before they became famous. He therefore discounted any idea that new types of industrial and clerical work could be authentic or health building and in fact, dismissed them as unhealthy and effeminising.

Those preparing for these new types of work, what Sargent called the 'studious class', had developed 'drooping head[s], flat chest[s], hollow back, and constricted ribs … spinal curvature, soft and flabby musculatures, pale faces, inert skins, cold hands and feet and other evidence of a feeble circulation and malnutrition'. These conditions were caused by 'the pressure of the desk against the body, the constriction of clothing during the growing period, the relaxed state of certain muscles, and the over-strained condition of others' (Sargent, 1889, 1906, 1912; Sargent & Sargent, 1927). These ailments had a name, 'desk diseases', and in order to prevent or cure these problems each Harvard student was required to meet with Sargent to learn how to improve their health and form (Thomas de la Peña, 2003; Zakim, 2018). To Sargent, the entire university system was a clinic where sickness was both created and cured.

Solutions for desk diseases and urban industrialisation were described in Sargent's 'popular handbook' titled *Health, Strength & Power* (1914a, originally published in 1904). Written for 'persons subjected to the strains of modern life', specifically 'students … business and professional men', the book taught readers how to 'retain our acquired Health, Strength, and Power under the conditions imposed upon us by modern progress'. Exercises 'were suggested by different forms of labor … which men in city life necessarily abandoned'. Some had titles like 'Striking the Anvil', 'Scooping Sand', 'Rope Pulling', 'Fire Engine', 'Teamsters' Warming', 'Paddling Canoe', 'Throwing the Lasso', 'Driving Stakes', 'Wood-Chopping', 'Mowing', 'Pitching Hay', 'Grinding Corn', 'Sawing Wood', 'Hoisting Sail' and 'Furrowing Sail' (Figures 4.1 and 4.2). Other books for students of many different ages also prescribed imitation of rural work (Colburn,

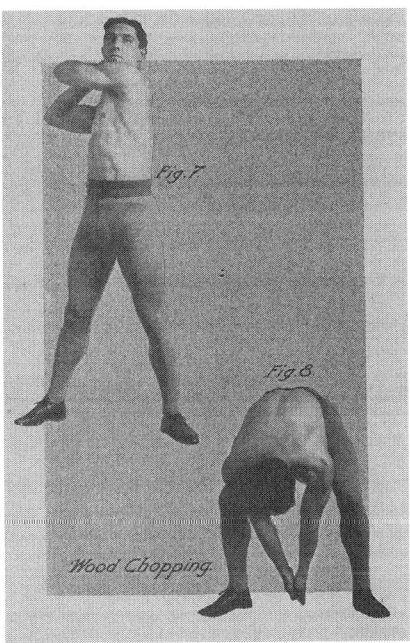

FIGURE 4.1 'Wood chopping' from Dudley Allen Sargent's *Health, Strength & Power* (1914a, p. 173).

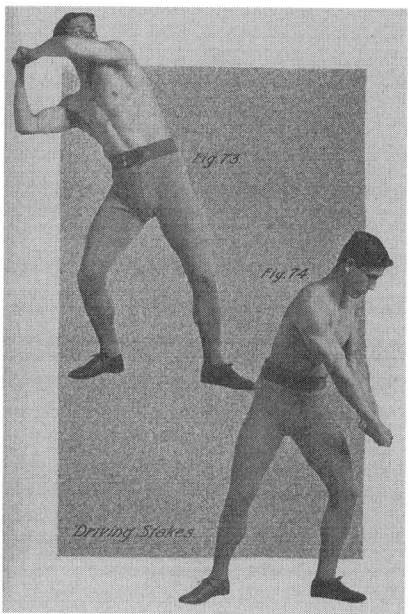

FIGURE 4.2 'Driving stakes' from Dudley Allen Sargent's *Health, Strength & Power* (1914a, p. 2).

1901). The performances of rural workers became exercises that thousands would perform so they could counter the effects of a future of industrial or clerical work.

Sargent's student: Accessing the American worker directly

While most of Sargent's students were content with exercises, some sought a deeper connection to workers (Park, 2007b). According to Walsh, Sargent desired to rid his exercises of connection to the lower classes. It was not that Sargent did not want his students to connect with rural people and environments, but that it simply was not practical for every student (Walsh, 2020). In fact, Sargent and other antimodernists encouraged students who could do so to seek out rural people and rural environments as part of the informal curricula of universities. This was particularly important for students of urban sociology and engineering students who needed connection with their subjects and underlings in order to do their jobs correctly.

Some students who were influenced by their antimodernist teachers 'rode the rails' with America's growing population of transient homeless known as 'hobos'. Others fought striking workers outside factory gates (DePastino, 2010; Norwood, 1994). One of Sargent's students, future American president Theodore Roosevelt, travelled to Maine while a student at Harvard in 1879. There Roosevelt hired as guides two working lumberjacks, William Sewell and

Wilmot Dow. Together, they hunted, tramped in the woods and up mountains and paddled (Harmon & Sewall, 1972; Meddybemps Philosophy, 1905). Sewall also took Roosevelt to a lumber camp where he slept, ate and even engaged in a wrestling competition with the workers (Brinkley, 2009; Sewall, 1919; Roosevelt 1879a, 1879b; Vietze, 2010).

After college Roosevelt continued associating with rural workers. In 1884, he opened a cattle business in North Dakota with the specific objective of connecting with workers and their environments (Hutchinson, 2015; Kidd, 2004; Townsend, 1996). Reflecting on Roosevelt's improved health over the course of his life, Sargent wrote: 'I am fully of the opinion that what Roosevelt did for his physical organism, thousands of other men may do by similar methods … ' (Sargent, 1919).

Conclusion

The turn of the century was a time of national self-reflection when academic and popular authors nostalgically contemplated the type of men, and type of masculinity, that had conquered the North American continent. At the same time, teachers scrutinised the middle-class body, judging it to be inferior compared to the imagined bodies of the past. The idea that industrial progress should continue and would improve and civilise the country was replaced by a pessimistic attitude towards modernity, and the idea that people needed to retard social progress to maintain personal and national health. Men needed to reestablish their natural masculinity. This was not a fad, it was instituted into Sargent's physical culture curriculum, which set a national standard and was propagated by thousands of Sargent's students. At this foundational moment in the history of mass schooling, Sargent and his students determined that outdoor work and outdoor activities were 'naturally' masculine. Sargent's influence would have a great effect on how schools systematically segregated males and females in terms of the types of lessons they received and the types of work they were being prepared to perform. It also systematically ostracised those people whose bodies and gender performances did not fit this sexual binary. While the antimodernist curriculum of Sargent was reactionary, it also showed that the American worker projected a type of power that forced elites to react. This projection of power shaped both mass schooling and the bodies of thousands of university students during this important period of American modernisation.

References

Adams, B. (1903). *The law of civilization and decay: An essay on history* (2nd ed.). Macmillan.

Baron, A. (2006). Masculinity, the embodied male worker, and the historian's gaze. *International Labor and Working-Class History, 69*(1), 143–160.

Beard, G.M. (1881). *American nervousness, its causes and consequences: A supplement to Nervous exhaustion (neurasthenia)*. Putnam.

Bederman, G. (1995). *Manliness & civilization: A cultural history of gender and race in the United States, 1880–1917*. University of Chicago Press.

Beiderhase, J. (1906). Athletics for girls and women: Discussed by the Public School Physical Training Society. *American Gymnasia and Athletic Record*, 2(8), 169–170.

Bennett, B.L. (1999). *Sargent, Dudley Allen*. American National Biography Online. https://doi-org.ezproxy.library.sydney.edu.au/10.1093/anb/9780198606697.article.1900191

Bishop, M. (1962). *A history of Cornell*. Cornell University Press.

Bjorkman, E. (1909). What industrial civilization may do to men. *World's Work, 17,* 11493–11494.

Black, J. (2013). *Making the American body: The remarkable saga of the men and women whose feats, feuds, and passions shaped fitness history*. University of Nebraska Press.

Brinkley, D. (2009). *The wilderness warrior: Theodore Roosevelt and the crusade for America*. HarperCollins.

Cabot, R. (1914). *What men live by; work, play, love, worship*. Houghton Mifflin.

Colburn, B.L. (1901). *Graded physical exercises*. E.S. Werner.

Cottrell, D.M. (1994). The Sargent School for Physical Education. *Journal of Physical Education Recreation & Dance*, 65(3), 32–37.

DePastino, T. (2010). *Citizen hobo: How a century of homelessness shaped America*. University of Chicago Press.

DeVault, I.A. (1995). *Sons and daughters of labor: Class and clerical work in turn-of-the-century Pittsburgh*. Cornell University Press.

Devlin, A. (2005). *Between profits and primitivism: Shaping white middle-class masculinity in the United States, 1880–1917*. Routledge.

Douglas, A. (1977). *The feminization of American culture* (1st ed.). Knopf.

Faculty Minutes. (1916, November 27). (Not catalogued). SUNY ESF Moon Library Archives, Syracuse, New York.

Foster, H.W. (2000). Physical education vs. degeneracy. In S.H. Smith & M. Dawson (Eds.), *The American 1890s: A cultural reader* (pp. 302–306). Duke University Press.

Gorn, E.J. (2010). *The manly art: Bare-knuckle prize fighting in America* (Updated ed.). Cornell University Press.

Gunn, J.C., Jordan, J.H., & Royce, C.S. (1868). *Gunn's new family physician: Or, home book of health, forming a complete household guide*. Moore, Wilstach & Baldwin.

Harmon, H.S., & Sewall, W.W. (1972). *Recollection of William Wingate Sewall (1845–1930) of Island Falls. Maine: Dedicated to the people of Island Falls in observance of Centennial Year 1972*.

Hutchinson, P.J. (2015). *Crafting an outdoor classroom: The nineteenth-century roots of the outdoor education movement*. (Publication No. 3714791) [Doctoral dissertation, Boston University]. Proquest Dissertations & Theses Global.

Jordan, B.R. (2016). *Modern Manhood and the Boy Scouts of America: Citizenship, race, and the environment, 1910–1930*. UNC Press Books.

Kasson, J.F. (2001). *Houdini, Tarzan, and the perfect man: The white male body and the challenge of modernity in America*. Hill and Wang.

Kidd, K.B. (2004). *Making American boys: Boyology and the feral tale*. University of Minnesota Press.

Kimmel, M.S. (2005). *The History of men: Essays on the history of American and British masculinities*. SUNY Press.

Lansing, M.J. (2009). 'Salvaging the man power of America': Conservation, manhood, and disabled veterans during World War I. *Environmental History, 14*(1), 32–57.

Lears, T.J.J. (1981). *No place of grace: Antimodernism and the transformation of American culture, 1880–1920*. Pantheon Books.

Lebergott, S. (1966). Labor force and employment, 1800–1960. In D.S. Brady (Ed.), *Output, employment, and productivity in the United States after 1800* (pp. 117–204). National Bureau of Economic Research.

Leonard, F.E. (1906). The introduction of manual labor as a system of exercise in educational institutions (1825–1835). *Mind and Body: A Monthly Journal Devoted to Physical Education, 13*(148), 97–103.

Leonard, F.E. (1915). *Pioneers of modern physical training*. Association Press.

Lewis, D. (1872). *Our digestion: Or, my jolly friend's secret*. Maclean.

London, J. (1911). *When God laughs, and other stories*. Macmillan.

Macleod, D.I. (2004). *Building character in the American boy: The Boy Scouts, YMCA, and their forerunners, 1870–1920*. University of Wisconsin Press.

Meddybemps Philosophy. (1905, December 24). *Boston Globe*, 20.

Merwin, H.C. (2000). On being civilized too much. In S. Smith & M. Dawson (Eds.), *The American 1890s* (pp. 306–318). Duke University Press.

Mills, W. (1951). *White collar: The American middle classes*. Oxford University Press.

Mrozek, D.J. (1989). Sport in American life: From national health to personal fulfillment. In K. Grover (Ed.), *Fitness in American culture: Images of health, sport, and the body, 1830–1940* (pp. 18–46). University of Massachusetts Press.

Newton, J.L. (2017). Forging titans: The rise of industrial capitalism in the Northern Forest, 1850–1950. (Publication No. 10621535). [Doctoral dissertation, Syracuse University]. Proquest Dissertations & Theses Global.

Norwood, D.R. (1982). The sport hero concept and the Louis Cyr. (Publication No. MK57271). [Masters thesis, University of Windsor (Canada)]. Proquest Dissertations & Theses Global.

Norwood, S.H. (1994). The student as strikebreaker: College youth and the crisis of masculinity in the early twentieth century. *Journal of Social History, 28*(2), 331–349.

Park, R.J. (1987). Edward M. Hartwell and physical training at The Johns Hopkins University, 1879–1890. *Journal of Sport History, 14*(1), 108–119.

Park, R.J. (2007a). Biological thought, athletics and the formation of a 'man of character': 1830–1900. *The International Journal of the History of Sport, 24*(12), 1543–1569.

Park, R.J. (2007b). Muscles, symmetry and action: 'Do you measure up?' defining masculinity in Britain and America from the 1860s to the early 1900s. *The International Journal of the History of Sport, 24*(12), 1604–1636.

Park, R.J. (2007c). Science, service, and the professionalization of physical education: 1885–1905. *The International Journal of the History of Sport, 24*(12), 1674–1700.

Park, R.J. (2012). 'Soldiers may fall but athletes never!': Sport as an antidote to nervous diseases and national decline in America, 1865–1905. *International Journal of the History of Sport, 29*(6), 792–812. 10.1080/09523367.2011.642553

Prescott, H.M. (2007). *Student bodies: The influence of student health services in American Society & Medicine*. University of Michigan Press.

Proctor, H. (2020). Curriculum, history, and 'progress'. In T. Fitzgerald (Ed.), *Handbook of historical studies in education* (pp. 439–451). Springer.

Putney, C. (2001). *Muscular Christianity: Manhood and sports in Protestant America, 1880–1920*. Harvard University Press.

Roosevelt, T. (1879a, September 14). *Letter From Theodore Roosevelt to Martha Bulloch Roosevelt*. Ms Am 1541.9 (107). Harvard College Library. Retrieved 29 May 2016, from http://www.theodorerooseveltcenter.org/Research/Digital-Library/Record.aspx?libID=o283359.

Roosevelt, T. (1879b). *Personal diary of Theodore Roosevelt, 1879*. Theodore Roosevelt Papers at the Library of Congress. Library of Congress Manuscript Division. Retrieved 9 June 2023, from https://www.theodorerooseveltcenter.org/Research/Digital-Library/Record?libID=o288505

Rotundo, A. (1993). *American manhood*. BasicBooks.

Rudolph, F. (1962). *The American college and university: A history*. University of Georgia Press.

Sargent, D.A. (Ed.). (1889). *The System of physical training at the Hemenway Gymnasium*. G.H. Ellis.

Sargent, D.A. (1906). *Physical education*. Ginn & Co.

Sargent, D.A. (1912). Defects in the school curriculum in physical training as shown by the disabilities of college students. *American Physical Education Review, 17*(8), 602–607.

Sargent, D.A. (1914a). *Health, strength & power* (Unstated 2nd ed.). Dodge Publishing.

Sargent, D.A. (1914b). The relation of physical education to race betterment. In *Proceeding of the First National Conference on Race Betterment* (pp. 104–106). Gage.

Sargent, D.A. (1919). Roosevelt's physique. *Sargent Quarterly, 4*(1), 1–3.

Sargent, D.A., & Sargent, L.W. (1927). *Dudley A. Sargent: An autobiography*. Lea & Febiger.

Sewall, W.W. (1919). *Bill Sewall's story of T.R.* Harper & Brothers.

Slavishak, E.S. (2008). *Bodies of work: Civic display and labor in industrial Pittsburgh*. Duke University Press.

Srole, C. (2012). *Transcribing class and gender: Masculinity and femininity in nineteenth-century courts and offices*. University of Michigan Press.

Strong, J. (1907). *The challenge of the city*. Young People's Missionary Movement.

Sullivan, J.L., & Sargent, D.A. (1892). *Life and reminiscences of a 19th century gladiator*. Alfred Mudge & Son.

Thomas de la Peña, C. (2003). *The body electric: How strange machines built the modern American*. New York University Press.

Townsend, K. (1996). *Manhood at Harvard: William James and others*. W.W. Norton.

Turner, F.J. (1920). *The frontier in American history*. Hold Rinehart & Winston.

Vietze, A. (2010). *Becoming Teddy Roosevelt: How a Maine guide inspired America's 26th president*. Down East Books.

Walsh, S.L. (2020). *Eugenics and physical culture performance in the Progressive Era: Watch whiteness workout*. Springer International Publishing.

Weider, B. (1976). *The strongest man in history: Louis Cyr, 'amazing Canadian'*. Mitchell Press.

Winter, T. (2002). *Making men, making class: The YMCA and workingmen, 1877–1920.* University of Chicago Press.

Wood, H.C. (1880). Brain work and overwork. *Friends' Review: a Religious, Literary and Miscellaneous Journal, 33*(27), 425.

Wright, A.H. (1953). *Pre-Cornell and early Cornell.* Unpublished manuscript.

Zakim, M. (2018). *Accounting for capitalism: The world the clerk made.* University of Chicago Press.

Zarnowski, F. (2013). *American work-sports: A history of competitions for cornhuskers, lumberjacks, firemen and others.* McFarland & Co.

5

DETERMINING BIOLOGICAL CITIZENSHIP

Creating and effacing difference in Puerto Rico's education

Bethsaida Nieves

On 5 February 1900, the United States Senate held the Senate Bill 2264 Hearings in order to determine a new form of government for Puerto Rico after the Spanish-American War of 1898. Joseph B. Foraker, a Republican representing Ohio, was the chairman of the hearings committee, and several military generals, businessmen as well as local leaders working in Puerto Rico testified at the hearings. The hearings centred on the practices of government, which included the administration and management of the system of rule for Puerto Rico. Of special concern were acts of governing, which considered the moral character of Puerto Ricans and their ability to properly control and influence the institutions of government. Judge H.G. Curtis, a member of the Insular Commission, pointed out that after the Treaty of Paris was signed, Puerto Ricans in Puerto Rico were 'inhabitants of an island' and yet citizens of neither the United States nor Puerto Rico (Foraker & US Government, 1900, p. 101). Puerto Rico's liminal legal status provided the opportune condition to decide what type of education would be implemented on the island. This is significant because it provided policymakers with the opportunity to construct a citizen that could act and participate in both Puerto Rican and American society.

This chapter examines the predictions and calculations of difference that defined the Puerto Rican child as one that needed to be reformed. The primary objective of this chapter is to elucidate the discontinuities within the history of discourses that 'constructed' the Puerto Rican student as an object of reflection and action. To this end, this chapter considers the discursive formations of difference that were made possible in Puerto Rico's education at the turn of the 20th century. Secondly, it analyses how institutional practices gave both legitimacy to those conceptualisations of

DOI: 10.4324/9781003288671-8

difference and to what counted as valuable knowledge. Thirdly, it examines how these discourses of difference provided educators with information about whom the Puerto Rican child was, is or could become. These epistemological and ontological reference points shifted under the first years of civil colonial rule, which constructed a state of liminality in Puerto Rico's education and society.

The following discussion focuses on how discourses of difference in terms of 'race' and 'intelligence' present in the Senate Bill 2264 Hearings of 1900 'travelled' to Puerto Rico via a teachers' manual and educational reports. It first considers how senators in the United States constructed discourses of difference to rationalise the need for education reforms in Puerto Rico. While these lawmakers conceptualised education reforms as a necessary aspect of voting rights and citizenship production, part of their rationale included racially segregating schools in Puerto Rico. Second, it looks at how discourses of difference and reform evident in the Senate Bill 2264 Hearings were mobilised in Puerto Rico's education system via emerging discourses and practices of psychology and statistics. Specifically, it delves into how educators and administrators began to use emerging discourses of psychology and statistics to predict and calculate difference in terms of 'race' and 'intelligence', and in turn, use those numbers to legitimise the need for education reforms in Puerto Rico, which included establishing schools in Puerto Rico similar to the Tuskegee Normal and Industrial Institute in Tuskegee, Alabama (Tuskegee Institute), and the Hampton Industrial and Agricultural School in Hampton, Virginia (Hampton Institute). Documents analysed include the *Teachers' Manual* (Puerto Rico, 1900) that was created by Victor S. Clark, an economist who served as the President of the Insular Board of Education for Puerto Rico from 1899 to 1900; and the educational reports (Puerto Rico, 1901, 1902, 1903) written for the Secretary of the Interior for the United States by school administrators and educators working in Puerto Rico between 1901 and 1903.

Constructing 'reason' via social epistemologies of difference

This analysis examines the constructions of 'reason' that 'make' the objects of schooling possible (Popkewitz, 1998, 2008), specifically investigating how scientific reasoning about the Puerto Rican child was a social production that becomes part of cultural theses of Puerto Rican schooling and society. For example, the concept of the Puerto Rican child is a discursive *event*, understood as part of a system of thought and cultural practices, or *archive* (Foucault, 1972). The *event* and *archive*, in turn, inform the *episteme* (Foucault, 1994), which is the language of reason and production of knowledge. For example, by examining Puerto Rican education at the turn of the 20th century, we can begin to understand how the concept of the Puerto

Rican child becomes the subject and object of educational reforms. In using the history of the present, the system of thought is the discourse, so that the discourse is not an analytic of the words of a text, but an analytic of the system of ideas that make a particular concept possible. The analysis of the social, political and epistemological conditions that make the construction of particular concept possible is a social epistemology (Popkewitz, 1997). In this chapter, I examine the construction of the politics of knowledge in the social and educational sciences that made the concept of the Puerto Rican child possible at the turn of the 20th century.

My approach to a history of the present and analysing discursive formations and recursions relies on a Foucauldian approach to discourse analysis. According to Veyne (2010), Foucault considered discourse as a culturally constructed representation of reality, not a universal truth about reality. Foucault's objective was, 'to "problematize" an object, find out how a human being was envisaged in a particular epoch [and] describe the various social practices—scientific, ethical, punitive, medical and so on—that determined how a human being was envisaged' (Veyne, p. 107). In this sense, Foucault sought to understand the discourses that made it possible to construct and locate what it was to be, and what it was possible to do within a particular time period. Foucauldian discourse analysis, then, looks at how discourse constructs knowledge and governs, through the various social practices (Foucault, 1980, p. 200), what is and is not possible to talk about at a particular historical moment (Foucault, 1972). As Foucault argues:

> The analysis of statements, then, is a historical analysis, but one that avoids all interpretation: it does not question things said as to what they are hiding, what they were 'really' saying … but on the contrary, it questions them as to their mode of existence, what it means to them to have come into existence … what it means to them to have appeared when and where they did—they and no others.
>
> (Foucault, 1972, p. 109)

When considering how power and knowledge are constructed and circulated in society, a Foucauldian discourse analysis provides a way to see how particular classifications of thinking and being have come to be seen as common sense ways of thinking, acting and participating in society.

By also drawing on Foucault's conceptual framework of the history of the present, I problematise the proclaimed truths and historical facts about Puerto Rican schooling by examining the multiple discursive rationalities and historical trajectories used to order and classify what is 'seen' and 'acted upon' as the objects of schooling in Puerto Rico at the turn of the 20th century. Uncontested truths of Puerto Rican society are questioned and examined, and multiple fields of relationships are considered in the constructions of history and of the Puerto Rican subject. By decentring the subject, societal constructions of knowledge and culture are the focus of history, and not the subject. Decentring the subject in this way repositions the historical argument in two ways. First, it repositions the historical subject: as being the discourse itself rather than the individual. This changes the focus of the historical discussion from one in which history is seen as a natural and causal progression with definitive results, to one in which a system of statements functions in the construction of knowledge and culture (Foucault, 1991, p. 55). Such an analysis is meaningful because it breaks with the belief that a body of knowledge, or an episteme, is a grand narrative or theory and instead looks at the episteme as a discourse tied to societal investments in politics and morality. For example, I look at the discourse of citizenship as an epistemic construction tied to notions of exceptionalism grounded in a rationalisation of science and morality that circulated between Puerto Rico and the United States.

Secondly, by decentring the subject, the subject no longer becomes the historical carrier and conveyer of universal essences of truth, experience and being. Rather, there is a break with these 'transcendental teleologies' (Foucault, 1972, p. 131)—the 'polymorphous interweaving of correlations' that make up a particular episteme becomes the focus on inquiry (Foucault, 1991, p. 58). This allows me to examine the formation and transformations of statements within a discourse. It also allows me to examine how particular societal practices enable discursive statements to continue to exist, be modified or even become transmogrified. In doing so, I am problematising the historical origins and essences about truth, experience and being in Puerto Rican education and society.

Discourses of difference and reform in the United States Senate Bill 2264 Hearings of 1900

Although the line of questioning during the Senate Bill 2264 Hearings focussed on the legal, political and economic conditions in Puerto Rico, there was a concerted effort to define the 'race' and 'intelligence' of Puerto Ricans as a precursor to establishing the rules of government and governing for the island and its peoples. Among the questions debated extensively was whether restricted suffrage or universal suffrage in Puerto Rico should be tied to property ownership and education level. Intertwined with these discussions of voting rights and education was whether or not schools in Puerto Rico ought to be segregated by race, as in the US southern states. The exchange below between Chairman Senator Joseph B. Foraker (Republican from Ohio), Senator Knute Nelson (Republican from Minnesota) and Judge H.G. Curtis demonstrates how the idea of 'race' was becoming part of how Puerto Rico's societal relations were being discussed and conceptualised:

Mr. Nelson:	In those schools do the white and colored[1] children go together?
Mr. Curtis:	Yes, sir.
The Chairman:	Is there any race prejudice?
Mr. Curtis:	Very little. You will find a black woman with a white man, and a white woman with a black man and dark baby. It does not create the disturbance it would in this country, but still there is some prejudice.
Mr. Nelson:	In establishing any school system there, would it be necessary to make a double system—one for the colored people and one for the whites?
Mr. Curtis:	Oh, no, sir; not at all.
Mr. Nelson:	As has been the case in some of the Southern States?
Mr. Curtis:	I do not think they would require that at all. (Foraker & US Government, 1900, pp. 86–87)

Evident in this passage is the attempt to mobilise a discourse about 'race' in Puerto Rico by creating a parallel of difference based on the construct of 'race' between US southern states and Puerto Rico. Furthermore, the inquiry into racially segregating schools in Puerto Rico hearkened back to *Plessy* v. *Ferguson* (1896), which condoned the idea of 'separate but equal' in the United States (Erman, 2012, p. 10). This is important because while the Senate Bill 2264 Hearings sought to define aspects of government, governing and education in Puerto Rico, discourses of difference based on 'race' became central to those discussions. In this sense, Puerto Rico and the US southern states were being discursively conceptualised throughout the Senate Bill 2264 Hearings as similar, and the construct of 'race' was the defining metric.

These discourses are significant because they demonstrate the reasoning that US Senators and members of Puerto Rico's society used to define constructs of 'race' and 'intelligence', and in turn, attempted to adapt those rationalities to education and voting rights in Puerto Rico. For example, in constructing a parallel of discourses about 'race', 'intelligence' and voting rights between the postbellum southern US states and Puerto Rico, US senators rationalised that they could adapt legislation and education reforms being promoted in the US southern states to Puerto Rico. In this sense, voting rights based on literacy were tied to education and education reforms, but the rationale used to decide these educational reforms relied upon a particular reasoning about 'race' and 'intelligence' that travelled between the United States and Puerto Rico. Moreover, in the effort to 'make everyone the same' by creating a parallel between the US southern states and Puerto Rico, Puerto Ricans in effect were reinforced and (re)inscribed as the 'Other'.

Efforts to quantify people of 'colour' were evident in the following exchange about voting rights, property ownership and educational qualifications between Chairman Joseph B. Foraker (Republican from Ohio), Senator Chauncey M. Depew (Republican from New York) and Major Azel Ames. Senator Foraker asked Major Ames, 'Would you restrict the suffrage to property or educational qualifications?' Major Ames replied, 'Yes, sir; I think an alternative educational or property qualification is a good one' (Foraker & US Government, 1900, p. 191). Major Ames added that the literacy rate of the entire population of Puerto Rico was over 20% according to the 1897 Spanish census, with the lowest literacy rates recorded among farmers with small landholdings. This particular point is significant because, throughout the Senate Bill 2264 Hearings, there was an effort to determine how much money and resources were needed to rebuild Puerto Rico's agricultural industry, roads and schools after the destruction of Hurricane San Ciriaco of 1899 (Foraker & US Government, 1900, p. 223).

In continuing their inquiry to determine the voting rights for Puerto Ricans, the US senators shifted their focus to morality and 'race':

The Chairman: If allowed a restricted suffrage, do you think there would be any difficulty in electing, by districts, good men to a legislative assembly?

Major Ames: Not the least. I have had too much association with men whom you would like to see in the legislature to doubt it.

The Chairman: Good men?

Major Ames: Yes, sir; men who would represent their districts as well as any in New Hampshire or Massachusetts.

Mr. Depew: What proportion is negro?

Major Ames: Quite small. This census will give it very accurately, but it has been supposed from the census of 1897, the last one the Spaniards took, that was somewhere the neighborhood of 60% native blood; but that is, I think, not right. I think it is much less myself. I think it will be nearer to 30%. I include in that all Berbers, Corsicans, etc. – all who have color. (Foraker & US Government, 1900, p. 191)

In this exchange, the phrase 'good men' take on a markedly racial undertone with the response, 'as well as any in New Hampshire or Massachusetts', especially when considering that Hiram Revels (Republican from Mississippi) who was a Senator from 1870 to 1871, and Blanch K. Bruce (Republican from Mississippi) who was a Senator from 1875 to 1881 (and who also worked in education), had been the first two African American senators elected in the state of Mississippi.

Moreover, there was a focussed attempt to define how much of the Puerto Rican population had 'colour'. With respect to government and governing, this focus on 'colour' and morality was also a decision on the 'ability' and 'fitness' of Puerto Ricans. The subtext of the above exchange highlights the idea that those with 'colour' either were, or could become, a threat to governance in Puerto Rico. Senator Depew (Republican from New York) continued the above discussion on defining 'negro' by responding to Major Ames with the following statement:

Mr. Depew: I mean Africans.

Major Ames: We have almost no pure Africans, and what we have there are from the United States or St. Thomas. ... I should say from 50,000 to 80,000 people would cover the distinctly negro population, but we have an enormous number of those who appear to be negroes, but who, if you will examine closely, you will find are not, but are from the Barbary coast, and oftentimes these peoples are in various shades of color. ... I found the Berber class was very large and a great number of Malay origin and some Corsicans. Some of these were brought there very early in its history, and there was a mixture of the Barbary coast man and the French Corsairs and those dealing along the Spanish main, and the Spanish continued the mixture, and then came the 'flotsam and jetsam' of Hawkins's and Drake's and Morgan's fleets who remained there, and in that way we have got, ethnologically, the most mixed mass I ever saw in the same area. (Foraker & US Government, 1900, pp. 191–192)

While the statement by Major Ames frames and normalises the conquest and colonisation of Puerto Rico as 'exploration', the key focus of this exchange is to construct and define a racial hierarchy of people in Puerto Rico via 'various shades of colour' and declaring the island's inhabitants as an ethnological 'mixed mass'. In this sense, the idea of creating and effacing difference becomes critical to understanding how the construct of 'race' was being conceptualised in and for Puerto Rico at the turn of the 20th century. By trying to quantify a 'racial pureness' for Africans in Puerto Rico, Major Ames mobilised a discourse of ethnology that in effect, 'made everyone the same' through the extensive, forced and violent mixing of peoples through conquest and colonisation. This is significant because the full exchange above (Foraker & US Government, 1900, pp. 191–192) reinforces the dehumanising idea of 'Self' and 'Other' through the constructions of a racial hierarchy and a racial provenance in which America was conflated with 'whiteness' and moral goodness, and thus served as the default standard of both 'race' and racial 'purity'. By the same token, Major Ames attempted to define the 'Other', the Puerto Rican, as a conglomeration of races, which was incapable of attaining the ambiguous scientific and statistical ideal of racial 'purity'. Moreover, the attempt to establish a racial provenance for Puerto Ricans is also important because it would be used by US senators to determine the 'fitness' and 'ability' of Puerto Ricans to participate in the government and governing of Puerto Rico in the next two decades (Erman, 2012, p. 33, p. 41).

Overall, the above excerpts from the Senate Bill 2264 Hearings demonstrate a concentrated effort by US senators to define the 'Other' through the constructs of 'race' and 'intelligence' in Puerto Rico as determinants for voting rights and education reforms. In doing so, US senators began to parallel the postbellum US southern states with Puerto Rico after the Spanish-American War of 1898. These parallels were also echoed in the discourses of 'race' and 'intelligence' found in the educational reports that school administrators and educators working in Puerto Rico wrote for the Secretary of the Interior for the United States between 1901 and 1903. These reports included school laws that determined the number of Puerto Rican students that were to be sent to the Carlisle Indian Industrial School in Carlisle, Pennsylvania, the Tuskegee Normal and Industrial Institute in Tuskegee, Alabama and the Hampton Industrial and Agricultural School in Hampton, Virginia. The education reports also include a particular language and usage of psychology and statistics to predict and calculate differences in Puerto Rico's education. The convergence and assemblage of these discourses of difference sought to reform Puerto Rico's education in order to reform Puerto Rico's children and society. This discussion is important because it demonstrates how discourses of difference about 'race' and 'intelligence' present in the Senate Bill 2264 Hearings 'travelled' to Puerto Rico and influenced how educators at the turn of the 20th century talked about, defined and mobilised discourses of 'race' and 'intelligence' in Puerto Rico's education.

Using psychology and statistics to predict and calculate difference in Puerto Rico's education

At the turn of the 20th century, educators in Puerto Rico began to rely on psychology and statistics to predict and calculate the 'normalcy' and 'difference' of children. The emergence of concepts such as plasticity, total, average and percentages was beginning to shift the ontological and epistemological reference points used to define who the Puerto Rican child was, and what the

Puerto Rican child could learn. Education reforms during this period also emphasised critical thinking over rote memorisation and focussed on what children could produce with their hands. Not only did the education reforms change the type of knowledge that was valued in Puerto Rico's education, but they also redefined the ways in which Puerto Rican children were to act and participate in society.

The idea of plasticity became central to the emerging discourse of psychology in the *Teachers' Manual,* which emphasised the following:

> The responsibility which the teacher assumes in the practice of his profession is as great as that which the practitioner in any other profession assumes. To him is entrusted the mental development of the child. He guides the mind in its first steps toward knowledge; he molds it and gives it fixed and permanent form while it is still plastic.
>
> (Puerto Rico, 1900, p. 332)

Victor S. Clark's effort to professionalise teacher education in Puerto Rico included introducing modern scientific methods and practices to the teacher education curricula. For example, teachers were to evaluate hearing and sight tests to determine if a child was 'eye-minded' or 'ear-minded' (Puerto Rico, 1900, p. 456). Clark emphasised, however, that a teacher's lack of training in collecting psychological data could lead to errors. He cautioned, 'Of course where a number of teachers untrained in scientific methods are suddenly entrusted with original investigations without skilful [*sic*] supervision or direction, the practical value of much of the data they collect may be questioned' (Puerto Rico, 1900, p. 456). This emphasis on accuracy, observation and recording would also be emphasised in the statistical data that Puerto Rico's teachers were to gather about their students.

Although the new teacher education standards outlined in the *Teachers' Manual* required that Puerto Rico's teachers have a trained eye for psychological observation and data collection, Clark cautioned teachers that 'it must be remembered that it is not the sole object of child-study to collect psychological data' (Puerto Rico, 1900, p. 458). On the contrary, Clark posited, 'We want to know the child in order to enter into a fuller sympathy with him, not to let the knowing, however scientific, stand as the sole thing in view' (Puerto Rico, 1900, p. 458). Clark made this cautionary note in the *Teachers' Manual,* but child psychology studies continued to play an increasing role in teacher training in Puerto Rico between 1901 and 1903 (Puerto Rico, 1901, pp. 42–43; Puerto Rico, 1902, p. 93, p. 163; Puerto Rico, 1903, p. 167). During the same period, educators and administrators working in Puerto Rico also began to increase their reliance on statistics to evaluate and 'know' more about the Puerto Rican child.

In conjunction with collecting psychological data on students, the *Teachers' Manual* also instructed Puerto Rico's teachers to learn school statistics and to maintain a roll-book containing the data for their yearly statistical reports, which was to include the following, '1. The name of each pupil. 2. His age. 3. The date of enrollment. 4. The number of days attended. 5. The number of minutes tardy. 6. It should give some data as to the pupil's progress in his studies' (Puerto Rico, 1900, pp. 502–504). Puerto Rico's teachers were instructed to use the data collected in the teacher's roll-book to make general summaries about 'the total enrollment of the school, the total attendance of the pupils in days, the average number of days attended by each pupil, the average age of the pupils and such other points as may be specifically required' (Puerto Rico, 1900, pp. 502–504). The importance of collecting this statistical information about totals and averages was that it provided a basis for calculating and predicting 'normalcy' and 'deviance' for children based on enrolment, attendance, tardiness and academic progress.

In 1901, the yearly education report submitted by the Commissioner of Education of Puerto Rico to the Secretary of the Interior for the United States included a new school law mandating the collection of statistical data on Puerto Rico's schools (Puerto Rico, 1901, p. 168). Collecting statistical data on the conditions of schools in Puerto Rico was meant to 'throw the most light upon the actual conditions prevailing in our schools' (Puerto Rico, 1903, p. 22). Statements like this demonstrate an emerging discourse about the truth and reliability of numbers by Puerto Rico's educators, and between 1901 and 1903, English Supervisors/Superintendents of Schools did indeed increase their reporting of statistics data in their yearly education reports. For example, in 1901, Paul G. Miller's 'Supervisor Report' for School District No. 10 in San Germán, Puerto Rico was the only report submitted that year that included statistics data. Miller collected data on the population of students, the population of students enroled, rural barrios without schools and the number of teachers teaching in the towns and rural areas (Puerto Rico, 1901, p. 108). In 1902, Miller added a comparison between the total number of students enroled in rural and town schools, as well as the total number of boys and girls enroled between 1899 and 1902 (Puerto Rico, 1902, p. 88). In general, by 1902 there was a gradual shift in the languaging about school statistics by some English Supervisors/Superintendents of Schools. John Mellowes, the supervisor for School District No. 11 in Mayagüez, Puerto Rico, was among the first English Supervisors to describe his own use of statistics in the yearly reports as a type of 'comparative statistics' (Puerto Rico, 1902, p. 91). By 1903, nearly all of yearly supervisor reports from the 19 school districts across Puerto Rico included statistical data that focussed on population, enrolment and attendance numbers. A notable shift in the languaging and thinking about statistics is also demonstrated in the wording of Daniel F. Kelley, the English Supervisor for School District No. 13 in

Aguadilla, Puerto Rico, who believed that the use of statistics allowed a 'true view' of what was transpiring in Puerto Rico's education (Puerto Rico, 1903, p. 145). This emerging belief in the 'truth' in numbers by the school supervisors provided educators with a numeric metric for determining what was 'normal' and 'abnormal' within a given population of students.

Most notable was the growing use of statistics to collect information about the racial makeup of Puerto Rico's schools. Statistical data based on the construct of 'race' began to appear in Puerto Rico's educational reports in 1901. The 'Statistical Report on Teachers' for 1901 and 1902 included a question about the 'race' of teachers. The form read, 'Full name of teacher; address, where born, year, single or married, white or colored, where educated, what diplomas are held, grade of certificate held in P.R., has certificate ever been canceled or teacher suspended, where taught, years taught... ... ' (Puerto Rico, 1901, p. 203; Puerto Rico, 1902, p. 171). This shift in the type of data collected by government administrators is significant because the very act of categorising teachers by 'race' provided administrators with a basis to compare and predict the trends of teacher performance across Puerto Rico's school districts. In sum, changing the type of data collected about Puerto Rico's teachers helped to mobilise discourses of difference in terms of 'intelligence' and 'ability' based on 'race'.

Similarly, the 'Teacher's Monthly Report' from 1901 included forms containing questions that divided and categorised students by 'race'. As argued previously, the act of including the construct of 'race' in the yearly education statistics reports opened the discursive space for rationalising the intelligence and ability of students in terms of a fabricated construct of 'race'. Moreover, the questions provided educators with a seemingly neutral and logical system of reasoning to explain *why* particular groups of students were present or absent, which could be used to define the moral character of students and their families. Collecting student data based on totals by 'race' also opened the discursive space for determining and predicting the successes and failures of students in schools across Puerto Rico (Puerto Rico, 1901, p. 186).

In 1902, forms for the 'Teacher's Monthly Report' included the following additional question regarding the racial makeup of students in Puerto Rico's schools: 'Total number of pupils enrolled from the beginning of the school year up to the end of the month: white-males and females; colored-males and females' (Puerto Rico, 1902, p. 171). The added question provided a longitudinal view for collecting data on Puerto Rico's students, and in turn, gave educators a statistical tool to predict the presence and absence of students in the classroom over an extended period of time. Moreover, the idea of predicting presence and absence becomes important in this discussion about educational statistics because it also provided educators with a basis for assessing who was or was not learning, and beyond that, for predicting trends regarding who *could* or *could not* learn. Coupling the data collected on the racial makeup of teachers and students, administrators could also rationalise that there was a correlation between student and teacher performance based on 'race'. In addition, by including 'race' as a comparative metric for determining and predicting academic success and failure of students and teachers, the rationale for proposing education reforms based on 'race' could be made possible.

Between 1901 and 1902, the 'Supervisor's Report' shifted its focus as well to include data on 'race'. In 1901, the directions for the report stated that, 'The remarks of the supervisor shall cover at least the following points: Enrollment, progress, order, method, cleanliness, neatness, sanitary arrangements, condition of room, furniture, and results of inspection' (Puerto Rico, 1901, p. 201). In 1902, the 'Supervisor's Report' forms made an additional request to include information about the racial makeup of Puerto Rico's schools, which included 'Number of teachers employed during this month: Colored-males, females; White-males, females; Total number of pupils re-enrolled during the month: White-males, females; Colored-males, females' (Puerto Rico, 1902, pp. 172–173). The shift in the language of this report is remarkable because by including 'race' as a determinant for student and teacher success, it did two things: first, it changed the boundaries of inclusion and exclusion in the context of system expansion and new developments; and second, it changed the narrative of 'intelligence' and 'ability' from being about that which could be learned, to that which was inherent in the bodies of particular 'races'. Collecting data about attendance and enrolment also opened the discursive space of using presence and absence as a factor for assessing and predicting the ability and likelihood for effective teaching and learning based on 'race'. While these discourses of statistics provided a seemingly impartial metric to compare students and teachers, they provided the basis for constructing the 'Other' in the languaging and practices of Puerto Rico's education system. Moreover, it provided a rationale for predicting how the 'Other' would or could act and participate in Puerto Rico's schools and society.

As in other statistical reports, collecting school statistics based on 'race' provided education administrators with a basis for identifying, classifying and organising difference. Moreover, the collection of statistical data based on 'race' may have provided education administrators with a rationale for racially segregating schools in Puerto Rico. For example, Arthur D. Dean, an expert agent from the Department of Education of Porto Rico, toured Puerto Rico in 1903 to collect information for his government report, 'Possibilities of Industrial and Agricultural Education in Porto Rico' (Puerto Rico, 1903, p. 175). Dean suggested that the US government create a Tuskegee or Hampton Institute in Puerto Rico (Puerto Rico, 1903, p. 186). In his view, an agricultural and mechanic arts college in Puerto Rico could be established under the Morrill Acts of 1862 and 1890 (Puerto Rico, 1903, p. 186). Dean also suggested that schools in Puerto Rico be segregated by race if monies were equally allotted between them. He argued, 'No distinction is made for race or color, but there can be separate schools, provided that the money be equally divided' (Puerto Rico, 1903, p. 186).

The idea of racially segregating schools in Puerto Rico, however, was not supported by Commissioner of Education for Puerto Rico Martin G. Brumbaugh (1900–1901), nor by his successor, Samuel M. Lindsay (1902–1904). Both Commissioners rebuffed the idea of racially segregating schools in Puerto Rico. In Brumbaugh's 1901 annual report to the Secretary of the Interior for the United States, he advised not raising the 'color question' with respect to Puerto Rico's schools:

> The color question has not been raised. It will not be if good sense and ordinary discretion prevail. About 9 per cent of the teachers and 28 in 1903 of the pupils are colored. They attend all schools with perfect quality. No friction has arisen; no protest has been openly made … . the colored children do about as well as the other pupils, and are not at all a disturbing influence in the schools.
>
> (Puerto Rico, 1901, pp. 37–38)

In a similar vein, Commissioner of Education for Puerto Rico Samuel M. Lindsay argued that idea of 'the color line' prevalent in the United States was not applicable to Puerto Rico. In his annual report to the Secretary of the Interior for the United States, Lindsay argued that collecting exact data on the 'color distribution' of students in Puerto Rico's schools was not possible:

> In summarizing the school statistics from our records it is not always possible to give the summaries by color distribution, as the color line is not so sharply drawn in our schools, and the statistics of this subject are considered less exact than they would be in the States. I have, however, been able to give the total number of pupils enrolled by color and sex, but not excluding the duplicates or reenrollments. The summary of pupils enrolled, excluding duplicates and reenrollments, can be given only for the total enrollment and not by color and sex distribution.
>
> (Puerto Rico, 1903, p. 4)

Commissioner Lindsay's response provides a counter-narrative to the Senate Bill 2264 Hearings, which attempted to create a racial hierarchy and a racial provenance of 'race' and 'colour'. In responding to a request by officials in Washington, D.C. to identify the attendance of school buildings in Puerto Rico by race, Lindsay remarked that schools in Puerto Rico were open to children of all races:

Also, question No. 4 can be answered only by giving the number of building used as schoolhouses, separating the buildings rented and not separating the buildings used for white schools and the buildings used for colored schools, because all the schools in Porto Rico are open alike to white and colored pupils.

(Puerto Rico, 1903, p. 5)

Commissioner Lindsay's statement points to the underlying assumption by administrators in Washington, DC that schools in Puerto Rico could be separated by race. Schools in Puerto Rico, however, did not become racially segregated. What occurred instead was a focussed effort to train Puerto Rico's students in manual training and agriculture.

Between 1901 and 1903, school laws were passed for sending Puerto Rican students to the United States to study at the Carlisle Indian Industrial School, the Tuskegee Normal and Industrial Institute, and the Hampton Industrial and Agricultural School. In 1901, Colonel Pratt, superintendent of the Indian Industrial School at Carlisle, Pennsylvania admitted 30 Puerto Rican students to the school (Puerto Rico, 1901, p. 74). Educators and administrators also relied on two newly passed laws to send Puerto Rican students to the Hampton and Tuskegee Institutes. House Bill 35 was enacted to enable students to attend schools 'selected by the president of the senate, the speaker of the house, and the commissioner of education, of 25 young men, each of whom is given $400 for his year's maintenance and education' (Puerto Rico, 1901, p. 74).

By 1903, the school laws outlining the conditions for sending Puerto Rican students to the United States had expanded to ten sections (Puerto Rico, 1903, p. 246). Of special note is section 73 which stated, 'The colleges or institutions designated to which the said students shall attend are Hampton Institute, Hampton, Virginia, and Tuskegee Institute, Tuskegee, Alabama, and such other similar educational institutions as the commissioner of education may from time to time specify' (Puerto Rico, 1903, p. 246). Manual training and agriculture education had expanded to the University of Puerto Rico, which in 1903 established teacher-training programs in the departments of mechanical and agricultural education (Puerto Rico, 1903, p. 252), and was a central component of the elementary education reforms that were put into place in Puerto Rico between 1900 and 1903.

Conclusion

This chapter has investigated the forms of 'reasoning' about Puerto Rican education by considering: (a) how epistemic shifts help us understand the production and organisation of knowledge; (b) how a history of the present can be used to problematise the structuring of historical reason; (c) how the epistemological decentring of the subject can provide a way to problematise how the social construction of knowledge becomes an effect of power; and (d) how both a history of the present and an epistemological decentring of the subject can provide an interpretive way to think about how the social sciences were used to order, classify and construct 'difference' with regard to Puerto Rico's education at the turn of the 20th century.

Applying this reasoning to the legal discourses, teacher-training materials and educational reports that are analysed in this chapter, a view of how a scientific reasoning about Puerto Rican citizenship and the Puerto Rican child in Puerto Rico begins to emerge. This chapter has focussed on how narratives of 'race' and 'intelligence' in the Senate Bill 2264 Hearings in 1900 'travelled' to Puerto Rico and influenced both the use of statistics in education reports and the rationale educators used to make education reforms in Puerto Rico. The objective has been to show how discourses of 'race' and 'intelligence' were mobilised in Puerto Rico through the emerging discourses and practices of psychology and statistics. This chapter's investigation of the organisation and circulation of a system of thought speaks to the scientific assemblage of knowledge about Puerto Rican education, as well as to how multiple trajectories 'constructed' what it was possible to know and speak about with respect to education in Puerto Rico at the time.

These assemblages of discourses about difference in Puerto Rico's education and society highlight the conditions that made it possible to construct difference and act upon the conduct of the 'Self' and 'Other'. Put another way, these assemblages of discourses made difference intelligible and informed how people governed themselves and governed others. In Puerto Rico's case, sustained avoidance has become a strategy or tactic for governing, which has maintained the practices of liminal governmentality that has kept Puerto Rico in a state of suspended sovereignty since the turn of the twentieth century.

Note

1 In discussing racist and racialising categorisations and classificatory practices from the past, it is necessary to quote terminology that is offensive for the purposes of facing history, deconstructing the historical meanings and intents of the offensive terms, and creating new spaces for languaging that is humanising and anti-racist.

References

Erman, S. (2012). Reconstruction and empire: Legacies of the U.S. Civil War and Puerto Rican struggles for home rule, 1898–1917. *SSRN Electronic Journal.* 10.2139/ssrn.2036696

Foraker, J.B., & US Government. (1900). *Industrial and other conditions of the Island of Puerto Rico, and the form of government which should be adopted for it: Hearings before the Committee on Pacific Islands and Puerto Rico of the United States Senate on Senate Bill 2264, to provide a government for the Island of Puerto Rico, and for other purposes, February 5, 1900.* US Government Printing Office.

Foucault, M. (1972). *The archaeology of knowledge; and, the discourse on language.* Pantheon Books.

Foucault, M. (1980). History of systems of thought. In D.F. Bouchard (Ed.), *Language, counter-memory, practice: Selected essays and interviews* (pp. 199–204). Cornell University Press.

Foucault, M. (1991). Politics and the study of discourse. In G. Burchell, C. Gordon & P. Miller (Eds.), *The Foucault effect: Studies in governmentality: with two lectures by and an interview with Michel Foucault* (pp. 53–72). University of Chicago Press.

Foucault, M. (1994). *The order of things: An archaeology of the human sciences.* Vintage Books.

Popkewitz, T.S. (1997). A changing terrain of knowledge and power: A social epistemology of educational research. *Educational Researcher, 26*(9), 18–29.

Popkewitz, T.S. (1998). *Struggling for the soul: The politics of schooling and the construction of the teacher.* Teachers College Press.

Popkewitz, T.S. (2008). *Cosmopolitanism and the age of school reform: Science, education and making society by making the child.* Routledge.

Puerto Rico. (1900). *Teachers' manual for the public schools of Puerto Rico issued under the authority of the Insular Board of Education.* Silver, Burdett & Company.

Puerto Rico. (1901). *Report of the Commissioner of Education for Porto Rico to the Secretary of the Interior, U. S. A., 1901.* Government Printing Office.

Puerto Rico. (1902). *Report of the Commissioner of Education for Porto Rico to the Secretary of the Interior, U. S. A., 1901.* Government Printing Office.

Puerto Rico. (1903). *Report of the Commissioner of Education for Porto Rico to the Secretary of the Interior, U. S. A, 1903.* Government Printing Office.

Veyne, P. (2010). *Foucault: His thought, his character.* Polity.

6

HOME ECONOMICS AS A SCHOOL SUBJECT IN DENMARK

From disciplining girls in the kitchen to providing general knowledge about public health

Annette Rasmussen and Karen E. Andreasen

The first part of the 20th century involved revolutionary changes—technological and political—that influenced schooling and social life for many people throughout the world. New technologies changed the existing economic structures and facilitated greater wealth in many countries, which led to new organisational and state forms. New welfare regimes aroused and led to a greater focus on public health and schooling, which aimed both at expanding knowledge on health matters through education and reaching new and more groups of people.

In Northern Europe, where the dominant occupations had previously been within agriculture, industry took over and with this followed an intense urbanisation of society (Danmarks Statistik, 2000, p. 15; Jespersen, 2011; Rasmussen & Andreasen, 2020). While within agriculture, the family had been the main context for production, reproduction and the primary social functions, the new times of industrialisation caused changes to these functions of the family and a societal need to develop social and welfare reforms. In the Nordic countries, this gave rise to the welfare state in its early development (Esping-Andersen, 1990). Health and education gradually shifted from being a purely household matter to being a matter of the state, a shift that during the 20th century was considered important to the education of women, allowing them to move beyond 'domestic' spaces and into the public world (Rogers, 2006).

To disseminate the requisite enlightenment among the population at large necessitated the training of personnel, which also involved the introduction of a new school subject in home economics. From the state's perspective, home economics played a key role in ensuring the health of families, thereby keeping expenses low for the state in relation to citizens' illness and maintenance. Political initiatives aimed at promoting education in home economics as well

DOI: 10.4324/9781003288671-9

as health among citizens as part of the nascent welfare state went hand in hand with and contributed to developing education in home economics.

Denmark is particularly interesting as a case on this matter, since the home economics movement developed early in this country (Petri & Kragelund, 1980). From around 1895 and onwards, home economics developed as an educational area and as a professional field with its own curriculum, methods, textbooks and educational institutions in Denmark (Dahlsgård, 1980; Petri, 1981). However, proponents from the home economics movement were not only concerned with these issues in relation to adult women's education and occupation, but also argued for the importance of the teaching and enlightening of children as well, and therefore for the introduction of home economics in basic education. In 1899, the National Education Act introduced home economics as a school subject, although very few schools had school kitchens at the time (Thisted, 2001).

In this chapter, we address the development of home economics schooling in a welfare-state perspective with a particular focus on gender. Thus, the chapter will trace the historical conditions for the development of home economics as a school subject as well as its contribution to the development of public health and the social position of women, which we analyse in relation to power and welfare-state theories, paying special attention to gender.

Methodology: Theories of biopolitics and curriculum studies

In asking how home economics as a school subject developed in the Nordic welfare state and how it contributed—by means of educating women—to reproducing genders, we aim to identify the underlying rationalities and power structures behind this. This means that we begin with a post-structural thinking about discourses and power, which, drawing on Foucault, takes aim at contradictions and what is privileged in relation to something else (Foucault, 2008). It emphasises the close relationship between power and knowledge and is conceptualised as governmentality, which expresses how governing became manifest as a way of thinking and disciplining the body. Governmentality consists in the specific forms of discourse that rationalise the unfolding of power within an area (home economics), specify the objectives of it (e.g. a healthy population) and identify its objects (education of the population, especially women).

The concept of governmentality involves systematic reflections and practices that concern both governance of the self and governance of others (i.e. the state governing the citizens). It is particularly relevant to the first part of the 20th century, since in this period the state increasingly based its activities on a variety of calculations aimed at optimising the safety, welfare and well-being of its population. Society as an economic system constituted a new reality, as did the discovery of the population as an object of governance and the development of new sciences about this (Foucault, 1991; Rose, 1996). A new means of biopower was developed that aimed at optimising resources through the disciplining of the population.

The biopower on which governmentality is based took two forms: regulation of the population's life processes and disciplining of the individual body (Foucault, 1978). The regulation power is directed towards the population, which forms the object of regulation through the explicit calculations and regulating norms. For this, the biopower depends on and conditions the development and budding of different life sciences, home economics exemplifying one of these. Accordingly, biopolitics concerns the handling and introduction of measures that regulate the lives of citizens and disciplines the citizens through education to make them behave in such ways that, seen from the state's perspective, are the most rational (Foucault, 2008, p. 317). The disciplining of the body thus optimises its resources to make it more useful, productive and obedient.

As outlined above, biopolitics in many ways stands as equivalent to the ideas of the Nordic welfare state, which, by using biopower, links to gender as a basic organising principle of society. Through the concept of biopower and the forms of regulation and discipline it depends on, our analysis is carried out in two steps. First, we focus on the *regulating principles and programmes* behind the development of home economics as a school subject and field of knowledge. Second, we focus on the aspect of *disciplining* by connecting the dissemination of knowledge through home economics education and consider how the curriculum of the body thus disciplined especially the female part of the population into specific roles of care.

The capacity to form and maintain a household embodies what some have called 'the right to a family', which reflects the character of laws regulating sexuality, marriage and household formation (Orloff, 1996). The right to a family was very much directed towards preparing women for an 'occupation' at home, which, preventing them from wider participation in the public sphere, carried an inherently anti-feminist notion. However, the education in home economics was also considered a prerequisite for the strengthening of women's position as wage earners and their integration into the public sector as a permanent part of the labour force. As such, it is the story of 'reproduction going public' (Hernes, 1987, p. 52ff).

We approach this by studying the subject's curricula, supported by the writings of women entrepreneurs in this field, their contribution to the development of the subject and the influence this had on women's lives and social positions. The empirical basis of the analysis is historical materials, including the curriculum text of the subject in the consecutive school laws of the 20th century, ministerial reports dealing with women's occupations, employment and education in Denmark, archival material, historical publications on the schools of home economics in Denmark and analyses from our previous writings on the theme (Andreasen & Rasmussen, 2020; Rasmussen & Andreasen, 2020, 2022).

Welfare-state policies of education

In the early 20th century, the welfare-state development in Denmark was a result of both extensive poverty and powerful social movements of labour, women and the folk high school. Following long periods of war, the population experienced scarcity of resources, starvation, malnutrition and health problems, which in different ways put pressure on the national finances (Rasmussen & Andreasen, 2022). The period was characterised by numerous welfare initiatives and is widely known for its framing of the modern welfare state. Even so, many initiatives can be rooted as far back as the preceding century, in which the Danish state—as in other countries at the time—had established some public support for citizens who, due to age, illness or other circumstances, were not able to fend for themselves. Thus, following the dominant 'universal model', welfare became characterised by the state provision of health, education and care as pivotal points (Esping-Andersen, 1990; Hernes, 1987), which relied on biopolitics for its effectuation (Foucault, 2008).

In Denmark, there was an expansion of the education system in general, especially after World War II, to provide educational opportunities for as many as possible. This was a consequence of political initiatives aimed at, on the one hand, supplying the population with the necessary academic skills in a changing labour market, and, on the other hand, assisting citizens in obtaining economic independence. This was important at a time when the state, based on the universal principle that every citizen was entitled to free welfare services, took on increasing economic responsibility, which was financed through taxation (Jespersen, 2011, p. 82).

The general expansion of education, and with this the socialisation of citizens into new public functions, laid the foundation for implementing policies of education that also targeted areas that had hitherto been located in the domestic sphere (Dahlsgård, 1980; Lützen, 2000). The 'education' within home economics had until then typically taken place as the informal training of girls within the home. Until the late 1800s, there was very little formal education for women, whether in home economics or in general. The knowledge in use for keeping homes and taking care of children's upbringing did not generally have the character of official knowledge of any (or much) academic status but was primarily disseminated through socialisation and training (Hernes, 1987; Zahle, 1873). However, several factors and developments at the time played a role in changing this and contributed to the emergence of home economics as an academic field, around which schools, education and new subject knowledge developed.

Such development enjoyed support and influence—in Denmark as well as in the Nordic countries in general—from contemporary ideas of education for all, labour market reforms and a general transition from agricultural to industrial society (Rasmussen & Andreasen, 2020). This included social and economic movements such as the struggle for equal rights for women, the labour movement's struggle for social democracy, and the increasing focus on issues relating to health and disease (Petri & Kragelund, 1980). On this basis, ideas and initiatives of welfare-state politics that supported a healthy population and a stable workforce developed to ensure low costs for the public budget. By disseminating knowledge about health and healthy lifestyle in the population through education, the government expected to keep social expenses low (Foucault, 2008; Hernes, 1987; Liversage, 1972). These merged with ideas of the Danish folk high school movement, in which education and 'enlightenment' played key parts (Dahlsgård, 1980).

The idea of a 'school for all' (the 'folk school' as it is called in the Nordic countries) was a welfare political ideal, which had been part of the Danish social democratic programme since its very beginning (Esping-Andersen, 1990). The core of this was to create a comprehensive and coherent school system that could ensure better possibilities of education for all—regardless of one's socio-economic background or whether one lived in an urban or rural area. However, up until the 1960s, the education system remained socio-economically strongly differentiated along the dimensions of rural–urban and public–private schools, and the possibilities of continued education—vocational or higher—were confined to the very few. The then main function of the education system was arguably to socialise children into the pre-existing structures of classes and genders and the occupational and social fields of activity linked to these. Most people had less than seven years of schooling, and often even less in the rural areas of the country (Haastrup, 1987; Jespersen, 2011). There appeared to be a need for strengthening the education of girls, since less than half of them obtained schooling after the age of 14 (Jørgensen, 1943, p. 16). Home economics appeared as an obvious area for the continued education of this group, since many women had their primary occupation within this area, whether within or outside their own homes. This matched well with disseminating knowledge about home economics through other kinds of education, including public folk schools.

In the development of the comprehensive folk school in Denmark, important educational reforms of the 20th century occurred in 1899, 1903, 1937, 1958, 1975 and 1993 (Nielsen, 2001; Nørgaard, 2001). The reforms resulted in new educational acts accordingly dated to the same years that formed the legal basis for the school subjects. These will be the main documents on which we base our analysis. Thus, we focus analytically on the national curricular intentions and understand that they have materialised in different ways in school practice.

The proponents' argumentation for 'housecraft' as a school subject

From the 19th century—when knowledge about health and hygiene and their significance began to develop in a more scientific sense—the argument for introducing and developing such a subject area also developed, with women primarily being the dominating proponents. The argumentation was communicated in many different contexts. One of these proponents in Denmark, Birgitte Berg-Nielsen (1861–1951), describes how the question of 'home economics as a school subject' was raised in the Danish Women's Society in 1885 (Berg-Nielsen, 1900, p. 26). In 1891, the Pedagogical Association also took up the matter and held a meeting on the question, where Berg-Nielsen presented a plan for such teaching, which she had submitted to the school director in Copenhagen (Berg-Nielsen, 1900, p. 27). However, such teaching required special school kitchen facilities. Based on the interest in the case, school kitchens had been set up at a few schools in municipalities with a strong economy. Frederiksberg was one such municipality and became the first Danish municipality to introduce home economics in the folk school in May 1897, before the subject was introduced by law (Berg-Nielsen, 1900, p. 27; Hansen, 1933, p. 149).

In an 1899 inquiry aimed at the 'Government and Parliament', many proponents from across the country expressed their arguments for the teaching (of girls) in home economics to the Danish government. Their inquiry also addressed the socialisation of girls, as can be seen in the following:

> It is our aim to establish school kitchens … . We need not point out the extraordinary importance which the housewife's skill, her insight and practical knowledge in home economics, has for the home, in the upper social classes as well as in the working class, and thereby for society as a whole. But also for the school, the admission of home economics as a school subject will be of the greatest value. It thereby becomes a means of arousing the children's interest and reverence for the work of the home, of developing their sense of order and economy, of meeting their sense of business. At the same time, the school kitchen offers great advantages in hygienic terms by breaking with the school's sedentary work.
>
> (Winteler et al., 1899, p. 13)

Such a subject and its potentials to disseminate knowledge about health and healthy lifestyle and thus to socialise women and the population as a whole—fits with the nascent ideas on the welfare state of the time. This idea that it breaks up the 'sedentary' work seems to speak to the nature of this subject as applied rather than theoretical. In this practical form, the subject of home economics was introduced as 'housecraft' in the folk school education act in Denmark in 1899. Housecraft (*husgerning*) was the name of the subject, which was for girls only. Thus, the Education Act, § 10, stated: 'Besides, on recommendation by the school commission and further provisions in the curriculum, instruction in nature study, woodwork, physical education for women, and female housecraft could be given'. Due to the lack of facilities such as school kitchens at many schools, and the corresponding costs of these, the subject was defined as an opportunity that the local school commissions could provide if they wished to do so.

The subject and its regulation

From the earliest implementation, the subject was taught from grade six, which remained unchanged throughout the 20th century. The number of lessons per week was suggested to be two to three in the ordinary curriculum, a number that remained unchanged during the different reforms of the folk school (Undervisningsministeriet, 1960, pp. 30–39; Holm-Larsen, 2014).

However, making it possible for schools to teach such a subject was not enough to make this happen in schools. A precondition for the implementation of the subject was access to the necessary facilities in the form of the school kitchen. Such facilities had, as mentioned, only been established in a few schools in areas with a strong economy (Hansen, 1933, p. 149). Establishing school kitchens required funding, and in the beginning the law was primarily aimed at schools in the metropolitan area (Copenhagen) that had the necessary teaching facilities (school kitchens) to be able to implement such teaching (Sthyr, 1899, p. 6).

Also, it was necessary to have teachers who were educated to conduct teaching in the subject, and in 1899 Berg-Nielsen received a grant from the Danish government to start an education of teachers for school kitchens (Berg-Nielsen, 1899). She appreciated the money, and as she wrote in *Woman and Society*—a journal published by the Danish Women's Society—it also expressed recognition of the cause that she and many other women had been fighting for:

> With these 6000 Kr. the education of women for the specific female deed— home economics—has been recognised by the state and found worth its support. It is the domestic woman, the future housewife, who by this has been recognised.
>
> (Berg-Nielsen, 1899, p. 72)

Here, she expresses hope that the state will establish a school for home economics, which she defines as 'a mission for life' for women, as she describes:

> We are thousands of women, who during our daily work at home feel the lack of a serious and versatile education for the deed, which is our life's task,

and on whose fortunate solution not only the cosiness and happiness of the individual home depends, but which also has decisive significance for the health and socio-economic development of the whole population. Therefore, we hope that the 6,000 kr. will not become a single standing grant; but that we should find benevolent understanding when we meet in the autumn with prayer and request for state support for the establishment of a school of home economics.

(Berg-Nielsen, 1899, p. 72)

The school kitchens represented a key factor and context in the regulation of the teaching in the subject. From the beginning, the kitchens on the one hand formed an idealised copy of those the girls knew from their homes or would meet later in life—the common and dominant female workspace, so to say, the central space for any home economics activity (Benn, 1995). On the other hand, the design of school kitchens also gave authorities and politicians the opportunity to provide teaching on the behaviour that was expected in a kitchen (e.g. regarding equipment and hygiene) by instructing and disciplining students. In this way, the subject materialised traditions, history and norms by 'building them into the room', so to speak. The practice (learning how) and its corresponding subject knowledge (learning about) were reflected in the curriculum and had the kitchen facilities as a necessary precondition.

Disciplining through the curriculum

In the first half of the century, all the previously mentioned teaching had women as their primary or only target group (Haastrup, 1987). This was in line with the dominant gender perspective of the time and elsewhere in Europe, which emphasised education for motherhood and positioned women in the home. However, in addition to this, it also proclaimed the importance of the home and family in society and thereby represented an enhancement of the domestic role of women (Rogers, 2006, p. 107). This is apparent in the very importance that the movements attach to the educational development of the area.

One of the Danish pioneers in the field, Eline Hansen (1859–1919), who was active in developing the so-called 'School Kitchen Instruction' (*Skolekøkkenundervisning*), described her views on the form and content of this, stating that:

It is not the intention to educate fully trained maids or housewives, this is not within the scope of the school kitchens. The objective is to arouse feelings and interests of the young (women) and provide them with an understanding for the importance of orderly housekeeping for human life, and through this deeper understanding increase bodily work.

The children are trained in keeping things punctually tidy, as each thing must be put in each place, and this is so much more necessary since every day it is a new group of children who work in the kitchen. The strictest tidiness needs to be impressed on them, both as to themselves, all foods, and kitchen ware. Likewise, they will be informed how they through cleanliness can fight the bacteria and the illnesses they may result in.

This instruction is particularly well-suited for the opposing of slowness and dullness. As there are four who will be doing the same work, this will provide ample opportunity to compare, give rise to competitive spirit, and be encouraging for their work.

Since the children will always have to help themselves, also at a pinch, their quick-wittedness and practical skill will be developed. And that not least in this respect a lot can be attained within one year, I experienced by comparing a final class with a beginning class.

Finally, one aims at arousing the children's feeling of responsibility and independence, by entrusting them with a task that they must solve on their own. They are allowed to make mistakes and learn from the mistake.

(Hansen, 1897, p. 205)

From the quote, it appears that the qualification as maid or housewife is said not to be the primary purpose. Rather, the description emphasises how the importance of housekeeping as bodily work must be understood and acknowledged. For this, the children need to be informed about the necessity of order and cleanliness. More important though is the development of personal and practical characteristics such as *cleanliness, swiftness* and *resoluteness,* which the participating women will develop, it is anticipated, through bodily *training* and *learning from making mistakes.*

One of the earlier-mentioned pioneers, Birgitte Berg-Nielsen, noted that 'by teaching Home Economics Chemistry, we must get to know the composition of the foods we are dealing with' (Berg-Nielsen, 1899, p. 74). And furthermore, she specified that they must learn about economics, health, the child's life and development, nursing, salting, nutrition, poultry breeding, brewing, baking, cleaning and decorating (Berg-Nielsen, 1899, pp. 72–78). Here, we find a somewhat more academic approach to the field, emphasising the instruction in chemistry as a basis for *learning about* economics and health issues. This is presented as necessary knowledge for the practical handling of matters within the field.

The content of *female housecraft* as a school subject was described in sentences like these, advising that 'the exercises must consist of preparing simple dishes' and support the learning of 'cleanliness, order and thrift' (Ministeriet for Kirke- og Undervisningsvæsenet, 1904, p. 14). In the classes, the pupils:

are divided into families of 5 Members each. ... the children must, as far as possible, pay for themselves and also eat the food they make themselves. They also learn table setting, and they learn not only what to eat, but how to eat.

(Ministeriet for Kirke- og Undervisningsvæsenet, 1904, p. 14)

Here, we notice that the lessons primarily take the form of training rather than instruction. This training consists of the preparation of simple meals that allow the children (girls only) to experience a progression of difficulty. It is aimed at the characteristics of *cleanliness, orderliness* and *thriftiness*. Some theoretical instruction is provided as a basis for the latter, in which the girls are to learn the accounting and calculation of expenses. The training of this is given a strongly realistic dimension, since the groupwork is organised in 'families', and the girls *themselves* must, whenever possible, pay for and consume the food they prepare. Thus, they are disciplined in traditions of performance and expectations of behaviour—as girls.

In 1937, the name of the subject remained the same and so did the general purpose of 'disciplining' girls into specific social roles (Foucault, 1978). This resonated well with the Educational Act of 1937, giving stronger emphasis in general to the practical elements of school life. With this act, the government tried to provide school opportunities for those children, especially from the rural areas, whose occupational destinations did not demand academic qualifications and exams. Besides, the strengthening of practical elements assumed that manual and practical elements have stimulating and pedagogic functions (Nielsen, 2001). Again, this speaks to the theme of applied learning with its specific embodiment and materialisation.

Following the Educational Act of 1958, the subject name was changed in the curriculum so that it no longer contained the word 'female' but only housecraft (Thisted, 2001). The purpose of the subject was then described as providing:

the pupils with basic knowledge about nutrition and thereby give them an understanding of what a well-prepared and properly composed diet means for the family's health and well-being.

Through exercises in cooking, pupils are trained in using the available nutrients in the right way and through cleaning work to keep a home proper and clean, considering current hygienic rules. ... knowledge of the economic side of good house crafting for the individual and society. ... home technical aids (e.g. heating sources, pressure cookers and washing machines).

(Undervisningsministeriet, 1960, p. 188)

The new curriculum had more theoretical content that concerned knowledge on nutrition, its importance for health and well-being, economics and safety in connection with the use of technical appliances in the home. Exercises in cooking ensured that there was still a strong element of practical training in how to practice clean and efficient housekeeping.

This curriculum made it clear that the subject could be provided for boys (Undervisningsministeriet, 1960, p. 188), in that case emphasising that:

> it is advisable that the plan be organized so that the boys are able to participate in domestic work. Through theoretical teaching and practical practice, the boys are trained to understand as many of the housewife's various tasks as the number of hours allows. ... The plan for cooking may be the same as for girls in 6th grade. If time permits, a plan of a day's diet and a week's dinners can be made jointly. When preparing the dinners, whole and semi-finished products are used to the extent deemed necessary.

It is remarkable that the theoretical elements are much more pronounced in the curriculum targeting boys. They are to be prepared for participating in housekeeping, not primarily but also through exercises. However, the main purpose of the subject appears to be providing them with an understanding of the different tasks of the *housewife*. It may include the planning of dinners, which may consist of the use of finished or semi-manufactured articles. This seems to be taken for granted that the boys will not have much time for housekeeping, as their main occupation will be outside the home.

In the 1975 revisions of the subject, which was now compulsory for both girls and boys (Thisted, 2001), its name changed from housecraft to 'home knowledge' (*hjemkundskab*). The content was described in the subsequent curriculum of 1976 as emphasising that:

> pupils acquire knowledge and experience in areas that may be of importance to them as consumers and in planning and managing the work at home. ...

> The lessons must help the pupils to understand the importance of the right diet composition and that they develop an aesthetic attitude with regard to hygiene and to the interior design and maintenance of the home.
>
> (Undervisningsministeriet, 1976, p. 7)

The subject is given a much more theoretical tone than in the earlier curricula. It mentions nothing about exercises, and the practical elements have been reduced to techniques and work processes that can rationalise tasks in the home. Its core is to make the pupils (both boys and girls) understand the importance of a *proper diet* and that they develop an aesthetic view to the *hygiene, practical arrangements* and *maintenance of the home*. The practical parts of the curriculum (i.e. the way in which it is carried out as instruction) are barely visible.

In the law from 1993, the purpose of the subject is described with these words:

The purpose of teaching home economics is that pupils acquire knowledge and skills so that they are able to take co-responsibility and show care for the activities that take place in the home, and that they gain insight into the conditions and values this area of life has in interaction with nature, culture and society.

(Børne- og Undervisningsministeriet, 1994)

Here, the subject of home economics is defined with a purpose, which is basically to provide the pupils with theoretical knowledge. The core elements of the content focus on developing students' capacities of taking responsibility and showing care in activities of the home. In addition to this, they obtain knowledge about the interaction between this activity and nature, culture and society. It is remarkable in this description that the curriculum of the body has disappeared.

Conclusion

When the subject of home economics was introduced in the Danish folk school in 1899, under the name 'female housecraft', it was aimed only at girls. Through a detailed curriculum of the body, it contributed to disciplining them into specific gender roles. Thus, they were specifically disciplined into kitchen routines of being tidy, clean and efficient.

Some of the arguments in support of the subject emphasised its importance for 'the home' and, as they argue, 'thereby for Society as a whole' (Winteler et al., 1899, p. 11). This underlined the initial conceptualisation of the school subject as an applied rather than abstract or theoretical subject. The descriptions of the subject that later followed express the subject knowledge in a more academic sense as well as the knowledge related to socialisation. The descriptions changed at different times during the 20th century, becoming more and more theoretical and less practical.

In terms of socialisation, the subject of home economics reflects notions of what a home and a family are, how to act together at meals in a family, norms of good hygiene and who is responsible for this. In this latter respect, the responsibility was clearly placed on the women, as the subject disciplined them into specific roles as housewives (Lützen, 2000) and a thinking of themselves as subjected to the governance of men (Foucault, 1991). The school kitchen thus represented a materialisation of home economics, established the context for lessons and was an important means of communicating norms and knowledge. However, as a result of this, the subject in the first instance could only be implemented in schools that could afford to establish school kitchens, and in this way, schools in wealthy municipalities had an advantage here. Like elsewhere in Europe, improvements in children's—and girls'—schooling remained strongly class-based and tied to geographic location well into the 20th century (Rogers, 2006, p. 111).

In the 19th century and well into the 20th century, the dominating agents and leading proponents of teaching the subject were women. Many of these women were also active in relation to the establishment of, for example, schools of home economics, home economics colleges and courses in various contexts—an area of education that grew quickly in Denmark in the first half of the 20th century. Women thus, so to say, took (or gained) 'ownership' of the subject, its definition, its practice and the understanding of its unwritten rules and expectations that the school kitchens in implicit ways belonged to them. The domesticating of the public sphere was very much in line with the Nordic welfare-state idea that the state is the 'home of the people'. Thus, it assisted the development of the welfare state, in which the biopolitics played an important role in supporting the physical and social health of the population (Foucault, 2008).

When it later became a subject for boys as well, it was in the early years with a curriculum formulated differently from the girls', with a greater emphasis on theory. The curriculum never directly involved them—through the curriculum of the body—as had been the case with the girls. The fact that the subject was tied so closely to women gave them a kind of monopoly in the managing of home matters, which has lasted well into modern times. Thus, as stated by Foucault, knowledge is power, which in this case has involved numerous backlashes. Not least, it led to women becoming loaded with double work—still doing the main tasks in the home in the 'right' way—when entering the labour market.

References

Andreasen, K.E., & Rasmussen, A. (2020). Magdalene Lauridsen (1873–1957): Danish pioneer in the field of home economics. *Social Pedagogy Quarlerly/ Pedagogika Społeczna, 1*, 141–154.

Benn, J. (1995). Skolekøkkenet—et rum for husgerninger—for disciplinering og udfoldelse. In: V.O. Jensen (Ed.), *Skolefag i 100 år* (pp. 91–104). Danmarks Pædagogiske Bibliotek.

Berg-Nielsen, B. (1899). Husøkonomi som statssag. *Kvinden og Samfundet, 15*(5), 72–78. https://www.kvinfo.dk/side/444/?action=4&itemid=4672&searchtext= berg%20skolek%F8kken

Berg-Nielsen, B. (1900). Husøkonomi som undervisningsfag [Home Economics as a School Subject]. Birgitte Berg-Nielsen. Kbh.

Børne- og Undervisningsministeriet. (1994). *Bekendtgørelse om formålet med undervisningen i folkeskolens fag og obligatoriske emner med angivelse af centrale kundskabs- og færdighedsområder.* https://www.retsinformation.dk/eli/lta/1994/482

Dahlsgård, I. (1980). *Women in Denmark: Yesterday and today.* Det Danske Selskab.

Danmarks Statistik. (2000). *Befolkningen i 150 år.* Danmarks Statistiks Trykkeri.

Esping-Andersen, G. (1990). *The three worlds of welfare capitalism.* Princeton University Press.

Foucault, M. (1978). *The history of sexuality, vol. 1: An introduction.* Penguin.

Foucault, M. (1991). Governmentality. In G..Burchell, C. Gordon, & P. Miller (Eds.), *The Foucault effect: Studies in governmentality* (pp. 87–104). Harvester Wheatsheaf.

Foucault, M. (2008). *The birth of biopolitics: Lectures at the Collège de France, 1978–79.* Palgrave Macmillan.

Haastrup, L. (1987). Skolekøkken og arbejderfamilie. In S.A. Andersen, H. Caspersen, H.R. Christensen, N.F. Christiansen, H.T. Jensen, & L. Torpe (Eds.), *Årbog for arbejderbevægelsens historie* (vol. 17, pp. 119–156). Selskabet For Arbejderhistorie. https://sfah.dk/assets/uploads/aarbog/1987-17/1987-17-06-lisbeth-haastrup.pdf

Hansen, E. (1897). Huslig økonomi og skolekøkkenundervisning. *Kvinden og Samfundet, 13*(10), 200–204. https://www.kvinfo.dk/side/444/?action=4&itemid=4526

Hansen, T. (1933). Statens uddannelse af skolekøkkenlærerinder. In N.A. Larsen, & E.H.C. Mikkelsen (Eds.), *Dansk skole-stat, bd. 1* (pp. 149–150). Arthur Jensen. https://slaegtsbibliotek.dk/910457.pdf

Hernes, H.M. (1987). *Welfare state and woman power: Essays in state feminism.* Norwegian University Press.

Holm-Larsen, S. (2014). Elevtimetal i folkeskolens fag fra 1960 til 2014: Fra den Blå Betænkning til heldagsskolen. In B.R. Larsen, C. Larsen, J.E. Larsen, L.R. Rasmussen, & S. Wiborg (Eds.), *Uddannelseshistorie 2014* (Appendix: 1–16). https://uddannelseshistorie.dk/wp-content/uploads/2020/08/timetalsanalyse1960-2014.pdf

Jespersen, K.J.V. (2011). *A History of Denmark* (2nd ed.). Palgrave Macmillan.

Jørgensen, A. (1943). Den ufaglærte ungdom. In J. Novrup, A. Jørgensen, L.H. Petersen, & A. Lading (Eds.), *Den ny ungdomsskole.* Nyt Nordisk Forlag.

Liversage, T. (1972). *Kvinden og historien. Kønsroller og familiemønstre i økonomisk betydning [Woman and history. Gender and family patterns in an economic perspective].* Gyldendal.

Lützen, K. (2000). The cult of domesticity in Danish women's philanthropy, 1870–1920. In P. Markkola (Ed.), *Gender and vocation: Women, religion, and social change in the Nordic countries, 1830–1940* (Studia Historica, no. 64, pp. 147–176). Suomalaisen Kirjallisuuden Seura.

Ministeriet for Kirke- og Undervisningsvæsenet. (1904). *Bekendtgørelse om undervisningen i mellemskolen.* https://library.au.dk/materialer/saersamlinger/skolelove?tx_lfskolelov_display%5Baction%5D=displayLaw&tx_lfskolelov_display%5Bcontroller%5D=Display&tx_lfskolelov_display%5Blawid%5D=397&cHash=5c01bb1e0d476416ffb4550121670ea5

Nielsen, V.O. (2001). Socialdemokratiet, velfærdssamfundet og folkeskolen. In L. Kettel (Ed.), *Skolen i samfundet: Analyser og perspektiver* (pp. 30–40). Billesø & Baltzer.

Nørgaard, E. (2001). Noget om tidligere skolereformer. In L. Kettel (Ed.), *Skolen i samfundet: Analyser og perspektiver* (pp. 10–18). Billesø & Baltzer.

Orloff, A. (1996). Gender in the welfare state. *Annual Review of Sociology, 22*(1), 51–78.

Petri, G. (1981). Huslig uddannelse: Socialisering omkring århundredskiftet. In M. Winge (Ed.), *Pigeopdragelse* (pp. 38–41). Emmeline.

Petri, G., & Kragelund, M. (1980). *Mor Magda—og alle de andre: Husholdning som fag fra 1900 til i dag.* Komma.

Rasmussen, A., & Andreasen, K.E. (2022). Education of women homemakers in postwar Denmark: Home front alliances and rearmament in a welfare state perspective. In S. Engelmann, B. Hemetsberger, & F. Jacob (Eds.), *War and education: The pedagogical preparation for collective mass violence* (pp. 323–347). Brill.

Rogers, R. (2006). Learning to be good girls and women. Education, training and schools. In D. Simonton (Ed.), *The Routledge history of women in Europe since 1700* (pp. 93–133). Routledge.

Rose, N. (1996). 'Governing' advanced 'liberal democracies'. In A. Barry, T. Osborne, & N. Rose (Eds.), *Foucault and political reason: Liberalism, neo-liberalism and rationalities of government* (pp. 37–64). UCL Press.

Sthyr, V. (1899, March 24). *Lov om forskellige forhold vedrørende folkeskolen.* https://library.au.dk/materialer/saersamlinger/skolelove?tx_lfskolelov_display%5Baction%5D=displayLaw&tx_lfskolelov_display%5Bcontroller%5D=Display&tx_lfskolelov_display%5Blawid%5D=41&cHash=2c9ea85e0d200e7a2f0cbf5e6b9d4aa8

Thisted, E. (2001). Hjemkundskab i 100 år. In K. Arvedsen (Ed.), *Fagenes historie—skole og seminarium: Del 2.* Københavns Dag- og Aftenseminarium.

Undervisningsministeriet. (1960). *Undervisningsvejledning for folkeskolen: Betænkning afgivet af det af undervisningsministeriet under 1 September 1958 nedsatte læseplansudvalg* [Betænkning nr. 253]. S.L. Møllers Bogtrykkeri. https://www.betænkninger.dk/wp-content/uploads/2021/02/253.pdf

Undervisningsministeriet. (1976). *Undervisningsvejledning for folkeskolen 9: Hjemkundskab 1976.* https://library.au.dk/fileadmin/lfskolelov/1976-09-hjemkundskab.pdf

Winteler, L. et al. (1899). Til Regering og Rigsdag. *Kvinden og Samfundet, 15*(1), 13–14. https://www.kvinfo.dk/side/444/?action=4&itemid=4638&searchtext=skolek%F8kken

Zahle, N. (1873). *Om den kvindelige uddannelse her i Landet.* Th. Linds Forlag.

7

IN THE NAME OF HEALTH AND COMPREHENSIVE EDUCATION

Historicising contemporary school health in Chile[1]

Felipe Hidalgo Kawada

As it has been seen throughout this book, the 'curriculum of the body' operates in various forms in schools (Burns et al., 2020; Proctor & Burns, 2017) and has been taken up and administered in diverse ways in different contexts and nations. This chapter continues to examine these deployments in specific contexts, offering a critical and historical analysis of contemporary school health in Chile through the exploration of a contemporary policy called *Decree 381, Other Indicators of Educative Quality* (*Otros Indicadores de Calidad Educativa*, in Spanish).

The focus on the *Other Indicators of Educative Quality* (*OIEQ*, hereafter) is not about offering an exclusive analysis of this policy. Instead, the analysis moves beyond the belief of this policy as a static, stable and predefined artefact (Prior, 2004; Tight, 2019); it is used as a lens to historically and critically comprehend the ways in which health is being taken up in Chilean schools. Specifically, the discourses and practices around bodies, health and childhood and how they intersect with ideas around becoming a 'healthy student' and 'healthy school' are analysed. In this way, the aim is to move beyond analyses that link contemporary educational reform solely to the project of neo-liberalism and also to see how the project of medicalisation conjoins with market logics in and through schooling.

The chapter begins by providing a brief overview of colonial legacy, private charity and public initiatives that have marked the developments of health during the history of schooling in Chile. Next, the contemporary context is examined, focussing on mobilisations for education, medicalisation processes and the instalment of neoliberal practices in schools. The chapter then provides a critical analysis of how the ideas around becoming a healthy student and healthy schools are presented in the *OIEQ*, and how

DOI: 10.4324/9781003288671-10

it sheds light on contemporary health discourses and practices in Chilean schools.

Mapping school health in Chile: Colonial legacy, private charity and public initiatives

Over more than four centuries—first as a colony of Spain, and later as an independent republic—a plethora of health discourses and practices have circulated and been deployed into Chilean schools. During the colonial era (16th–18th centuries), Catholic influence, mixed with scientific and modern European medicine, defined the boundaries of how health was understood. Topics such as health, illness, life and death observed in texts used for learning and praying (Copin, 1784) show how religious orders played a fundamental role in the few schools founded in this period, and how other understandings of health were valued to a lesser extent or outright suppressed (Copin, 1784; Frontaura, 1892; Labarca, 1939). Throughout the 19th century, in the now independent republic, the educational project was based on a colonial religious continuity and the aspiration of pursuing a scientific-technical education, understood as a way of accessing modernity (Hirmas, 2016; Toro-Blanco, 2019a). In this context, medicine began, by different institutionalised mechanisms, to be legitimised as hegemonic in both knowledge and practice (Fuster, 2013). However, it was from the late 19th century that health began to play a much more significant role in schools (Illanes, 2010). In the context of illnesses and epidemics and the need to reinforce national identity, hygienic, patriotic and eugenics discourses were justified in schools (Acuña, 2020; Caffarena, 2016; Martínez, 2017). These discourses continued being deployed in schools over the 20th century through various initiatives. Thus, physical education, school sports (Acuña, 2020), residential school excursions that prioritised healthy living (Villalobos, 1905), school breakfast (National Council of Nutrition, 1939), mental hygiene (Fuentes, 2018), and medical inspections, among others, were integrated into school life and led by various professionals, such as doctors, psychiatrists, psychologists, school counsellors, nurses and teachers (Fuentes, 2018; Hidalgo Kawada & Martínez, 2020; Martínez, 2017; Toro-Blanco, 2019b).

These practices were run initially by private providers and then gave way to a much more active engagement of the state in these matters. These private interventions conducted especially over the 19th century in Latin America were, according to Pedraza (1999), mainly performed by upper-class people. This was the propitious scenario for the bourgeoisie to install their ideas around hygiene, feeding and sexuality, among other health-related issues. In Chile, meanwhile, private charity was the main way to assist poor people during the 19th century, a model inherited from the colonial period (Fuster, 2013).

On the other hand, from the end of the 19th century, in the context of a nascent idea of public health, and in a much more visible way during a large part of the 20th century, the school space constituted a fundamental place to deploy state interventions. These were focussed mainly on poor children (Serrano et al., 2012). For the state and its institutions (e.g., schools), engaging with poor children and their families was a priority. Schools looked for different strategies to attract them, although the attendance, especially over the 19th century, constituted a significant issue, despite the promulgation of laws related to free-of-charge schools (Hirmas, 2016).

The main political purpose of state interventions within the school space was related to producing, in children (students) and their families, an adherence to and compliance with the norms that the state proposed to them. In this sense, the purpose was related to feeling identified with the project of nationhood (Serrano et al., 2012). Thus, the school as a space of mandatory learning, and the medical *dispositif* as an apparatus of expert knowledge and power, constituted a powerful way of regulating and managing marginalised segments of society. Likewise, school students signified a way to access and regulate their own marginalised families and communities (Fuster & Hidalgo, 2020).

This public approach, or 'Chilean-Welfare' state spirit (Acuña, 2020) was preponderant, especially from the 1920s to 1973. During the Popular Unity period (1970–1973), marked by the first socialist government democratically elected in the world, health was an important part of the political agenda. President Salvador Allende, as a doctor and an adherent of the so-called Latin American social medicine (Waitzkin et al., 2001), proposed to change social and health inequities for children and adolescents by, for example, tackling hunger and promoting sports and recreational activities for poor children (Hidalgo Kawada, 2022).

Many of these practices developed over a large part of the 20th century were rejected under the dictatorship of Pinochet (1973–1990), in favour of developing an education model based on a neoliberal agenda (Connell & Dados, 2014). The health initiatives of the dictatorship included advocating 'temperance' and changing the 'deep-rooted Chilean culture' around alcoholism, promoting a patriotic, hard-working, obedient and depoliticised subject to construct the New Homeland—'Chile on the right track', far from Marxism (Servicio Nacional de Salud, 1979).

The ideas historically approached in this section serve as a prelude and facilitate the comprehension of a long history of school health in Chile, providing a backdrop to analyse more clearly contemporary scenarios, which are presented in the next sections. To contextualise contemporary health school scenarios in Chile, the following sections will consider three key ideas: medicalisation, marketisation and mobilisations for education.

Contemporary scenarios: Medicalisation, marketisation and mobilisations for education

The idea of the medicalisation of society (Conrad, 2007) is pertinent to understanding current school health issues. Initially, medicalisation can be understood as the myriad ways in which science has shaped the administration and regulation of populations settled in industrial European cities between the 17th and 19th centuries (Fuster, 2013). The social panic about poor hygiene and illnesses related to these conditions gave rise to a set of techniques and tools to regulate populations in the name of health. In these specific contexts, concepts such as 'biopower' and 'biopolitics' have been useful to understand the relationships between health—configured by medical knowledge—and the politics of bodies (Thompson & Coveney, 2018; Wright & Harwood, 2009). In general terms, biopower is constituted by the construction of a set of 'truths' regarding human life, and consequently, a body of experts focussed on managing and spreading these truths. It is constituted by strategies of intervention in the name of health and life, and it is composed of modes of subjectification, or 'practices of self', which are centred on the compelling of individuals to work for themselves (Wright & Harwood, 2009). Biopolitics refers to the point of entanglement between politics and biological life. From this perspective, the body is understood as a terrain of dispute in relation to the ways of regulation and control of bodies (Thompson & Coveney, 2018).

In contemporary medicalised society, non-medical problems are often now defined, administrated and treated as medical problems, labelled in the form of 'illness' or 'disorder' (Welch et al., 2012). At the school level, medicalisation is observed in diverse ways, such as establishing problematisations, labelling school experiences and proposing ways of actions according to medical knowledges. Some of the most commonly analysed emergent school health issues have been the call for schools to intervene in the obesity epidemic, and the rise of psychopathology in school curricula and practice (Harwood & Allan, 2014; Gard & Wright, 2005; Rich, 2012; Rich et al., 2020; Wright & Harwood, 2009). Rich et al. (2020) argue that obesity has arisen as a school health issue over the last three decades and has intensified in recent years. The focus is placed on the body weight of students, configuring a 'weight-centred health paradigm' or a 'weight normative approach', where body weight and shape emerge as central school health goals (Rich et al., 2020). In the same vein, Harwood and Allan (2014) affirm that 'schools are sites of significance in the contemporary production of psychopathology'

(p. 1), where a wide range of mental health disorders (i.e., ADHD, Asperger syndrome, etc.) are constituting common diagnoses for children at school (Harwood & Allan, 2014).

In Chile, since the late 1980s and early 1990s, obesity and sedentary lifestyles have been recurrent discursive themes in the field of school health. Mobilising catastrophic language, it was proclaimed that the population, especially school-aged children, are succumbing to overweightness and obesity and that the situation was becoming increasingly dire, especially after reaching one of the highest levels of prevalence in the world (Organisation for Economic Cooperation and Development [OECD], 2019). Since then, a series of programmes and campaigns to 'fight obesity' have been put into practice, such as the Against-Weight Plan and the National Zero Obesity Strategy, among others (Ministry of Social Development and Family of Chile, 2019).

This focus on obesity in school-aged children in Chile is not unrelated to international school health trends. Shilling (2010) noted more than a decade ago that health had reached unprecedented levels of relevance and had become a central aim in the education systems of several countries in Europe, North America, Asia and Australia. Obesity, sedentary lifestyles, psychopathologies, mental disorders and others health issues have been the main target of school interventions (Rich et al., 2020, Wright & Harwood, 2009). Accordingly, a series of policies, programmes and curricular reforms have been deployed in schools, justified through discourses of health promotion and holistic education (Bekerman & Zembylas, 2018; Camacho-Miñano et al., 2019).

However, although current Chilean school health is situated in a context of global trends, these must not be understood as just a replica of international health reforms. The process of recontextualisation (Rich, 2012), in terms of how schools incorporate, translate and deploy these health reforms must be considered. It must be recognised that current health policies in Chile are inexorably intertwined with a long and situated school medicalisation history as well as other struggles and disputes in the national education arena, including the historical specificity of national school health policies and practices. A key argument here is that the emergence of the *OIEQ,* which will be analysed later in this chapter, reflects a new policy logic that appeared as a response to the ongoing student protests initiated in 2006 against marketisation installed during the 1980s.

In the middle of these massive protests, the response of government was to promulgate new laws that introduced more sophisticated control systems and accountability processes (Falabella, 2020). According to Falabella (2020), this consolidated a 'performative school market model' by the creation of the National Quality Assurance Education System (Law 20.529)

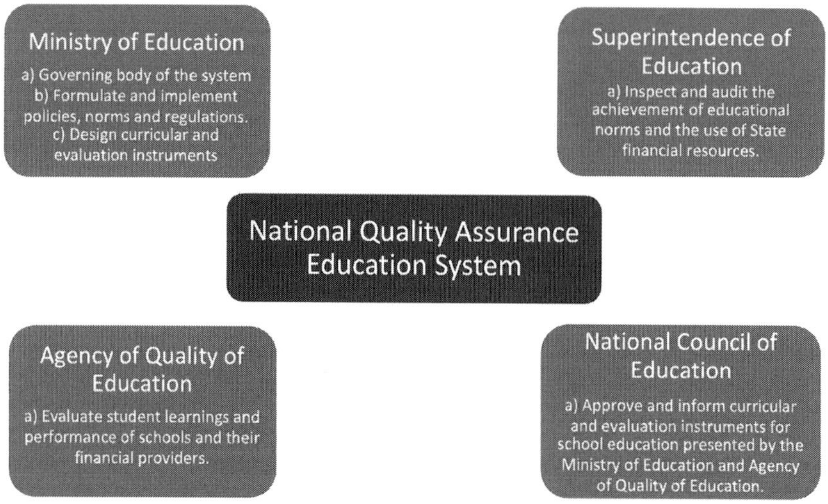

FIGURE 7.1 National Quality Assurance Education System in Chile. Retrieved and adapted to English from the official website of the National Council of Education of Chile [CNED]: https://www.cned.cl/sistema-nacional-de-aseguramiento-de-la-calidad-de-la-educacion-escolar-sac

(Figure 7.1), where, in the name of 'educational quality and equality assurance', standardisation, tests, accountability practices in general and a new moral—concomitant with these values—were validated as the best way to improve the Chilean education.

In the context of a new National Quality Assurance Education System (see Figure 7.1), and following international trends related to providing a broad and comprehensive education, the traditional Quality of Education National Measuring System (SIMCE, in Spanish), which historically evaluated learning in 'Mathematics' and 'Spanish Language', was expanded to include new indicators. These new indicators, comprising eight dimensions, were called *Other Indicators of Educative Quality* (Decree 381, 2013). This set of compulsory assessment indicators started to be tested from 2014 in all schools officially recognised by the Ministry of Education (see Figure 7.2). As the Agency of Quality of Education (2014) highlights, the goal of these new indicators is to evaluate the 'personal and social development' of students, with the purpose of reaching a 'comprehensive' education.

The sections that follow provide a closer examination of the *OIEQ* document to show how health is understood and managed, as well as how it interplays with the dynamics of the Chilean education system.

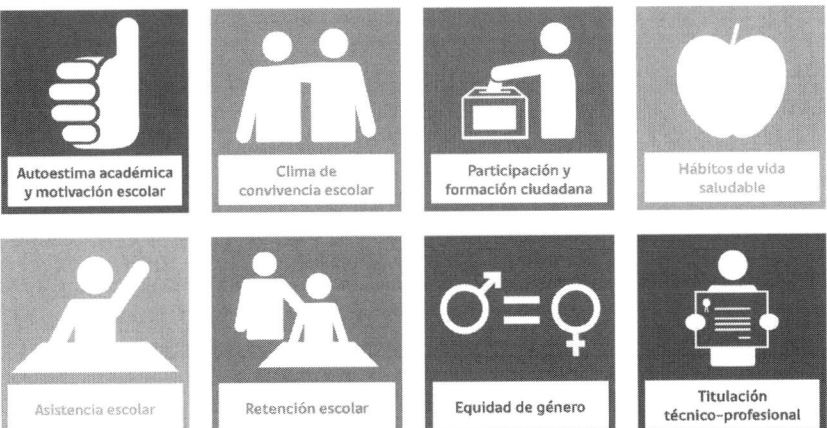

FIGURE 7.2   Other Indicators of Educative Quality. From left to right: academic self-esteem and school motivation; school mediation; participation and citizenship formation; healthy lifestyles; school attendance; student retention; gender equity; and vocational promotion. Agency of Quality of Education (2014, p. 5).

Becoming a healthy student

According to Rabello (2020), global capitalism has not only imposed a new global mode of production, but also new global ways of being and living. In this context, Rabello (2020) suggests the emergence since the 1990s of the idea of the *global child*. This point is especially relevant for thinking about the processes experienced in Chile or Latin America, considering that these global ideas have historically been produced and legitimised in the Global North and then spread to the peripheries (Mignolo & Walsh, 2018; Resende, 2018).

Concomitantly, in the process of constructing the *OIEQ*, the first move made in this universalised and globalised direction was to adhere to the traditional definition provided by the World Health Organisation [WHO] in 1948, which defined health as 'a complete state of physical, mental and social wellbeing, and therefore … extended beyond the mere absence of illness' (Agency of Quality of Education, 2014, p. 46). The *OIEQ* discursively built the idea of a (global) *future healthy student* as a child/adolescent with adequate body contours, active, happy, open to meeting others, with developed social abilities visible in their capacity to respect rules and work in a team; and with the ability to self-control their impulses and emotions, and consequently perform well in school.

Healthy lifestyles are discursively justified in the *OIEQ* based on understanding the body as a biological machine, taking the Cartesian metaphor of a machine made up of bones, muscles and a number of systems (Le Breton, 2017). From this modern, western and medical perspective, the body would need to be trained for its optimal performance, in other words, to reach health. Thus, it is pointed out that healthy lifestyles contribute towards an 'appropriate body weight, to develop strong bones and muscles, and to have an immunological system that can actively protect them of viral cases that commonly are transmitted at schools' (Agency of Quality of Education, 2014, p. 48).

In medicalised scenarios, psychological knowledges are also a key approach for framing the healthy child expected to be built. For example, it is justified that healthy lifestyles would contribute towards having mentally(emotionally) prepared children, observed as students with 'better mood states, greater self-confidence and self-esteem, and greater impulse control and frustration tolerance, among others' (Agency of Quality of Education, 2014, p. 48). These 'psycho-emotional' goals are expanded to the terrain of reaching social competencies as well. Some scholars (Binkley, 2011; Brunila, 2014) suggest that these movements can be understood as part of a contemporary therapeutic culture, where emotions, feelings, but especially personal happiness are positioned as highly relevant matters, being the target in different fields, and now justified through the use of objective measures, methods and procedures, that is to say, justified by knowledges with scientific status.

However, the focus on happiness has indeed not only been a feature of contemporary times in Chile. During the first part of the 20th century, schools looked for new ways of regulating children and young bodies (Toro-Blanco, 2018). Following North American-inspired pedagogical models, such as the New School, ideas related to a comprehensive education were promoted. Likewise, and making use of psychological and psychiatric knowledges, various bodily practices began to be linked to the need to generate joy and pleasure in students (Toro-Blanco, 2018), somehow involving a focus on accessing the *child's interiority*. This child-focussed component, with happiness as a goal, was a discourse that circulated widely throughout much of the 20th century. For instance, in the 1970s ideas related to the 'comprehensive development of the child', or the 'happiness of children and young people' were recurrent in speeches of the socialist Popular Unity government (Hidalgo Kawada, 2022; Rojas, 2010). Happiness, which throughout all these decades appeared as a quest, a horizon to reach—mainly linked to providing better material conditions for the country's children—presents some nuances in contemporary scenarios.

One of its particularities is that happiness now is not seen as a horizon to hypothetically reach as society, but an optimal individual emotional performance (Binkley, 2011) that is concomitant with neoliberal values, where happiness is not defined precisely as a horizon or utopia, but rather as a *compulsory* emotional state of the contemporary subject. Thus happiness, understood as one of the mechanisms in the contemporary subjectification process (Binkley, 2011; Vintimilla, 2014), is observed in different ways throughout the *OIEQ*. One of the rationales is based on the value of having healthy lifestyles, which would make a change on—or be in tune with—body weight/shape/size, and consequently, on a variety of psychological dispositions and happiness. This is exemplified in the following way:

> For example, a student who is physically fit and eats in a way that allows him/her to have a normal weight is more likely to feel comfortable with his/her physical appearance and confident to live new experiences, to cope constructively with difficulties and to develop a good self-image. It should also be noted that physical activity causes the human body [to] release endorphins, a hormone that makes people feel happier, more vital and fulfilled, which contributes to good mental health.
>
> (Agency of Quality of Education, 2014, p. 48)

This approach, along with showing the relevance of psychological knowledges and happiness, now scientifically explained under physiological principles, produces and normalises the expectations of contemporary subject formation: the possibility that students can reach the 'optimal human emotional performance' (Binkley, 2011, p. 384).

Along with happiness and a number of emotional and social competencies, the *OIEQ* is supported by a neoliberal approach to the student subject, based on a belief that individuals are responsible for the management of their health. Burns (2008) maintains that being an 'entrepreneurship of self' has been intensified in the context of globalisation and neoliberalism, organising schooling and health. This can be observed, for example, in the way in which all these views and expectations on student bodies are expressed through a formula in the *OIEQ* that allows schools to 'calculate' students' healthy lifestyles. This formula reinforces the contemporary biomedical and neoliberal logic of understanding health as an objective and measurable matter, and something that can be managed by individuals and managed by schools. As they affirm in the *OIEQ*, 'there is a close relationship between the health state of a person and her/his lifestyle, which is conditioned mainly by their nutritional habits, physical activity and selfcare' (Agency of Quality of Education, 2014, p. 46). Thus, a student's health is evaluated by inputting information about nutritional habits, physical activity and self-care (which is referred to as the prevention of risk behaviours and promotion of self-care and hygiene in relation to sexuality, hygiene and consumption of alcohol, tobacco and drugs): all of which is entered input into a formula (see Box 7.1), which adds the score of each dimension, and divides this result by three. Thus, eating well, doing exercise and prioritising self-care results in the ideal performance for becoming a healthy student.

Box 7.1   Formula to calculate the student's healthy lifestyles indicator.

$$HV_i = \frac{HVal_i + HVau_i + HVva_i}{3}$$

Another problematic dimension of a health perspective focussed on young people's management of their bodies and emotion, measured and reported through formulas of this kind, is the overlapping of other understandings of bodies and health. Positioning from what Mignolo and Walsh (2018) call geopolitics of knowledge, it seems that peripheric health understandings and experiences from children and youth from 'remote' territories away from the capital city, such as Rapa Nui Island, the Andes Mountains and Patagonia, are not yet sufficiently valid and valuable knowledges to be considered. The curriculum of the body in the context of Chilean schools is being subject to a series of mandates, expectations and performance frameworks, which, in this case, function as 'colonialist operations' (Bard Wigdor & Vergara, 2018), where neither the Mestizo, Indigenous, *altiplánico* and immigrant nor other bodies that inhabit these territories, seem to live up to this global child body. It is precisely in the colonising process of promoting a global and universal child that there is a denial of the corporealities, skins, textures, smells, desires and feelings of non-metropolitan or 'other' peoples. As Rabello (2020) provocatively states, the point of issue seems to be that 'someday people from the Global South will reach the humanity and health of people from the Global North and developed countries. It is just a matter of time' (p. 52).

Becoming a healthy school

As has been observed in different national contexts, school health has moved to surveillance practices and accountability frameworks (Macdonald, 2011; Rich, 2012). In the same way, it has been observed that these practices are positioned, in different educational settings, as the best ways to solve education systems issues or 'problems' (Palacios et al., 2019). The creation of the *OIEQ* is consistent with this approach. In the *OIEQ*, it is not only students evaluated using healthy lifestyles' indicators, but also schools, which are sorted and classified according to their performance of being healthy. Evaluation, classification and sorting schools are relevant practices in the context of a performative school market model (Falabella, 2020), where it is common to proclaim the need to have well-informed parents and families to make good decisions about the education of their children (Hofflinger et al., 2020;

Box 7.2 Formula to calculate the school's healthy lifestyles indicator.

$$HV_k = \frac{\sum_{i=1}^{n_k} HV_i}{n_k}$$

Proctor & Aitchison, 2015). Specifically expressed in the National Quality Assurance Education System, this process, and making results public for everyone, is positioned as beneficial in terms of allowing for the 'greater empowerment of parents regarding the education their children are receiving'. Accordingly, the results of the *OIEQ* are publicly provided.

In terms of evaluation, a healthy school is calculated using the formula given in Box 7.2. The school's healthy lifestyle (HVk) is calculated simply by averaging the number of students who attend the same school and have been categorised under the healthy lifestyle score (*nk*).

The categorising process of healthy schools is divided into three steps. Firstly, the data collection is developed, using SIMCE questionnaires which are responded to by students. These questions are related to attitudes and behaviours perceived by the students themselves, as well as their perceptions of the promotion of healthy lifestyles in their schools. Secondly, the score calculation by student, by grade and by cycle (primary and secondary) is obtained, using the formula in Box 7.2. Finally, after obtaining the results, one of three rankings of categorisation is possible for schools: (a) promotes actively healthy lifestyles; (b) promotes moderately healthy lifestyles; or (c) does not promote healthy lifestyles.

Thus, health, happiness and the search for the emotional optimisation of the contemporary subject have led to new and creative ways of understanding schooling and its processes. For example, this case shows how parents and guardians would have more bases, now related to health and soft competencies, for making 'informed' decisions in the Chilean market of education—and it would be interesting to explore to what extent these new categories, like a 'healthy school', are being utilised as advertising mechanisms to captivate students/families under the idea of providing a 'comprehensive' education.

The political decision to make schools and students compete for rankings of social and educational health in Chile is certainly worthy of critical examination, especially in the context of Chile's schooling systems and structures. As many scholars have noted (e.g., Bellei et al., 2020; Falabella, 2020; Gayo et al., 2019), the Chilean school system presents historical problems in terms of stratification, peripherical segregation and spatial concentration patterns (Gayo et al., 2019) and a number of socioeconomic inequalities and segregations, in which a large percentage of 'vulnerable students' attend public schools, while 'middle-class' and 'upper-class' students are consumers of subsidised private and private schools, respectively (Bellei et al., 2020). It is in this context of structural inequality that the *OIEQ* attends to what is interpreted as the key problem of individual 'vulnerability' in relation to health and wellness. The proposal is that the current education system can fix these unfair components of competition among schools, affirming that this emphasis on wellness will over time break the correlation between the socioeconomic characteristics of schools and academic attainment.

Conclusions

This chapter has analysed how health and wellness have become mobilised in national education policy metrics that increasingly make schools accountable for social as well as academic development outcomes and has located contemporary school health within neoliberal governmental modalities. These developments can be seen as a product of contemporary global forces, mediated locally, and with deep histories of homogenisation and colonisation in the name of health. By such calculations and processes as those set out by the *OIEQ*, diverse corporealities and their multiple deployments are called into question from within the school space, inviting (or forcing) them to be part of this new profile of childhood and youth, as a global subject, who manages their body shape, their body contours and their emotions in order to enjoy a fullness of health, leaving behind—apparently, although it is not possible—the legacy embodied in histories of oppression, Blackness, miscegenation, and rootedness with the land, the majestic mountains, the sea and the cosmos.

The necessity of measuring and classifying bodies/health is not new in Chile. In the beginning of the 20th century, anthropometric measures operated to produce a racialised discourse, as when for example the school teacher Leotardo Matus sought to prove the existence of a 'Chilean race', conducting more than 100,000 observations of children 10 and 20 years of age, which concluded not only the existence of a particularly Chilean race, but also a superiority of this Chilean race over the European. (Hidalgo Kawada & Martínez, 2020; Martínez, 2017). In that sense, this policy and contemporary school health practices might be understood as a continuity of a historical school medicalisation pathway, now intertwined with contemporary contexts of accountability processes, market-oriented education system and new health concerns.

Note

1 This work was supported by the National Agency of Research and Development of Chile [ANID] under the Becas–Chile Grant No. 72200081.

References

Acuña, P. (2020). ¡Formemos espartanos chilenos! Políticas y campañas deportivas durante la dictadura de Carlos Ibáñez, 1927–1931. *Cuadernos de Historia, 52,* 233–261.

Agency of Quality of Education. (2014). *Otros indicadores de calidad educativa.* Ministerio de Educación de Chile. https://hdl.handle.net/20.500.12365/10447

Bard Wigdor, G., & Vergara, L. (2018). La (neo) colonización de los cuerpos: (Re) existir frente al heteropatriarcal capitalista. *Observatorio Latinoamericano y Caribeño, 2*(1), 40–57.

Bellei, C., Orellana, V., & Canales, M. (2020). Elección de escuela en la clase alta chilena: Comunidad, identidad y cierre social. Archivos Analíticos de Políticas Educativas, *28*(5), 1–23. 10.14507/epaa.28.3884

Bekerman, Z., & Zembylas, M. (2018). *Psychologized language in education: Denaturalizing a regime of truth.* Palgrave Macmillan.

Binkley, S. (2011). Happiness, positive psychology and the program of neoliberal governmentality. *Subjectivity, 4,* 371–394. 10.1057/sub.2011.16

Brunila, K. (2014). The rise of the survival discourse in an era of therapisation and neoliberalism. *Education Inquiry, 5*(1), 7–23. 10.3402/edui.v5.24044

Burns, K. (2008). (re)Imagining the global, rethinking gender in education. *Discourse: Studies in the Cultural Politics of Education, 29*(3), 343–357. 10.1080/015963 00802259111

Burns, K., Proctor, H., & Weaver, H. (2020). Modern schooling and the curriculum of the body. In T. Fitzgerald (Ed.), *Handbook of historical studies in education* (pp. 1–21). Springer. 10.1007/978-981-10-0942-6_34-1

Caffarena, P. (2016). *Viruela y vacuna: Diffusion y circulación de una práctica médica: Chile en el contexto hispanoamericano, 1780–1830.* Universitaria.

Camacho-Miñano, M., MacIsaac, S., & Rich, E. (2019). Postfeminist biopedagogies of Instagram: young women learning about bodies, health and fitness. *Sport, Education and Society, 24*(6), 651–664.

Connell, R., & Dados, N. (2014). Where is the world does neoliberalism come from? The market agenda in southern perspective. *Theory and Society, 43,* 117–138.

Conrad, P. (2007). *The medicalization of society: On the transformation of human conditions into treatable disorders.* Johns Hopkins University Press.

Copin, M. (1784). *El libro de la infancia, ó Ideas generales y definiciones de las cosas de que los niños deben estar instruidos.* La Imprenta del Real y Supremo Consejo de Indias.

Falabella, A. (2020). The seduction of *hyper-surveillance*: Standards, testing, and accountability. *Educational Administration Quarterly, 57*(1), 113–142. 10.1177/ 0013161X20912299

Frontaura, J. (1892). *Noticias historicas sobre las escuelas públicas de Chile á fines de la era colonial.* Imprenta Nacional.

Fuentes, J. (2018). Higiene mental escolar: Discursos y prácticas médico-pedagógicas para vigorizar la psiquis infantil: Chile, 1890–1950. *Cuadernos Chilenos de Historia de la Educación, 10,* 101–143.

Fuster, N. (2013). *El cuerpo como máquina: La medicalización de la fuerza de trabajo en Chile.* Ceibo.

Fuster, N., & Hidalgo, F. (2020). Moral, educación y medicalización en Chile (1872–1927). In F. Hidalgo (Ed.), *Educación física en Chile: Discursos, performatividades y posibilidades de los cuerpos* (pp. 41–68). Kinesis.

Gard, M., & Wright, J. (2005). *The obesity epidemic. Science, morality and ideology.* Routledge.

Gayo, M., Otero, G., & Méndez, M. (2019). Elección escolar y selección de familias: Reproducción de la clase media alta en Santiago de Chile. *Revista Internacional de Sociología, 77*(1), e120.

Harwood, V., & Allan, J. (2014). *Psychopathology at school: Theorizing mental disorders in education.* Routledge.

Hidalgo Kawada, F. (2022). Reflexiones en torno a la salud y la educación en el periodo de la Unidad Popular. In C. Matamoros, & S. Neut (Coords.), *Nuevas historias de la educación durante la Unidad Popular* (Vol. 1), (pp. 199–228). Sole.

Hidalgo Kawada, F., & Martínez, F. (2020). En el nombre de la salud: Contextos, discursos y prácticas en la escuela en la educación física en Chile (1889–1920 y 1998–2019). In F. Hidalgo Kawada (Ed.), *Educación física en Chile: Discursos, performatividades y posibilidades de los cuerpos* (pp. 69–126). Kinesis.

Hirmas, E. (2016). Transformaciones del capital cultural y conformación del capital social: La escuela, los preceptores, los alumnos y sus familias: Norte Chico de Chile, 1860–1920. *Tiempo Histórico, 7*(12), 59–83.

Hofflinger, Á., Gelber, D., & Tellez, S. (2020). School choice and parents' preferences for school attributes in Chile. *Economics of Education Review, 74,* 101946. 10.101 6/j.econedurev.2019.101946

Illanes Oliva, M.A. (2010). *'En el nombre del pueblo, del estado y de la ciencia, … ': Historia social de la salud pública en Chile 1880–1973.* Ministerio de Salud de Chile.

Labarca, A. (1939). *Historia de la enseñanza en Chile.* Imprenta Universitaria.

Le Breton, D. (2017). *Anthropologie du corps et modernité.* Presses universitaires de France.

Macdonald, D. (2011). Life a fish in water: Physical education policy and practice in the era of neoliberal globalization. *Quest, 63,* 36–45.

Martínez, F. (2017). *Hacia una pedagogía del cuerpo: La educación física en Chile, 1889–1920.* Ministerio de Salud de Chile.

Mignolo, W., & Walsh, C. (2018). *On decoloniality.* Duke University Press.

Ministry of Social Development and Family. (2019). *Estrategia Nacional Cero Obesidad: Para detener el aumento de la obesidad en Chile al año 2030.* Ministerio de Desarrollo Social y Familia.

National Council of Nutrition (1939). *¿En qué consiste el desayuno escolar?* Ministerio de Salubridad, Previsión y Asistencia Social.

OECD. (2019). Tackling obesity, unhealthy diet and physical inactivity. In *OECD Reviews of Public Health: Chile: A healthier tomorrow* (pp. 81–110). OECD Publishing. 10.1787/9789264309593-6-en

Palacios Diaz, D., Hidalgo Kawada, F., Cornejo Chavez, R., & Suárez Monzón, N. (2019). Análisis Político de Discurso: Herramientas conceptuales y analíticas para el estudio crítico de políticas educativas en tiempos de reforma global. *Archivos Analíticos de Políticas Educativas, 27*(47), 1–34. 10.14507/epaa.27.4269

Pedraza Gómez, Z. (1999). Las hiperestesias: Principio del cuerpo moderno y fundamento de diferenciación social. In M. Viveros, & G. Garay (Eds.), *Cuerpo, diferencias y desigualdades* (pp. 42–53). Utópica Ediciones.

Prior, L. (2004). Doing things with documents. In D. Silverman (Ed.), *Qualitative research: Theory, method and practice* (pp. 76–94). SAGE.

Proctor, H., & Aitchison, C. (2015). Markets in education: 'School choice' and family capital. In G. Meagher, & S. Goodwin (Eds.), *Markets, rights and power in Australian social policy* (pp. 321–339). Sydney University Press.

Proctor, H., & Burns, K. (2017). The connected histories of mass schooling and public health. *History of Education Review, 46*(2), 118–124. 10.1108/HER-06-2 017-0012

Rabello, L. (2020). Why global? Children and childhood from a decolonial perspective. *Childhood, 27*(1), 48–62. 10.1177/0907568219885379

Resende, V. (2018). Decolonising critical discourse studies: for a Latin American perspective. *Critical discourse studies.* 10.1080/17405904.2018.1490654

Rich, E. (2012). Beyond school boundaries: New health imperatives, families and schools. *Discourse: Studies in the Cultural Politics of Education, 33*(5), 635–654.

Rich, E., Monaghan, L.F., & Bombak, A.E. (2020). A discourse analysis of school girls engagement with fat pedagogy and critical health education: Rethinking the childhood 'obesity scandal'. *Sport, Education and Society, 25*(2), 127–142. 10.1 080/13573322.2019.1566121

Rojas, J. (2010). *Historia de la infancia en el Chile republicano, 1810–2010.* JUNJI.

Serrano, S., Ponce de León, M., & Rengifo, F. (2012). *Historia de la educación en Chile (1810–2010).* Taurus.

Servicio Nacional de Salud (1979). *Alcohol y alcoholismo. Texto guía para profesores.* Programa de prevención primaria del alcoholismo en la comunidad escolar.

Shilling, C. (2010). Exploring the society-body-school nexus: Theoretical and methodology issues in the study of body pedagogics. *Sport, Education and Society, 15*(2), 151–167.

Thompson, L., & Coveney, J. (2018). Human vulnerabilities, transgression and pleasure. *Critical Public Health, 28*(1), 118–128.

Tight, M. (2019). *Documentary research in the social sciences.* SAGE Publications.

Toro-Blanco, P. (2018). De fortificar la voluntad a desarrollar la personalidad: Cuerpo y emociones en la educación chilena (c.1900–c.1950). *Cad. Cedes Campinas, 38*(104), 49–62.

Toro-Blanco, P. (2019a). Entre modulaciones de afecto y autoridad en episodios de la historia de la educación chilena (c. 1820–c. 1950). *Revista de Historia da Educação, 23*, e88795. 10.1590/2236-3459/88795

Toro-Blanco, P. (2019b). Orientación escolar, reforma, circulación de modelos para el conocimiento de las emociones juveniles (Chile, c.1946–c.1965). In C. Vieira, D. Osinski, & J. Gondra (Eds.), *História intelectual e educação: Reformas educacionais, estado e sociedade civil* (pp. 343–363). Paco editores.

Villalobos, D. (1905). *La Primera Colonia Escolar.* Imprenta, Litografía i Encuadernación Barcelona.

Vintimilla, C. (2014). Neoliberal fun and happiness in early childhood education. *Journal of the Canadian Association for Young Children, 39*(1), 79–87.

Waitzkin, H., Iriart, C., & Estrada, A. (2001). Social medicine then and now: Lessons from Latin America. *American Journal of Public Health, 91*(10), 1592–1601.

Welch, R., McMahon, S., & Wright, J. (2012). The medicalisation of food pedagogies in primary schools and popular culture: A case for awakening subjugated knowledges. *Discourse: Studies in the Cultural Politics of Education, 33*(5), 713–728.

Wright, J., & Harwood, V. (Eds.). (2009). *Biopolitics and the 'obesity epidemic': Governing bodies.* Routledge.

PART 3

Architecture and spatialities

8

THE CLASSROOM AS HEALTHY PAVILION

Fresh air, natural light and student bodies in 19th- and 20th-century American schools

Dale Allen Gyure

Educators throughout the world in the early 20th century, tasked with managing and protecting student bodies during the rise of mass schooling, faced an epidemic of childhood illnesses that frequently interfered with their educational aspirations and threatened community health. In imagining the school as a healthier space, they joined with politicians, physicians and architects to devise a two-pronged strategy influenced by a set of beliefs about the impact of physical surroundings on children's bodies. On the one hand, a series of institutionalised health practices, including mandatory vaccinations and medical inspections, helped to eventually gain control of most of the deadliest diseases. On the other hand, a parallel intervention focussed on the classroom's physical environment. In consultation with architects, educational reformers altered the classroom to make its air healthier to breathe and its light adequate for reading.

This chapter explains how American educators concerned with healthy student bodies implemented this strategy in the 20th century, with a focus on changes to classroom design that attempted to improve air circulation and lighting. Although the history of the worldwide sanitary movement and the importance of new regulations appearing around the turn of the century has been well documented, the role of architectural changes in managing and protecting student bodies is an emerging field, largely unknown outside of architecture. At the centre of these changes is the concept of the classroom as a healthy pavilion, flooded with natural light and circulating fresh air, in stark contrast to the prevailing 'closed box' classroom with few windows and a stifling, dangerous atmosphere.

DOI: 10.4324/9781003288671-12

The pavilion concept

As defined in this chapter, a pavilion classroom is a classroom that has the dominant characteristic of openness to the outdoors and a commitment to facilitating the circulation of fresh air and the inclusion of abundant natural lighting. Debuting in the first decade of the 20th century, typical features of pavilion classrooms included large windows on more than one wall and windows on opposite walls. Its origins, as this chapter will show, lay in the efforts of educational and medical reformers to combat rampant illnesses, particularly in two areas: special open-air schools for sick children that appeared throughout the world prior to the First World War, and the efforts of educators and physicians to develop healthier public-school classrooms for the masses. These endeavours combined to advance the cause of student health in the form of the pavilion classroom.

Terminology can be tricky in this area. Open-air schools matched their name—they were schools that emphasised fresh air to such an extent that walls were removed from a standard classroom layout, or in some cases structures were erected with little more than four columns supporting a roof and no walls to enclose interior space (like a park pavilion). Open-air school activities (instruction, dining and resting) often were conducted entirely outdoors. Most open-air schools used some form of pavilion classroom. A 'pavilion school' denotes a more traditional one-storey school building, where most or all learning spaces are pavilion classrooms. Finally, 'pavilion' was an often-used term, but so were 'cottage', 'unit plan' and 'California Plan' in the United States.

Nineteenth-century classrooms and student health

The 20th-century pavilion classroom developed as a reaction to the appalling conditions of its 19th-century predecessor. Although they varied in size, materials and quality of finish, almost all 19th-century classrooms shared a notorious commonality: they were harmful to children's bodies. The most dangerous aspects of the classroom environment were inadequate or non-existent ventilation and meagre lighting. Small-windowed rooms packed with children's bodies were ideal breeding grounds for contagious diseases. The health problems caused or exacerbated by badly designed classrooms were compounded by the unprecedented number of students attending public schools, due in part to compulsory education and child labour legislation and a rapid expansion of the country's urban population caused by rural migration and international immigration. Simply put, increasing public school enrolments and the inadequate layout of classrooms facilitated the spread of dangerous illnesses.

By mid-century, Americans were fully invested in a public education system (Reese, 2005). Unfortunately, the public's enthusiasm for mass education at this time did not generate similar interest in the physical structure of the schoolhouse and its internal environment. Educators uniformly denounced public schoolhouses for their bad locations, poor quality of materials and craftsmanship and noxious air (Gyure, 2018). School officials described these schoolhouses as 'dirty, rundown, gloomy, fetid, crowded, and lacking in toilet facilities' (Duffy, 1990, p. 181).

The classrooms in which generations of American children received their education were unhealthy. Classrooms settled into a fairly standard form by the late 19th century: typically a rectangular shape with a teacher's desk on a platform at one end, faced by orderly ranks of desks, usually secured to the floor. Customarily the room's long sides were at least twice the length of its short sides. Most classrooms were probably around 30–50 feet long and 20–25 feet wide. Windows were necessary for reading light and air circulation but often were insufficient for both. In the early years, heat was usually provided by fireplaces or wood-burning stoves, and both were notoriously ineffectual. The shoddy nature of construction in most of these buildings added to the uncomfortable schoolroom atmosphere, with drafts regularly seeping through the crudely assembled walls. Brick buildings in urban areas were more solidly constructed but equally unhealthy. The teacher's only means of regulating room temperatures and the amount of fresh air was through manipulating doors and windows (Gyure, 2018).

Many American children's lives were miserable and brief during this time. In the early years of the new nation, nearly half of all children died before the age of five, and the remainder had short life expectancies (Duffy, 1979). Thousands of children succumbed to diphtheria, smallpox, measles and yellow fever. Survivors infected classmates in the cramped, stifling conditions of the average schoolroom. The reports filed by educators and physicians from this era are filled with references to the debilitating effects of measles, diphtheria, whooping cough and other illnesses on educational practices (Billings, 1893; Endemann, 1873; Larrabee, 1888). The unfortunate design and squalid air of classrooms were widely regarded as exacerbating these health problems.

Educational reformers' efforts to combat such illnesses were hindered by misconceptions about the nature of contagious illnesses. The germ theory of illness, which held that sickness was transmitted by microscopic bacteria, was gaining acceptance in terms of its explanation of the origins of disease, but effective treatments did not yet exist. And as late as the 1880s, many physicians remained skeptical about germ theory's explanation of illness. Instead, they held to the 'zymotic' theory of disease, which postulated that 'microzymas' contained in every human and animal body could spontaneously undergo a chemical reaction—similar to fermentation—that changed them into bearers of infectious diseases like typhus and typhoid fevers, smallpox, scarlet fever, measles, cholera, whooping cough or diphtheria (Tomes, 1998).

The lack of understanding of germ theory led to some bizarre conclusions. Many reformers, for instance, still believed that direct sunlight could kill germs. 'Direct sunlight is the most economical and practical of all germicides', wrote education professor and hygiene expert Fletcher Dresslar. 'Schoolrooms that are kept thoroughly clean and receive a thorough sunning each day are not likely to need much further attention in the matter of disinfection' (Dresslar, 1913, p. 359). Educators like Dresslar asked architects to design school buildings so that sunshine could penetrate corridors, closets and toilets. Beliefs such as these arose from the so-called 'dust theory of disease', which coupled germ theory to an escalating American obsession with cleanliness (Hoy, 1996). The dust theory held that infectious germs attached themselves to particles of dust or dirt that enter the human body through breathing or other contact. 'It has been amply proven', claimed educator Thomas D. Perry, 'that the infectious germs of both [tuberculosis and pneumonia] are "air borne," that is, may be transmitted or "caught" by means of the infinitesimal dry particles of dust or dirt … ' (Perry, 1910, p. 5). Dust theory evolved from an earlier model of disease transmission emphasising 'fomites', a term applied to any object capable of carrying infectious material. For example, the Massachusetts State Board of Health proffered the fomite theory in a publication on scarlet fever that warned about infectious transmission by 'air, food, clothing, sheets, blankets, whiskers, hair, furniture, toys, library-books, wallpaper, curtains, cats, [and] dogs' (Massachusetts State Board of Health, 1888). Whether educators viewed the problem as dust or fomites, the solution was a bright, clean schoolhouse.

The most feared disease was tuberculosis (TB), or 'consumption'. By the early 20th century, it was the nation's leading killer, with TB accounting for nearly 10% of all deaths, including almost 25% among young adults (Tomes, 1998). While the circulation of fresh air seemed to neutralise TB, its means of transmission remained mysterious. Many late 19th-century physicians questioned whether TB was even contagious, and popular opinion blamed the disease on inherent physical deficiencies in the infected person rather than germs (McCarthy, 2001). This ignorance, coupled with a lack of treatment options, intensified the public's fear of TB. Until scientists discovered streptomycin in 1943 there was no cure: the most common treatment was bed rest, abundant sunlight and maximum exposure to fresh air, often at a sanitarium. But the 'rest cure' was no real cure—at least 50% of patients died within five years of their visit to an open-air sanatarium, echoing the mortality rates of untreated patients (McCarthy, 2001).

The problem was compounded by the fact that children infected with TB, measles, diphtheria and other illnesses regularly attended schools throughout the country instead of quarantining. Many factors were involved in this situation. The absence of any useful treatments or alternative accommodations was significant—most infected people simply went on with their lives and hoped for the best. Additionally, a child in school, whether healthy or ill, generated no income. In an age of widespread child labour, many families needed to employ every able-bodied member to survive. For instance, the US Census Bureau reported that 1,750,000 children ages ten to 15 were 'gainfully employed' in 1900, although this estimate is low (Macleod, 1998). Beginning in the late 19th century, lawmakers restricted the hours children could work and the age when they could begin working, but child labour persisted for decades.

Child labour legislation often was paired with compulsory attendance laws requiring children to spend a certain portion of each year in school. By 1918, every state had mandated school attendance to some degree. These laws generally obligated children between the ages of 5 and 14 to spend most of their days in school. Massachusetts had instituted the nation's first compulsory attendance law in 1852, but by 1886 only 15 states, or 39% of the country, had enacted similar laws (Tyack et al., 1987). As the years passed, however, more states voted to create compulsory education. In 1918, Mississippi became the 48th and final state to pass such legislation (Katz, 1976).

Ventilation

By the late 19th century, classroom stoves and fireplaces had given way to complex mechanical ventilation systems in larger school buildings, but indoor air quality remained hazardous. Medical experts deemed classroom air harmful and evoked the infamous Black Hole of Calcutta as a cautionary tale (Buchan, 1891). Impure air was probably the greatest challenge encountered by children's bodies in public-school classrooms. For example, architect Charles Dwyer had addressed this in a mid-century book, in which he exclaimed:

> Want of pure air is the certain agent of destruction to our youth; and of all places its terrible effects are more potent and more certain in the schoolroom than in any other, because of the mass of exhalation from so many lungs, some already diseased and pouring forth their noxious vapors to be inhaled by the victims around.
>
> (Dwyer, 1856, p. 57)

Classrooms' flow of fresh air was hampered by numerous factors, ranging from simple overcrowding, to a lack of windows, to the opening or closing of windows by teachers, which interfered with the proper operation of mechanical ventilation systems and led to constant clashes between teachers and administrators (Rousmaniere, 1997).

As far back as the 1830s, when public schooling was still in its nascent stages, educators complained about improper ventilation in urban schools. Shortly thereafter, Boston formed a special Committee on Ventilation to investigate air quality in the city's public schools and was astounded by the results. Grammar school classrooms were receiving only 5% of the amount of fresh air considered necessary for a school day. And classroom air was described as a 'foetid poison' that hindered children's health and ability to learn (Schultz, 1973). Despite the alarm, the study had little immediate impact on the design of the city's schoolhouses. Late in the century, the Massachusetts Board of Health found almost 90% of Boston schools to have inadequate ventilation, while another survey again found serious defects in most school ventilation systems (Duffy, 1979; Pearmain, 1898). Boston was not unique in this regard. Health investigators found extremely high levels of carbonic acid in the air in New York City classrooms; an article in the *Journal of the American Medical Association* described the American classroom as 'a propaganda of contagion'; and in 1893, engineer John S. Billings complained: 'Of all classes of municipal buildings in the United States, public or private, there are probably none which have until recently, been in such an unsatisfactory condition, as regards their ventilation, as the public schools' (Billings, 1893, p. 410; Endemann, 1873, pp. 137–142; Larrabee, 1888, p. 614).

The exhaled air from 50-odd bodies in a classroom was difficult to expel. Those (mostly urban) school buildings containing heating and ventilating machinery prior to the 1890s used heated flues to induce airflow and regulate temperature. The alternative approach was to circulate air through the school building by mechanical means. Although expensive, mechanical ventilation systems generally were more reliable than furnaces. These plenum systems used large basement fans powered by steam or electricity to circulate heated air through the building. In some cases, exhaust systems placed the fans in the attic and pulled rather than pushed air through the ducts. Unfortunately, the newer systems often worked as poorly as their precursors (Rousmaniere, 1997). For example, despite improved ventilation technology, a study of New York City schools in 1924 found that only 2% of the city's classrooms had functioning ventilation equipment (School Survey Committee, 1924).

Lighting

While some sanitary movement leaders focussed on providing healthy air and eradicating dust, other reformers directed their attention to classroom lighting conditions, linking scientific studies on children's defective eyesight to inadequate or dangerous school lighting conditions. In the age before the widespread availability of reliable electric lighting, control of natural light in the classroom was considered essential for protecting children's eyes. Reformers touted decades' worth of supposed evidence that insufficient or misdirected lighting had damaged students' eyes, as seen in a book on schoolhouse lighting that began with three 'indisputable' statements based on decades of evidence: '1. A large percentage of the children in our schools have defective eyesight. 2. This percentage increases as the children advance from one school year to the next. 3. The cause has been traced in part to the school' (Rowe, 1904, p. 8). The state of Rhode Island's test of 1,000 schoolchildren found 33⅓% had 'defective vision' in one or both eyes, while a similar study of nearly 5,000 Chicago students found 35% with problems (Baker, 1910). In both cases, the amount and quality of lighting was deemed the culprit.

Furthermore, because experts agreed that all students should learn to write with their right hands, architects were encouraged to design classrooms so that all light entered the room from a bank of windows on the students' left side as they sat facing the teacher (Marble, 1892; Robson, 1874; Rowe, 1904; Wheelwright, 1901). Light coming from the student's right side would cast a shadow on the desk, while light from behind or in front of the students would shine in their eyes or those of the teacher, which was far worse. Additionally, architects were advised to avoid locating windows in more than one classroom wall lest they introduce 'cross-lighting', regarded as damaging to children's eyesight. In the absence of a contemporary term, I call this one-side-only standard the Unilateral Lighting Rule (ULR): it was followed religiously at the time by architects throughout the Western world (see Figure 8.1). In 1875, for

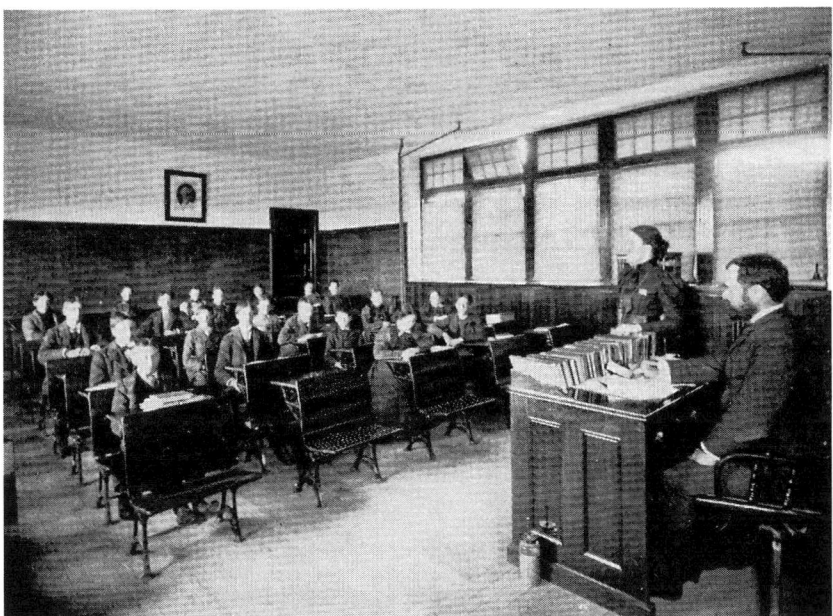

FIGURE 8.1 A traditional classroom following the ULR, with immovable desks arranged in orderly ranks, a bank of windows on one wall and poor ventilation. Barrington High School, Barrington, Rhode Island, 1898.

Source: T.W. Bicknell (1898), *A History of Barrington, Rhode Island*, opp. p. 528.

example, the Chicago Public Schools Superintendent Josiah L. Pickard alerted his colleagues to the need for proper lighting by emphasising the ULR. 'The tendency to assume such awkward and unhealthy positions [of the head], arises from the lack of sufficient light, in still many more from the admission of the light in the wrong direction', he wrote (Chicago Board of Education, 1875, p. 104). And according to Fletcher Dresslar, 'the results of careful examinations made in all progressive countries prove conclusively that school conditions are responsible for a large part of the nearsightedness prevalent among the children of the higher grades' (Dresslar, 1913, p. 221). When the Illumination Engineering Society (IES) published its *Code of Lighting School Buildings* in 1918, the nation's first standardised school lighting code, it reinforced the ULR and recommended windows 'located on one side of the room only' (Illumination Engineering Society, 1918).

Medical interventions

For much of the 19th century, attempts to rectify the classroom environment were sporadic and minimal. Boston became the first municipality to protect schoolchildren's bodies when it temporarily required all students entering the common schools to provide evidence of smallpox vaccination during an 1827 outbreak. The requirement became permanent in 1850. Boston in particular and Massachusetts in general would lead the nation in responsible approaches towards students' health. The Boston School Committee created the first body to investigate and report on classroom ventilation (1846) and authorised the first permanent system of medical inspections in public schools (1894). The state of Massachusetts passed the country's initial compulsory vaccination law for public school students (smallpox, 1855) and the first comprehensive sanitary code for school buildings (1888); soon after comprehensive codes for schools appeared in Chicago and New York (Duffy, 1990).

Following the American Civil War (1861–65), a nationwide sanitary movement flourished, and reformers exerted more pressure on educators to alleviate student health issues. Medical inspections of children and professional evaluations of classroom facilities and conditions became more common. But most classroom environments remained detrimental to student bodies because their physical spaces were not conceived and built with health in mind. Massachusetts found that 90% of its schoolrooms lacked ventilation equipment and relied on doors and windows for fresh air. Nearly two decades earlier, a Pennsylvania county school superintendent claimed there was not a single well-ventilated schoolhouse in his district, and hardly any in the entire state. His assessment was supported by the Pennsylvania State Superintendent, who found bad ventilation in almost half of the state's schools and called for a law requiring adequate air circulation in classrooms (Duffy, 1979).

Mandatory medical inspection of schools and students would prove a turning point in the war to protect children's bodies. Europe led the way in the late 19th century, followed by the United Kingdom in 1907 (Kirk, 1998; Roberts, 1917). The US lagged behind the rest of the world in this area, hindered by the nation's size and lack of a centralised educational authority. Progress here was measured in smaller steps. Boston's 1894 provision for medical inspections in the schools was unique, spurred by a diphtheria epidemic, but it encouraged reformers around the country and was emulated a few years later in Chicago and New York (Duffy, 1981, 1990). A snapshot of the turn of the century reveals a nationwide trend towards greater interest in students' health and an expanding roster of school inspection programs. Approximately half of the 45 states required some form of school building inspection by 1900, although implementation was the responsibility of local schools or medical boards, resulting in only a handful of cities with legitimate school inspection programs. A majority of states also implemented sanitary codes for school buildings, following Massachusetts's pioneering example. And throughout the nation, cities were winning the battle against smallpox thanks to legislation requiring vaccination for public school admission (Duffy, 1979, 1990).

Pavilion classrooms

The combined pressures of increasing enrolments and inadequate facilities reached a critical point in the early 20th century. At this juncture, since the rising tide of public school enrolments could not be stemmed, educators looked to physicians and architects to improve the classroom environment. The response was the pavilion classroom, inspired by two parallel inventions: the so-called 'open-air school' for children with TB, and the pavilion school. The openness and light associated with these special types would soon become the goal for designers of public-school classrooms.

In an effort to combat TB, European educators began to erect schools with few or no walls for children suffering from TB or related respiratory ailments; the goal was to maximise their exposure to sunlight and fresh air (Figure 8.2). The first of these 'open-air schools'—the 'Waldschule' (forest school)—appeared in the Berlin suburb of Charlottenburg in 1904. The Waldschule was inspired in part by so-called 'Nightingale pavilions' in contemporary hospitals, named for British nurse Florence Nightingale, who campaigned after the Crimean War to promote air circulation in hospital wards as a way to discourage infection from miasma (bad air filled with decomposing organic matter). Her efforts were effective, and since the 1860s physicians and architects had been designing such wards as long, narrow, partitionless, one-storey wings with large windows in opposing walls to facilitate air circulation and daylight (McDonald, 2022). The Waldschule, for pretubercular and 'weak' children, went even further than the

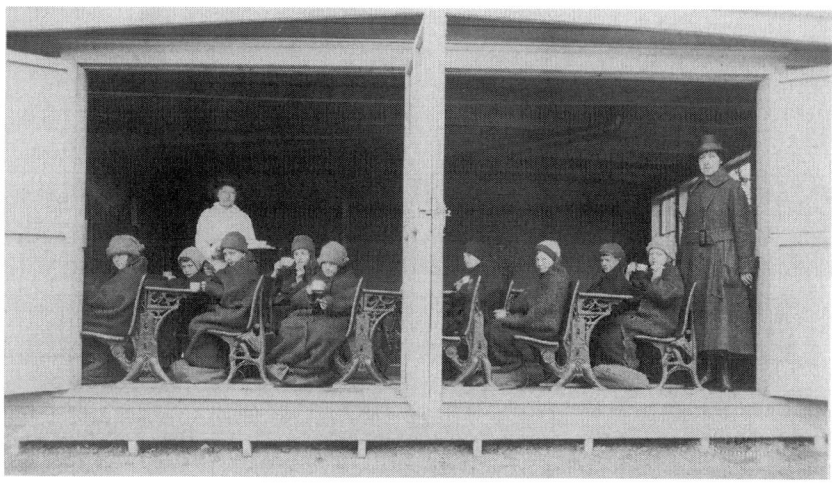

FIGURE 8.2   Open-air school, Larchmont, New York, early 20th century. Tuberculosis and other contagious diseases influenced the earliest efforts to bring more fresh air and sunlight into classrooms.

Source: Out Doors School of Larchmont Public Health Association, Larchmont, NY, (n.d.), [Photograph], Human Ecology Historical Photographs, Collection no. 23-2-749, item no. M-I-P-07, Rare & Manuscript Collections, Cornell University Library.

Nightingale pavilions towards eliminating barriers between inside and out. Its classroom structures with skylights and large windows in two walls, resting shelters with one wall entirely removed and dining pavilions made of only columns and a roof were all intended to guarantee that student bodies would receive continuous exposure to fresh air (Châtelet, 2008).

The popularity of open-air schools led many reformers to contemplate the beneficial effects of sunlight and fresh air on non-TB students. A major breakthrough in this regard actually occurred at the same time as the invention of open-air schools, when pavilion school pioneers conceived of public-school classrooms adopting the pavilion concept for the first time (Figure 8.3). Bilateral openings in the classroom walls would prove to be the crucial innovation. The pavilion ideal allowed for healthier school buildings in two ways. First, classrooms were cross-ventilated with constantly flowing air between large exterior windows on both long sides of the space. The second innovation followed the first. The increased illumination from these bilateral openings transgressed the ULR but improved the quality and quantity of light in the classroom (Figure 8.4).

The first American pavilion school was the Polytechnic School in Pasadena, California. Designed by architects Myron Hunt and Elmer Grey in consultation with school principal Virginia Pease and opened in 1907, Pasadena Polytechnic

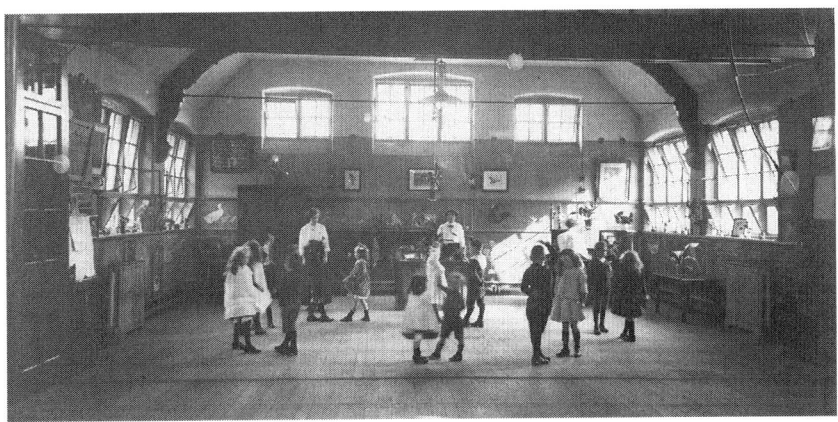

FIGURE 8.3 The pavilion classroom concept in action—flooding the room with light and fresh air from numerous windows.

Source: Holdsworth G., (1907), *Classroom, Ladycross Infants' School, Sandiacre, England, 1907* [Photograph]. Courtesy of Derbyshire County Council.

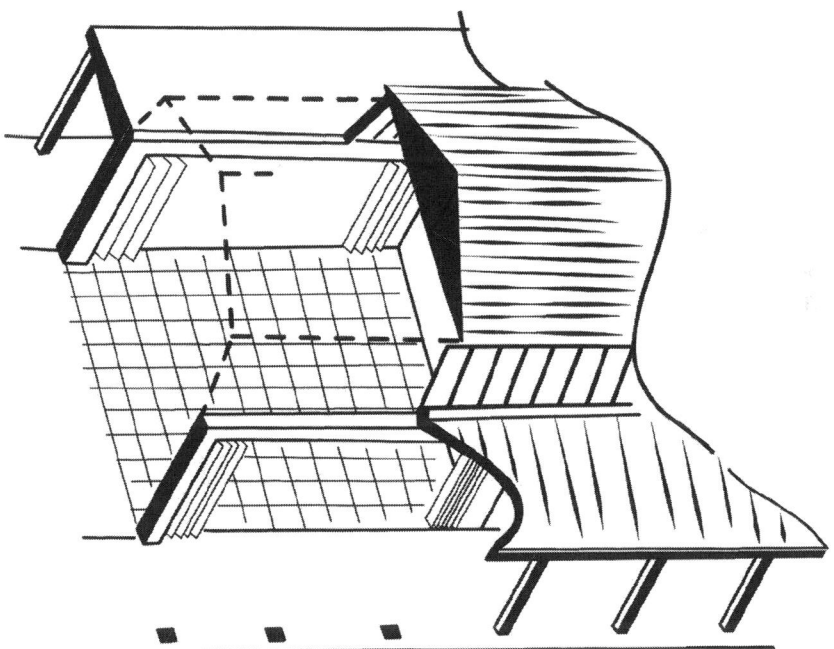

FIGURE 8.4 The pavilion classroom concept illustrated.

Source: Gunderson, M., (2020), *Derbyshire Type of Open-air Classroom*, [Drawing], redrawn from C.G. Stillman & R.C. Cleary (1949), *The Modern School*, Architectural Press.

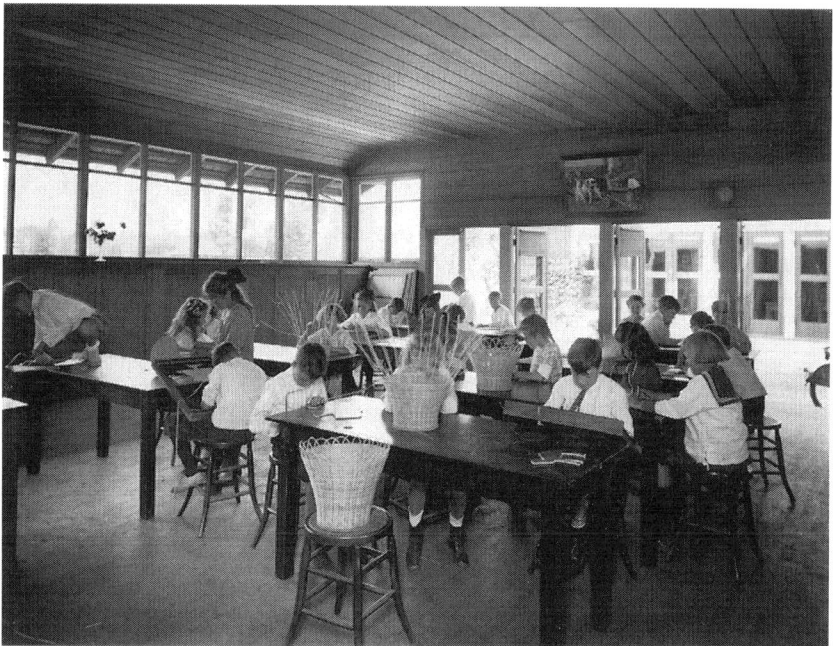

FIGURE 8.5 The first pavilion school for healthy students in America.

Source: Classroom, Pasadena Polytechnic School, Pasadena, California, early 1900s (n.d.), [Photograph], Polytechnic School Archives.

was intended to capitalise on Southern California's mild climate and abundant sunshine. Pasadena Polytechnic was a simple one-storey wooden building with an H-shaped ground plan. Hunt and Grey placed a large, multipurpose assembly hall in the centre of the plan, between parallel rows of classrooms. All classrooms were at ground level and opened directly to a covered verandah instead of an interior corridor, and each room had openings in multiple walls—including windows that reached to within a few inches of the floor—to promote daylighting and air circulation (Figure 8.5). The Pasadena Polytechnic School was greatly admired by the educational community; numerous publications touted its health benefits, and the school was inundated with requests for copies of its architectural plans (Shamble, 2017).

In Colorado, Dr Richard Corwin, chief surgeon of the Colorado Fuel and Iron Company and a member of his local board of education, merged his TB studies with his educational interests, and by 1906 had conceived of a 'Modern Model School House', which became better known as the 'Cottage Plan' school. Within a few years, Corwin and local architects had developed the prototype into several schools in Pueblo and Colorado Springs, Colorado. Corwin deconstructed the traditional schoolhouse into its component parts. A large multipurpose main building contained an auditorium, library and principal's office, while small, freestanding 'cottages' flanking the main building held the individual classrooms. Each rectangular cottage was one storey in height and contained only a classroom and small cloakroom. Corwin placed windows in all four walls of these cottages, contrary to the ULR, and from the beginning he uniquely extolled both the ventilation *and* lighting benefits of this arrangement (Cottage Schools, 1912).

The work of pavilion school advocates helped demonstrate the attractiveness of this new kind of design that focussed on keeping student bodies healthy. Their efforts were overshadowed, however, by the publicity surrounding open-air schools, which spread quickly through the Western world, aided by organisations of physicians, architects and educators. Shortly after it opened, the Waldschule was featured at the First International Congress on School Hygiene in Nuremberg, Germany. Three years later, the Second International Congress on School Hygiene convened in London. Reformers rallied around the cry for 'More air! More air! More air in the school room, more air in the lungs, more air in the curriculum!' (Kingsley & Dresslar, 1917, p. 196). By the time the fourth congress opened in Buffalo, New York in 1913, American reformers had demonstrated their support for open-air principles. Providence, Rhode Island became the first city to adopt the open-air approach in its schools in 1908. Boston followed Providence's lead later that year, and by 1910 more than a dozen cities operated open-air schools. Over 200 open-air schools operated in the United States by 1917 (Kingsley & Dresslar, 1917).

The combination of a burgeoning open-air school movement with the influence of the Pasadena Polytechnic School led to the first extensive use of the pavilion model for healthy public school students in the United States. In 1911, citizens in Oakland, California, took the extraordinary step of demanding open-air classrooms in public school buildings. The city issued a municipal bond and hired architect John J. Donovan to supervise the building campaign. Oakland's committee on school design concluded that there should be at least one open-air classroom added to all existing buildings, and in all new school construction every classroom had to be an 'open-air room' (i.e., the room needed a large exposure to the east and all windows and doors to be operable). In addition to larger windows in the exterior wall, the committee required transom windows in the wall separating the classroom from the corridor for cross ventilation. In 1913, the city opened four new open-air public schools constructed to these requirements (Donovan, 1915).

Oakland's investment was quickly matched by other California cities. Citizens of San Diego also requested open-air classrooms, and their board of education erected the first group of them in 1913. San Jose, Santa Clara, Berkeley and Sacramento all made the transition to open-air principles in new public school buildings by 1915 (Shamble, 2017). These so-called 'California

Plan' schools featured common characteristics: one-storey height for better fire safety, verandahs or covered walkways instead of interior corridors and window openings in more than one classroom wall to stimulate cross ventilation.

The popularity of Austrian-born architect Richard Neutra in the interwar era advanced the cause of the pavilion classroom in America. Neutra immigrated to the United States in 1923 and became known for his elegant minimalist houses; prior to that, during the First World War, he had spent nearly a year in various hospitals and sanitaria seeking a cure for malaria and TB (Hines, 1994). Neutra's contribution to school design emerged from his experiences: an emphasis on the close relationship between indoor and outdoor classroom space. The first project to demonstrate his ideas was the un-built Ring Plan School project (1928), a one-storey, oval-shaped structure with classrooms encircling an open-air common area that could be used for play, school gatherings or swimming. Neutra imagined outdoor covered walkways for the Ring Plan School rather than an interior hallway, and each classroom included a moveable glass wall that opened onto a patio with a grassy lawn beyond, eliminating any significant barrier between inside and outside and bringing open-air school principles fully into the mainstream (Neutra, 1930).

Neutra worked with educators to create an updated California Plan school, with classrooms aligned side-to-side along a covered walkway. Following the Pasadena Polytechnic model, natural light and fresh air were the driving forces. Neutra's familiarity with the early California schools can be seen in his own Corona Avenue School (1935) in Los Angeles. It relied on what Neutra labelled the 'In-Door Out-Door Classroom', which placed a small paved patio and short spur walls beneath an overhanging roof to define the area immediately outside the classroom's glazed, sliding wall, adjacent to a grass yard circumscribed by hedges and containing a garden section (Neutra, 1935). Never before in America had classrooms been so full of healthy fresh air and sunlight.

Post-war successes

Early 20th-century reformers encouraged bilateral openings in the classroom to protect students' health by circulating fresh air and allowing daylight to inundate the room. These suggestions were eventually incorporated into the mainstream of new school design and can be seen in the most publicised school buildings of post-war America—like the Crow Island (1941, Winnetka, Illinois) and Heathcote Schools (1953, Scarsdale, New York) (Hille, 2011). Neutra's notion of the 'In-Door Out-Door Classroom' became the model for many American educators and architects during and immediately after the Second World War. Articles and advertisements in educational and architectural journals depicted bright classrooms with huge windows (or window-walls in some cases), often with direct access to an outdoor area. This dream image of healthy student bodies in spacious rooms overlooking verdant courtyards was promoted to urban and suburban schools alike, despite size or location (Gyure, 2017).

Concurrently, public health initiatives demonstrated their effectiveness as diseases that once devastated schoolchildren were brought under control. A synthesis of medical discoveries, political pressure and public health programs created such momentum that a noted public health historian has claimed 'the battle against these disorders [smallpox, typhoid, and others] had essentially been won' in the 1930s such that 'what remained was a mopping up operation' (Duffy, 1990, p. 263). Furthermore, 'By the late 1940s, the major medical disorders that had plagued the United States throughout nearly all of its history had virtually disappeared' (Duffy, 1990, p. 280). This victory was accomplished by mass immunisation and environmental alterations. The results were often dramatic. New York City practically eradicated diphtheria within 20 years by vaccinating up to 60% of its children and expanded to vaccinating preschool children for smallpox. Chicago nearly eliminated typhoid within two decades by redirecting its sewer flow and chlorinating the public water supply. A national campaign for diphtheria vaccinations helped remove the disease as a threat to schoolchildren by the 1940s (Duffy, 1990). Finally, TB—the most feared of all diseases—became less of a threat. In 1920, for example, the national TB death rate was 113.1 out of every 100,000 citizens; two decades later that number had fallen to 45.9. Between 1940 and 1955, the TB mortality rate dropped by 80%, to a paltry 9.1 per 100,000 people (Duffy, 1990, pp. 263, 280).

Developments in electric lighting and mechanical ventilation allowed classrooms to become brighter and healthier. In 1923, as mechanical ventilation became more reliable, participants at the annual convention of the American Society of Heating and Ventilating Engineers even voted to delete the term 'fresh air' from their proposed ventilation code, due to its irrelevance (Cooper, 2002). Eventually, air conditioning sealed many classrooms from the outdoors, eliminating the need for cross ventilation. The improvements in ventilating equipment meant open windows on opposite sides of the classroom were no longer required to create appropriate air circulation to hinder students from passing germs to each other—and would actually interfere with the mechanically balanced airflow cycle. A leader of the National Council on Schoolhouse Construction optimistically stated, 'Heath and sanitation will not permit the return to open window ventilation dependent for operation upon the whim of one person, or of the outside wind-pressure … ' (Higgins, 1944, p. 90). The extensive availability of heating-ventilation-air conditioning (HVAC) systems by the 1960s closed many classroom windows for good. Better HVAC systems also inspired a post-war fad for windowless classrooms, with advocates extolling the virtues of distraction-free classrooms without windows and the extensive cost savings of no-glass construction (McDonald & Burts, 1961).

Lighting technology also improved, allowing most American schools to have some form of artificial illumination by the 1930s. Remarkably, the ULR's firm hold on some educators and architects meant that there was still some resistance to bilateral openings despite contrary evidence from existing pavilion-type and open-air classrooms. The 1918 IES lighting code, for example, reinforced the ULR (Illumination Engineering Society, 1918). When the IES updated its code in 1938, the ULR remained the ideal. 'For reading with a directional light source it is desirable that the unit be placed to the rear at one side of the reader in order that the specular reflection may be away from his eyes', it wrote; windows should be located along the classroom's left wall, and never 'at the right or in front of the pupils' (Illuminating Engineering Society, 1938, pp. 18, 20).

Conclusion

The ULR eventually lost support, as educators and architects were able to take advantage of medical advances in the understanding of vision and eye-related conditions, school systems developed better eyesight screening programs and electrical lighting became less expensive and more prevalent. A review of the most important American educational and architectural journals, such as *American School Board Journal, School Executive, The Nation's Schools, Architectural Record, Progressive Architecture*, and *Architectural Forum*, reveals that articles on dangerous classroom air, inadequate lighting or architecture's complicity in both had disappeared by the mid-1950s, replaced by advice on how to control glare, increase 'foot-candles' (a measurement of light intensity), use proper classroom colours and surface finishes and arrange desks to maximise proper airflow in terms of cubic feet per minute. In recognition of this mastery over the interior environment, American standards for the lighting and air movement and quality of classrooms have remained virtually the same since the late 1950s (Baker, 2012).

The pavilion classroom model emerged from efforts to protect the health of student bodies by implementing a simple idea: placing windows on opposite sides of the classroom. Once educators were assured that abundant light from more than one source would *not* damage children's vision, in contradiction to the ULR, there were repercussions for the classroom's internal organisation. If students no longer needed to be arranged in rigid, unidirectional rows to comply with the ULR, and light was equally distributed throughout the room, teachers could offer more informal classroom experiences. Together with a revolution in school furniture that introduced smaller-scaled, light-weight desks and chairs, the classroom's physical and material environment suddenly was more conducive to progressive 'active learning' techniques and the fostering of casual relations between teachers and children that had already proven effective at the preschool and kindergarten levels (Müller & Schneider, 2010). The ability to move desks in different directions or combine them into small groups—all unimaginable in the ULR-dictated classroom—helped create new opportunities for pedagogy and curriculum (Gyure, 2018). The non-directionality fostered by well-lit and ventilated pavilion classrooms thus formed a fundamental component of modern education. But its roots were firmly planted in early 20th-century reform movements aimed at protecting young student bodies from alarmingly high rates of dangerous illnesses by making classrooms healthier.

References

Baker, L. (2012). *A history of school design and its indoor environmental standards, 1900 to today.* National Clearinghouse for Educational Facilities.

Baker, N.R. (1910). Schoolroom fenestration. *American School Board Journal,* 40(May), 5.

Bicknell, T.W. (1898). *A history of Barrington, Rhode Island.* Snow & Farnham.

Billings, J. (1893). *Ventilation and heating.* The Engineering Record.

Buchan, W.P. (1891). *Ventilation: A text-book to the practice of the art of ventilating buildings.* Crosby Lockwood and Son.

Châtelet, A.-M. (2008). A breath of fresh air: Open-air schools in Europe. In M. Gutman, & N. de Coninck-Smith (Eds.), *Designing modern childhoods: History, space, and the material culture of children* (pp. 107–127). Rutgers University Press.

Chicago Board of Education. (1875). *Proceedings of the Board of Education of the City of Chicago.* Chicago Board of Education.

Classroom, Pasadena Polytechnic School, Pasadena, California, early 1900s. (n.d.). [Photograph]. Polytechnic School Archives.

Cooper, G. (2002). *Air-conditioning America: Engineers and the controlled environment, 1900–1960.* Johns Hopkins University Press.

Cottage schools in Colorado Springs. (1912). *American School Board Journal,* 45(September), 18–19.

Donovan, J.J. (1915). Problems that have been solved in Oakland's new school buildings. *The Architect & Engineer of California and the Pacific Coast,* 40(March), 42–70.

Dresslar, F. (1913). *School hygiene.* The Macmillan Company.

Duffy, J.J. (1979). School buildings and the health of American school children in the nineteenth century. In C.E. Rosenberg (Ed.), *Healing and history: Essays for George Rosen* (pp. 161–178). Neale Watson Academic Publications.

Duffy, J.J. (1981). Early days of the school health movement. *Conspectus of History,* 1(7), 46–61.

Duffy, J.J. (1990). *The sanitarians: A history of American public health.* University of Illinois Press.

Dwyer, C. (1856). *The economy of church, parsonage and school architecture, adapted to small societies and rural districts.* Phinney & Co.

Endemann, H. (1873). Chemical examination of the air of various public buildings. In *Third annual report of the Board of Health of the Health Department of the City of New York* (pp. 137–142). D. Appleton & Co.

Gunderson, M. (2020). *Derbyshire type of open-air classroom.* [Drawing].

Gyure, D.A. (2017). Creating friendly school environments: 'Casual' high schools, progressive education, and child-centered culture in postwar America. In J. Willis, & K. Darian-Smith (Eds.), *Designing schools: Space, place, and pedagogy* (pp. 68–82). Routledge.

Gyure, D.A. (2018). *The schoolroom: A social history of teaching and learning.* Greenwood.

Higgins, T. (1944). Mechanical equipment for the school. *Architectural Record, 95*(March), 89–90.

Hille, R.T. (2011). *Modern schools: A century of design for education.* John Wiley & Sons.

Hines, T.S. (1994). *Richard Neutra and the search for modern architecture: A biography and history.* University of California Press.

Holdsworth, G. (1907). *Classroom, Ladycross Infants' School, Sandiacre, England, 1907* [Photograph]. Derbyshire County Council.

Hoy, S. (1996). *Chasing dirt: The American pursuit of cleanliness.* Oxford University Press.

Illumination Engineering Society. (1918, April 30). Report on code of lighting schools. *Transactions of the Illumination Engineering Society, 13,* 185–200.

Illuminating Engineering Society. (1938). *American recommended practice of school lighting.* Illuminating Engineering Society and the American Institute of Architects.

Katz, M.S. (1976). *A history of compulsory education laws.* The Phi Delta Kappa Educational Foundation.

Kingsley, S., & Dresslar, F. (1917). *Open-air schools.* U.S. Government Printing Office.

Kirk, D. (1998). *Schooling bodies: School practice and public discourse, 1880–1950.* Leicester University Press.

Larrabee, J.A. (1888, November 3). The schoolroom a factor in the production of disease. *Journal of the American Medical Association, 11,* 613–617.

Macleod, D. (1998). *The age of the child: Children in America, 1890–1920.* Twayne Publishers.

Massachusetts State Board of Health. (1888). *Suggestions for preventing the spread of scarlet fever.* Massachusetts State Board of Health.

Marble, A.P. (1892). How to light school buildings. *American School Board Journal, 4*(July), 3.

McCarthy, O.R. (2001). The key to the sanatoria. *Journal of the Royal Society of Medicine, 94*(8), 413–417.

McDonald, E., & Burts, E. (1961). Opinions differ on windowless classrooms. *NEA Journal, 50*(October), 12–14.

McDonald, L. (2022). *Florence Nightingale and the medical men: Working together for health care reform.* McGill-Queen's Press.

Müller, T., & Schneider, R. (2010). *Die Klassenzimmer vom Ende des 19. Jahrhunderts bis heute.* Wasmuth.

Neutra, R. (1930). *Amerika: Die Stilbildung des Neuen Bauen in der Vereinigten Staaten (Neues Bauen in der Welt).* Anton Schroll.

Neutra, R. (1935). New elementary schools for America. *Architectural Forum*, 62(January), 25–35.

Out doors school of Larchmont Public Health Association, Larchmont, NY. (n.d.). [Photograph]. Human Ecology Historical Photographs, Collection no. 23-2-749, item no. M-I-P-07, Rare & Manuscript Collections, Cornell University Library.

Pearmain, A.U. (1898). The Boston schools: A sanitary investigation. *Municipal Affairs*, 2, (September), 497–501.

Perry, T. (1910). Dustless schools. *The American School Board Journal*, 41(November), 5.

Reese, W.J. (2005). *America's public schools: From the common school to 'No Child Left Behind'*. Johns Hopkins University Press.

Roberts, E.L. (1917). *Medical inspection of schools in Great Britain*. U.S. Government Printing Office.

Robson, E.R. (1874). *School architecture: Being practical remarks on the planning, designing, building, and furnishing of school-houses*. John Murray.

Rousmaniere, K. (1997). *City teachers: Teaching and school reform in historical perspective*. Teachers College Press.

Rowe, S. (1904). *The lighting of school-rooms*. Longmans, Green, & Co.

School Survey Committee. (1924). *Survey of public school system, City of New York*. Board of Education of the City of New York.

Schultz, S. (1973). *The culture factory: Boston public schools, 1789–1860*. Oxford University Press.

Shamble, C. (2017). *Growing children out of doors: California's open-air schools and children's health, 1907–1917* [Doctoral dissertation, University of Virginia]. Online Archive of University of Virginia Scholarship. 10.18130/V3F89H

Stillman, C.G., & Cleary, R.C. (1949). *The Modern School*. Architectural Press.

Tomes, N. (1998). *The gospel of germs: Men, women, and the microbe in American life*. Harvard University Press.

Tyack, D., James, T., & Benavot, A. (1987). *Law and the shaping of public education, 1785–1954*. University of Wisconsin Press.

Wheelwright, E.M. (1901). *School architecture: A general treatise for the use of architects and others*. Rogers & Manson.

9

ESCAPING INDOORNESS

Education and architecture in Italy's summer camps during the Fascist era

Paolo Sanza

Summer camps, known in Italy as *colonie estive* (singular: *colonia estiva*), *climatiche* or simply *colonie,* represent a fascinating chapter in the history of Italian architecture and youth education. During Fascist times in particular they offered an ideal setting to indoctrinate, or at least heavily expose, young minds to the ideals of fascism. As a result, the regime took a strong interest in the *colonie* and sponsored the establishment and construction of thousands of them.

The *colonia* concept continued to flourish after the Second World War as the value of its therapeutic, formative and recreational character was recognised. From the 1970s, however, the metamorphosis of Italian society, now wealthier and more inclined to entertain holidays with the whole family, prompted a profound crisis of the *colonia* concept that eventually led, for the most part, to its disappearance.

This chapter focusses on the re-framing and expansion of the *colonia* concept during Fascist Italy highlighting the role of architecture and its creators in responding to the challenges of fashioning spaces that could simultaneously educate, heal, facilitate play, foster friendship and respond to public and/or private ambitions. Drawing on archival documents, period publications, promotional materials and contemporary scholarly analyses, this chapter develops into five thematic sections: (a) the origin of the summer camps, (b) the rise of summer camps in Fascist Italy, (c) fascist pedagogy in the *colonie,* (d) the architecture of the *colonie* and (e) the *colonie* marine Agip and FIAT: two examples of architecture as a pedagogical machine.

The origin of the summer camps

The origin of the summer camps can be traced back to 18th- and 19th-century Europe and the development of early forms of health assistance to children.

DOI: 10.4324/9781003288671-13

It was considered therapeutic to send sick children to the seaside and expose them to sunlight, fresh air and salt water. Experiments in thalassotherapy (the use of seawater as a form of therapy) and heliotherapy (the exposure to daylight for the prevention and treatment of various diseases) were used to combat diseases such as tuberculosis, bone tuberculosis, scrofula and rickets that widely affected young people at the time. In the mid-18th century, British doctors were among the first to argue the benefits of seaside sojourns for both children and adults, and in 1791, the Royal Sea Bathing Hospital was founded in the English seaside town of Margate (Mira, 2019). A few decades later, another experiment aimed at the welfare of children (but not of a medical nature) found its origin in Switzerland. In 1876, Swiss pastor Hermann Walter Bion founded the first *colonie des vacanses* in the canton of Appenzell in the northeast of Switzerland as a response to the often unhealthy living conditions of children in overcrowded and filthy quarters that were surging in the expanding European cities of the late 19th century. Financed by donations, the two-week stay aimed to provide unprivileged city children aged 9–12 summer escapes to the countryside where they would be exposed to fresh air and sunlight (Pilat & Sanza, 2020) and open-air calisthenics for physical strengthening.

Similarly, in Italy, the summer camps were first born mainly as seaside sanatoria for the care of sick children. Their establishment can be attributed to a Florentine doctor, Giuseppe Barellai. Aided by donated funds and mimicking the British experiment, Barellai opened the first sanatorium in 1856 on the Tuscan coast for the treatment of children with scrofula through thalassotherapy. Notwithstanding the spread of the seaside sanatoria concept throughout Italy, the Swiss model also had its enthusiasts. In 1881 another doctor, the Milanese Malachia De Cristoforis, with the help of other philanthropists, founded the *Società per la Cura Climatica* and the first summer camp in the mountains surrounding Bergamo. Having predominantly a social purpose rather than a medical one, the beneficiaries of De Cristoforis's initiative were those children attending Milan's public schools who were identified as coming from low-income families and/or of weak constitution (Mira, 2019).

The rise of summer camps in Fascist Italy

Until the 1920s and the advent of Fascism (1922–1943), the *colonie* that had spread within the Italian peninsula were predominantly privately managed, and their funding came from doctors, teachers, bankers, nobles, wealthy individuals, religious and charity organisations, and other philanthropists. Under the Fascist government, the sponsorship of these structures morphed (Mira & Salustri, 2019).

Since its origin, fascism was mesmerised by the concept of youth. The movement was mainly composed of young people and presented itself as a newly established political formation, therefore, 'young'. For many fascists, however, the concept of youth was not solely associated with their age or the foundation date of their movement (Mira, 2019). It was rather linked to a mindset, possibly influenced by futurism, that regarded youth as a 'moral quality', and the 'synthesis of a daring and activist lifestyle: a passion for action, mystical sense of duty, dedication to the cause [of fascism] up to ultimate sacrifice, worship of power … and unlimited trust in man's ability to leave an indelible mark on history' (La Rovere, 2003, p. 53). Fascism's concept of youth was also intertwined with the concept of *uomo nuovo,* or new man. The *uomo nuovo*'s origins can be traced to the Italian Risorgimento, but the concept vibrantly ascended after the First World War in the wave of interventionist and futurist ideologies that advocated for renewal in the face of a stagnant political administration and the 19th-century customs that characterised the bourgeoisie, the nobility, the clergy and the aristocracy. The complex but fascinating concept of the *uomo nuovo* in Fascist Italy goes beyond the scope of this contribution. However, to comprehend the regime's interest in the *colonie,* it is sufficient to state that among the characteristics fashioning the *uomo nuovo fascista* were patriotic values and the physical strengthening of the body.

The moulding of the *uomo nuovo* and the fascists of the future could not have found a better setting than in children's education; particularly the *colonie estive,* where the pupils were more prone to absorb new pedagogic concepts and indoctrination as they resided for an extended time away from their family's influence. The *colonie* were also to be a privileged environment where the regime could manifest its welfare spirit while exhibiting an educational project targeted at the new generations (Orlandini, 2019).

The interest of Benito Mussolini's government in the *colonie* is revealed in the astonishing increase in their number: from approximately 170 registered *colonie* in 1926, four years after the ascendance of Fascism, to 1,195 in 1931, 4,357 in 1938, and eventually 5,805 hosting over 940,000 children in 1942 (Mira, 2019).

Colonie were constructed throughout Italy and across its diverse landscapes, from the Alps and the Apennines to the shores of rivers, lakes and seas, and within towns and cities. Some were tiny, no more than rudimentary shelters; others resembled luxurious resorts and small towns. Many would be known for 'their simple lines, profound conceptual gesture, and for fostering remarkable majestic experiences' (Pilat & Sanza, 2020, p. 109) for their young guests. Based on their site settings, they would be classified as *montane* (built on the mountains), *fluviali* (built along the shores of rivers), *lacustri* (built along the shores of lakes) and *marine* (built along the seacoast), and—depending on the occupied time—as permanent, short-term or diurnal.

Resembling hospitals, permanent *colonie* were open all year round and were reserved for children predisposed to tuberculosis as diagnosed by doctors, who also recommended the length of the sojourn, usually three months at the minimum. Short-term *colonie* were open only during the summer months, attended by boys and girls, commonly in separate turns, for at least a month to allow for a successful exposure to sunlight, and, when in *colonie marine,* to thalassic therapy. Short-term *colonie* could be further classified as private and public. Private summer *colonie* were attended solely by the children of employees of private or semi-private large industrial enterprises, such as FIAT, Piaggio or AGIP (the 1926 government-founded petroleum company, later ENI). Established with prophylactic aims, diurnal *colonie* were open from sunrise to sunset. For periods of 45 days, they welcomed otherwise healthy children who were in need of time spent outdoors and nutritious food, which was served at the *colonia* three times a day—for breakfast, lunch and *merenda,* the mid-afternoon snack (Mira, 2019).

Managed by Fascist party organisations, public *colonie* could be attended by children aged 6–13 who met various criteria. Admission to public *colonie* was predominantly reserved for children of unprivileged families, 'giving absolute preference to orphaned children of the Fallen, children of injured and disabled armed personnel who fought in WWI, for the [Fascist] revolution, and the East Africa and Spain campaigns, and children belonging to large families' (Rifugio Scout Vicenza, n.d.). Children's participation was regulated by a protocol illustrated in articles 33 and 37 of the GIL's *Regolamento delle Colonie Climatiche*. Article 33 stated that any child who met the participation criteria had to be carefully examined by a commission of no fewer than three medical professionals, one of whom had to be the medical health officer of the child's town. Article 37 noted that once the medical commission had examined and assessed the child's physical condition, it had to be very diligent in recommending which type of *colonia* suited the child best (*montana, fluviale, lacustre* or *marina*). A wrong diagnosis could send a child to a place with climate characteristics that at best offered no health benefit, and at worst actively harmed the child's health (Mucelli, 2009).

Fascist pedagogy in the *colonie*

At the dawn of the proclamation of the Kingdom of Italy in 1861, Italian politicians were well aware of the complexity of a reunified Italy, declaring: *Abbiamo fatto l'Italia. Ora si tratta di fare gli Italiani* (We have made Italy. Now we have to make the Italians). Indeed, since the collapse of the Western Roman Empire, Italy had endured the invasion of Germanic war tribes; it was conquered by diverse European and non-European powers; and it became the home of numerous city-states and maritime republics, which spurred the development of different languages and customs. At the time of reunification in 1861, Italy contained approximately 22 million people, but just 3%, roughly 665,000, spoke Italian (Gendel, 1966). The rest spoke 1 of more than 30 languages and dialects, which, despite sharing for the most part the same Latin roots, were very distinct from Italian.

When in late October 1922, King Victor Emanuel III asked Mussolini to form a new government, the Fascist leader inherited a nation united geographically, but still struggling to identify itself as the land of one people. Trento, South Tyrol and the Austrian Littoral had been annexed to Italy only a few years earlier, at the end of the First World War.

Mussolini understood the importance of patriotic education for a new and still fragmented country. The vigour with which the regime sought to link education and patriotism was, however, not unique to Italy. Already during the 19th century, many countries of the world felt obliged to respond to

> what appeared as the irresistible march of democracy, using all the tools at their disposal, public education, charismatic monarchs, 'invention' of traditions, monuments and statues, national holidays, etc., to 'educate' the people, make them faithful to the existing political order and out of the clutches of rival forces such as anarchy and socialism.
>
> (Duggan, 2009)

Even in contemporary democracies, although 'democratic procedures and ideals are, of their nature, universal and thus transcend the parochial demands of patriotism' (Patapan, 2014, p. 212), patriotic teaching is still ingrained in political agendas. In the United States, for instance, the pledge of allegiance is performed daily in public schools and even at private gatherings, and the national anthem is sung at the beginning of every sporting event and other public occurrences, regardless of their prominence.

To fulfil his desire to create the *fascists of tomorrow* and ensure the permanence and success of the Fascist revolution, in 1926 Mussolini established the Opera Nazionale Balilla (ONB) youth movement, an autonomous government agency under the umbrella of the Ministry of Education. The ONB became 'one of the most effective educational instruments that the world [had] ever known' (Cox, 1935, p. 267). At the helm of the ONB, Mussolini appointed Renato Ricci, a decorated First World War veteran, member since 1921 of the Partito Nazionale Fascista (PNF), or Fascist Party, and from 1924, member of the party's board of directors.

In broad terms, in shaping the ONB, Ricci looked to the theories of Robert Baden-Powell, the father of scouting, with whom Ricci had several contacts; Ricci also sought the advice of medical doctors, pedagogues, teachers and other experts. Furthermore, he immersed himself in reading texts on philosophy, pedagogy, architecture and anything that was somehow related to the creation of educational centres (Mucelli, 2009). His son Giulio recalled that

Ricci 'devoted the best of his life to the education of young people, doing everything possible to teach them moral values and a way of life very close to the bold models of classical antiquity' (Mucelli, 2009, p. 11).

The ONB's responsibilities were to: complement customary elementary to high school education with a variety of after-school programmes such as physical education, spiritual and cultural education, vocational and technical education, and assistance to religious education; instil in the youth the ethics of military training and discipline (Mucelli, 2009); and develop the awareness of their *italianità*, or of being Italian. In other words, the ONB was charged with handling everything related to the physical and moral education of youth (Cox, 1935). Supplementing after-school activities, the ONB organised excursions, camping trips and exhibitions. It was also charged with developing the organisation and programme of the *colonie* while also constructing new ones.

A little-known aspect of the ONB, advocated by Ricci, was the sponsorship of numerous trips abroad so that young Italians could meet peers from other countries and cultures. Towards that end, cruises were organised to the United States, South America, Africa, Asia and Northern Europe (Ricci, 1997).

In 1937, the ONB was folded into a new institution, the Gioventù Italiana del Littorio (GIL). The GIL absorbed the ONB's assets; it was placed under the direct control of the PNF and its secretary. Ricci was dismissed as president of the ONB and appointed first as the undersecretary of the Ministry of the Corporations and then, in 1939, as the Minister of the Corporations (Sanza, 2020). The absorption of the ONB into the GIL entailed predictable changes, including the reassessment of educational objectives, which now advocated for more pre-military education and stricter discipline than during Ricci's tenure.

The *Regolamento delle Colonie Climatiche,* or guidelines to the administration of the summer camps, published in 1938 by the GIL, outlined in a series of articles all aspects governing the *colonie,* from admission rules, as briefly exhibited beforehand, to spatial guidelines, daily rhythms, dress codes, dietary recommendations and more. Inside the *colonia,* the young guests were to follow an orchestrated daily routine marked by specific times for waking up and going to bed, dining, medical examination, therapeutic treatment, physical activity, playing, excursions, patriotic tales, Fascist culture, religious awareness, resting and body hygiene. Hence, the *colonia* was not solely to have a therapeutic and prophylactic purpose but was also meant to contribute to the formation of the *uomo nuovo* and the fascists of tomorrow. As Laura Marani Argnani wrote in *Per le Vigilatrici delle Colonie Climatiche* (1939, as cited in Orlandini, 2019, p. 151), 'The child's entry into a *colonia climatica*, saturated with the fascist spirit, is above all the [child-first] fully encounter with a concept of life that, in a particular fashion, mimics the [aspired] way and vision of life [dictated] by the [fascist] revolution'. To this end, daily activities included reading and conversing about patriotism and fascist culture, singing fascist and war-themed songs, praying and, twice daily, morning and evening, saluting the flag with the Roman salute, the gesture introduced by fascism in which the right arm was extended and raised upward with palm down and fingers touching.

Books available for reading were principally biographies of those individuals who had fallen for the fascist cause. Particularly appreciated at a later time was the book *Parlo con Bruno,* written by Mussolini and dedicated to his son Bruno (Orlandini, 2019), a pilot of the Royal Italian Air Force who, at just 23 years old, died in 1941 when the secret prototype Piaggio P.108B bomber he was piloting crashed due to an engine malfunction near the airfield of Pisa.

It was believed that, in addition to the strengthening of the body, physical education contributed to better intellectual development, greater self-confidence and self-esteem and the reinforcement of a national consciousness dotted with fascism's principles. Physical education exercises were, therefore, in part designed to contribute to the awareness of the merits and achievements of Italy and Fascism: imitating a rower's movement could be an occasion to emphasise Italy's prestige and power in the Mediterranean; the blacksmith's gesture could recall a hardworking Italy; and the movement of harvesting wheat by using a sickle could pay tribute to the Battle for Grain (Orlandini, 2019), the campaign launched in 1925 by the fascist regime aimed at self-sufficiency in the production of wheat. Calisthenics, however, was cautiously implemented. Different entities, including the GIL, advised against applying solely rigorous physical education exercises but rather allowed room for children's own desire to play and cultivate their natural body elasticity and vitality, without neglecting each child's development challenges (Orlandini, 2019).

Breathing exercises, considered of great importance for preventing lung diseases, were implemented daily. Upon their arrival at the *colonia,* children were educated on how to correctly breathe through the nose and provide adequate pulmonary ventilation. Connected to breathing exercises was singing. Singing was considered a very effective means of education and a 'vehicle for patriotic rhetoric and memory training', provided that the song's words were first explained because 'nothing must be entrusted to the memory of the child that is not first made clear to their intelligence' (Orlandini, 2019, p. 165).

Children's exposure to the sun or the amount of time in the sea's salty water was also regulated by the *Regolamento delle Colonie Climatiche.* Article 140 explicitly stated that the employment of the sun had to be 'direct, that is with bare skin … ; the whole body of the child has to be gradually exposed to the sun'. Yet, the exposure to the sun had to be measured against the child's physical condition.

For healthy children with the usual but moderate suffering triggered by living in cities and attending urban schools, the technique is simple: begin with an exposure lasting five minutes, increase it by five minutes every three or four days up to one hour. Best to keep the child lying down, alternating the supine position with the prone one. For less robust children, it is advisable to start the heliotherapy indoors, in a room facing east or southeast, with open windows and closed doors … . During therapy, provide children with good and abundant food, but not in excessive quantities.

Article 141 outlined thalassotherapy techniques and optimal meteorological conditions, such as allowing children to immerse themselves in the water on their own time, but initially only for a few minutes, to then be increased based on their individual tolerance; that the temperature of the water should not be less than 15°C and on a clear day, with no wind and calm sea; to bathe in the sea between 11:00 am and noon (Mucelli, 2009).

The child's physical well-being was at the centre of daily life in the *colonia*. However, this could not solely be achieved by orchestrating the child's therapeutic activities. Dietary and nutritional considerations played a considerable and complementary role in the development of healthy children and were likewise addressed at length in the GIL's regulatory handbook. It did not suffice, for example, that the ingredients to prepare each meal had to be genuine and coming from excellent sources, or that the meals had to vary daily, but that 'each and every dish' needed to be 'prepared with care and love by proficient personnel under expert supervision, and that special dietary needs for each child addressed' (Pilat & Sanza, 2020).

Among complementary daily activities was religion. Every morning, together with the raising of the flag, children recited a brief prayer. On Sunday, they attended Mass at a dedicated space of the *colonia*, and the conversation topics of the day were of a religious nature but simple enough for the children's comprehension, such as the explanation of prayers and parables (Orlandini, 2019).

Of great pedagogical novelty, and unlike the customs found in primary and secondary schools of the time across Italy and beyond, was dealing with children's bad or improper behaviour. The young *colonie* attendees were identified as subjects of weak constitution and in need of care and nourishment. Therefore, children's discipline had to be administered with care and love, admonishment had to be given by explaining the reasons, and punishment and threats had to be avoided because they 'hurt and offended children's souls, and could generate resentment, which would nullify the education effort and mark the child for life' (Orlandini, 2019, p. 173).

Except for medical duties and an array of manual work, the *colonie* were managed predominantly by women. The supervision of each group of children, comprising 25–30 pupils subdivided by gender, age and physical constitution, was assigned to a *vigilatrice, a* female supervisor (plural *vigilatrici*). Assigning such roles to women was not done casually. It was believed that experience had demonstrated that the female figure was the most suitable for the education of children aged 3–12 (Orlandini, 2019). In the *colonia*, in particular, where children sojourned away from their family for an extended period, the *vigilatrice* assumed a maternal character. Such positions were therefore advertised in the propagandist press, which stated that children in the *colonia* would find the 'sweet and intense smile of the mother left far away' (Orlandini, 2019, p. 155). The *vigilatrici*, however, were also expected to instil in the children a patriotic education in line with national policy. As was reported in Vittoria Calogiuri and Antonio Bonadies's *Scuola e Nazione per la difesa della razza*, the *vigilatrici*, as fascist women, could not forget that 'children aged six to twelve must have a sport and military education and discipline, as mandated by the fascist state. And this [could] not be difficult [to do] for women who live [in] and are being educated in the fascist state' (Orlandini, 2019, p. 156). Similarly, in her pamphlet, *Per le Vigilatrici delle Colonie Climatiche*, Laura Marani Argnani emphasised the importance of giving children a patriotic education, suggesting ideas and topics to the *vigilatrici*, so much that the secretary of the PNF recommended its adoption for the *vigilatrici's* training courses (1939, as cited in Orlandini, 2019).

The architecture of the *colonie estive*

The GIL, and the ONB before it, drew a general architecture programme outlining the various functions embedded in the *colonia* concept. Article 13 of the *Regolamento delle Colonie Climatiche* explicitly stated, among other recommendations, that all of the short-term *colonie*, whether *marine* or *montane*, had to provide for well-lit and well-ventilated dormitories with rooms having not more than 20–30 beds each; a large, well exposed, illuminated and ventilated refectory connected to the kitchen; an indoor or covered area to shelter the children during bad weather; a zone that could be transformed into a temporary chapel to celebrate the Sunday Mass; ample terraces or open spaces adjacent to those areas allocated to infirmary and quarantine; and sanitary and personnel facilities adequately designed to suit the total capacity of the *colonia*.

The GIL provided general spatial guidelines and relationships but did not dictate a specific architectural style for the *colonie*. However, during his premiership, Mussolini had often been sympathetic and even supportive of a modern architectural language (Pilat & Sanza, 2020) for the buildings to come. Among the directives for the 1932 exhibition *Mostra della Rivoluzione Fascista* held in Rome's Palazzo delle Esposizioni and commemorating the tenth anniversary of the coming to power of fascism, Mussolini, for instance, stated that:

The exhibition must reflect our time, therefore ultramodern, bold and audacious, without melancholy reminiscences of past decorative styles. We must discard projects of Ancient Rome flavor clad in false travertine, or of mannerism patterned on Baroque because great times cannot be weakened by imitating past styles but rather must create new forms and original expressions ... reflecting our dynamic, undocked and feverish age.

(Portante, 2015)

Specifically addressing the architecture of the *colonie*, on which he had placed great importance, Mussolini emphasised the need, while not directly referring to a contemporary architectural language, to make them 'noticeable even from a glance at the landscape' (de Martino & Wall, 1988, p. 8).

Colonie were predominantly built in remote areas and on the outskirts of seaside vacation spots and occupied large plots of land, often fenced. Isolating these structures and sitting them on vast acreage reflected their sanitaria origins, which advocated for plenty of air and sunshine. But alienating the *colonie* from their surroundings also supported the philosophical principles of the institution. Within the *colonia*, the young guests were to live a different reality than the one experienced at home or at school, and also quite distinct from the life of the inhabitants and vacationers of the nearby town(s) (Mira, 2019). The children were to experience a multi-dimensional, communal and, as previously noted, a highly structured existence choreographed in built environments quite different from those they were acquainted with.

Despite being erected across Italy, there was a preference to construct short-term *colonie* alongside the beaches of Tuscany and Emilia Romagna. The case of Tirrenia is particularly noteworthy. Located on the Tyrrhenian Sea, just a few kilometres north of Livorno and west of Pisa, Tirrenia was one of the many new towns founded by the fascist regime to become, in its founders' vision, a prominent beach resort and movie-production town, 'the Pearl of the Mediterranean Sea', as Mussolini stated. Renowned architects Adolfo Coppedè and Antonio Valente were among those called upon to plan the town. As a premier resort destination, Tirrenia was meant to attract wealthy individuals; consequently, several villas were built to satisfy such demand. Yet, neighbouring Tirrenia to its south, a plethora of *colonie* were planned and built, transforming the area into what can be viewed as a city of childhood.

In his book *Viaggio per le Città di Mussolini* (1939), documenting and narrating the new towns with poetic licence, Stanis Ruinas, the pseudonym of Italian writer and journalist Giovanni Antonio de Rosas, wrote (p. 352):

But the singing souls of green Tirrenia are and always be the children. The *colonie marine* of [the cities of] Livorno, Pistoia and Firenze, the splendid Villa Rosa, the *colonia* for the Italian children living abroad, and the new Pisa *colonia*, all built towards Calambrone, have not, and will not obscure the seaside resort town. Beach, sea, Mediterranean pine forests, there is something for everyone. These elements seem to partake in the joy of the little guests. Sand and water sparkle with joyfulness amidst the swarming and chirping of so much childhood. As evening approaches, the large avenue between the pine forest and the sea comes alive with songs and is streaked in white, blue, and pink [of the children's uniforms]. The flag that rises on the flagpole with the first sun and with the last descends finds all these children lined up like toy soldiers, with faces tense by the emotions, yet bodies firm as they perform the Roman salute.

Designed to accommodate anywhere from a few hundred to over a thousand children, short-term *colonie* were extensive structures. Those fashioned in modern style exhibited remarkable design ingenuity and an intrinsic dialogue with their natural environment. Mario Labò and Attilio Podestà in their 1942 book *Colonie Marine-Montane Elioterapiche,* described them as 'formidable in terms of technical elegance' and stated (p. 1):

> Everything in them, from the abstract lines and forms to the development of the plan... ... ; from the width and type of the windows to the design of the balustrades; from the plaster to the paving, colors, and material; from the refectory to the rooms for washing, dormitories, and gymnasia, comes together to produce an image which is realized and never forgotten in the minds of children: the memory of their stay in the *colonie.*

Arguably, well before the invention of environmental psychology—the branch of psychology that addresses the interplay between humans and the environment, including how architecture affects behaviour—the architects of the *colonie* were conscious of the positive effects on children of spaces thoroughly planned. For instance, in describing his design for the *Colonia Agip* located in the Adriatic Sea coastal town of Cesenatico, in the January 1939 issue of *Architettura,* Giuseppe Vaccaro stated how important it was to study the natural environment to best benefit the life of the children while at the *colonia.* Vaccaro concluded, 'sun and air must be rightly dosed to reap the maximum benefits; the panoramic views towards the sea and the countryside must be correctly balanced to nurture and cheer the spirit' (1939, p. 1). Other architects would abstractly transform political symbols or figures expressing the notion of mobility, speed and modernity so cherished at the time. Designs inspired by airplanes, ships or submarines aided in creating an architecture that would appeal to children's fantasies. The architect Clemente Busiri Vici called it *architettura parlante,* or 'talking architecture' (Pilat & Sanza, 2020, p. 116) when referring to his design for the 1932-built *colonia XXVIII Ottobre* in Cesenatico, which faced the Adriatic Sea and resembled a flotilla.

'Education and its exemplification in buildings and environments', writes Mark Dudek (2000, xiii), 'has always been concerned with radical ideas set in new and stimulating settings. It had to be radical because it was a system of mass education, constantly reinventing itself to provide more and more educational places of an ever-improving quality'. For Italian architects of the time, the theme of summer camps became a fertile ground for exploration. They interwove political ideologies, programmatic and medical directives, pedagogical sciences and notions of sustainability with their own design beliefs to create for children architecture of remarkable modernity and quality that was also well rooted in the landscape. Their designed spaces not only facilitated communal life, or augmented teaching and the cult of the body, but also allowed children coming from modest backgrounds to 'accept the influence of taste, to be stimulated for the first time, even if passively, by the experience of architectural form not only from the outside but adapted for living within' (Labo & Podestà, 1942, p. 1).

The *colonie marine Agip* and FIAT: Two examples of architecture as a pedagogical machine

Giuseppe Vaccaro's *Colonia Agip*, built between 1936 and 1938 and named after Sandro Mussolini, nephew of Mussolini, is an expression of high modernism. The *colonia* is situated on a bare plot of land that extends from the countryside to the beach and is bisected by the littoral road running north to south. Its 4,000 square-metre footprint, which occupies less than 8% of the lot area, exemplifies the importance of providing the building with plenty of fresh air and unobstructed sunshine to best benefit from heliotherapy. At the time of its construction, there were a few sporadic buildings around the *colonia*'s site. The place presented Vaccaro with a context of endless horizontality: on the one side, the Romagna plains; on the other side, the Adriatic Sea. Vaccaro responded to this highly emotive setting engulfed by the sun and inhabited by silence with a solution that captures and transforms in an architectural vocabulary all the perceived environmental forces of this strip of Romagna land.

The *colonia*, designed to welcome 300 children, is articulated in five structures organised to not interrupt the existing dialogue between land and sea but rather reinforce it. Two one-storey narrow wings, accommodating miscellaneous support services, are perpendicular to the sea and at a great distance from each other, at 150 metres apart. They embrace the land of the countryside while directing it to the sea and forming in the emptiness of the rural environment the quintessence of Italian urban life: the *piazza*. To the east, towards the sea, the two wings are connected by a portico open to both sides so as not to restrict the view of the sea nor the cool breezes emerging from it. The two wings are not furnished with a portico looking into the *piazza*, as an intuitive design solution would have stipulated; rather, the portico is flipped to the opposite side, facing recreational yet private gardens. It was a deliberate decision. Vaccaro's *piazza* is not a space for people of different ages as found in Italian urbanscapes—it is for children and their engagement with the sun and the other therapeutic forces of nature. Thus, the spaces for adults are secondary to the ones for children.

Placed symmetrically with respect to the *piazza*, a further portico rises above the lower one to support a three-storey-high and 100-metre-long parallelepiped hosting the dormitories. The porticos are not only the elements of an ingenious architectural composition but also those elements needed to provide shelter for outdoor activities when the day is too hot or on rainy days. The volume occupied by the refectory is centred in the composition and projects to the sea, bounded on three sides by the beach. Still, it is unperceivable from the landside as it is wedged in the lower portico.

Marking the axis and centred in the *piazza* is the extremely tall flagpole that rises well above the height of the dormitory block. On-axis, in a niche clad in marble and carved out from the glass box encompassing the dining hall, is an altar, which transforms the *piazza* into a gigantic outdoor place for religious ceremonies. There is a delightful classical soul under these choreographic episodes inscribed in highly refined architecture. It is possible to view in Vaccaro's composition the one organising the Papal Basilica of Saint Peter in the Vatican: the axis, the obelisk, the entry portico, the Basilica and the arms extending out to embrace and gather the pilgrims, which in Cesenatico were the children arriving from many parts of Italy for a time of physical, educational and spiritual growth.

The treatment of the dormitory's facades, parallel to the sea on one side and the countryside on the other, rises from the need to balance natural ventilation and protection from the sun to achieve optimal temperatures throughout the day within the chambers. Thus, the east and west facades have different aesthetics while implementing similar techniques to funnel the breezes and the sun's rays into the dormitories or stop them altogether.

Designed to house all the services required to isolate sick and potentially contagious children, the last structure is separated from the rest of the compound and sited at a distance, close to the northwestern edge of the site. But isolation is not alienation from the healing environment. If a white wall encloses the garden of the isolation pavilion, a long opening in it embraces once again the landscape, framing land, sea and sky, reunifying the natural elements with the sick children (Cao, 1994).

In an article published in the October 1938 issue of *Casabella-Costruzioni*, Raffaello Giolli summarised the building as follows (p. 6):

Freed of weight and cumbersome mass, even the walls have become crystal, and the sun and air have won … [T]he ground under the building is vacant not only for the views but for the *inhaling* of the sea and the mountains … [I]t is important that the children know that the architect has given freedom to the power of nature and the joys of free breathing.

The *colonia* FIAT in Marina di Massa on the Tyrrhenian Sea, named after Edoardo Agnelli, the son of FIAT founder Giovanni Agnelli, and designed to lodge 800 children of FIAT employees, was built in 1933 by the engineer

Vittorio Bonadè Bottino. The building conveys elementary simplicity, rising at the edge of the beach and sitting on a 54,000 square-metre parcel of land animated by a Mediterranean pine forest. But appearances can be deceiving. Contrasting with Vaccaro's horizontal forms and built in just 100 days, Bonadè Bottino's building rises to 17 floors for a total of 54 metres high. Symmetrically attached to the tower's circular base are two narrow rectangular wings parallel to the beach with their outer sides capped off by a semicircle. The wings, two storeys high and with a basement, are each 30 metres long and host the refectory and the kitchen on the ground floor. Various administrative spaces are divided between the basement and the second floor.

From a distance, the tower seems punctured by square openings with window seals at the same height marking each floor. Also evident are the round columns of the structural system. Flanking each window, they are placed partially outside the enclosing walls, accentuating the height of the building further. As one approaches the building, however, it becomes evident that the openings are not parallel but slowly step up. The reason is revealed inside, in the over 40-metre-high atrium that outlines the open dormitory. Bonadè Bottino invented an ingenious solution for this space. The dormitory is not segmented into individual floors or rooms but is a continuous helical ramp eight metres wide. It develops for 420 metres across the height of the building and opens to a lightwell whose skylight, or oculus, is composed of 14 sections filled originally with glass blocks. Resting on a windows-filled drum, the circular skylight appears engulfed in light and soaring over the deep space it encloses. From this bright element descends a 'soft light that rather illuminating highlights the volumes, making them almost incorporeal' (Giorni Rubati, 2015). Also singular is the solution to accommodate furniture on a continuously sloping floor; legs of two different lengths guarantee the needed horizontal surfaces for beds and other complementary accessories.

Though the continuous dormitory is open to the central space, the ingenuity of the design is such that noise does not penetrate beyond the ramps. Paradoxically, therefore, this immense continuous open-plan spiral offers the most intimate space for children (de Martino & Wall, 1988).

The children's daily ascent and descent of the spiral ramp filled with zenithal light must have been a joyful and memorable happening, one hard to forget despite their young age. Ninety years later, and although the once-open dormitory has been enclosed and subdivided into rooms to accommodate contemporary hostel standards, Bonadè Bottino's-ingenious solution for the 15-story atrium continues to amaze. In a 2010 Flickr post about the building, an anonymous viewer stated:

'What is that monster on the beach?' Then you discover it is from the 30s, that inside has a continuous spiral ramp, [it] was born as a summer camp and still is, and that it has a twin in Sestriere. Then you enter, and you fall in love.

Conclusion

'Fascist education', Mussolini argued:

> is moral, physical, social, and military. It aims to create men harmonically complete, therefore fascist, as we desire ... Childhood, as adolescence ... cannot be fed solely with concepts, theories, and abstract teaching. What we aim to teach our children must speak foremost to their fantasy, to their hearts, then to their minds.
>
> (Opera Nazionale Balilla, n.d.)

The *colonie* and their architecture formed an essential element in the education of children. Their construction transcended the mere objectives of a welfare policy to contribute to the task of forming the fascists of tomorrow, hence of the *uomo nuovo,* strong, patriotic and fascist.

'On the one hand', Laura Orlandini states:

> the *colonia* during fascist Italy had to be the place for personal development, the discovery of one's ability, physical and intellectual growth, and learning about community life through daily practice. On the other hand, this social community could not be free or develop freely because it followed predetermined paths as dictated by the fascist ideology.
>
> (2019, p. 166)

By having children involved in every moment of the day, the *colonia,* more than the school, offered the ideal environment to instil in the young guests the regime's ideals.

The architecture of the *colonie* was, therefore, entrusted with a double task: to house and facilitate the children's daily activities and to be the 'scenography in which the values of the regime [were] reflected' (Balducci, 2019, p. 119), that is an image of the power and modernity of Italy, as well as the efficiency and the welfare policies of the regime.

References

Balducci, V. (2019). 'Plasmare Anime!' L'architettura delle colonie per l'infanzia nel ventennio fascista. In R. Mira, & S. Salustri (Eds.), *Colonie per l'infanzia nel ventennio fascista* (pp. 107–129). Longo Editore.

Cao, U. (Ed.) (1994). *Giuseppe Vaccaro: Colonia marina a Cesenatico, 1936–38.* Clear.

Cox, P.W.L. (1935). Opera Nazionale Balilla: An aspect of Italian education. *Junior-Senior High School Clearing House, 9*(5), 267–270.

de Martino, S., & Wall, A. (Eds.) (1988). *Cities of childhood.* Architectural Association.

Dudek, M. (2000). *Architecture of schools: The new learning environments.* Architectural Press.

Duggan, C. (2009, May 24). Il significato di 'fatta l'Italia, bisogna fare gli Italiani'. *Il Piccolo*. https://ricerca.gelocal.it/ilpiccolo/archivio/ilpiccolo/2009/05/24/NZ_26_PIED.html

Gendel, M. (1966). *An illustrated history of Italy*. Weidenfeld & Nicolson.

Giolli, R. (1938, October). La Colonia Marina dell'A.G.I.P a Cesenatico. *Casabella-Costruzioni*, *11*(130), 6–19.

Giorni Rubati. (2015, February 15). Una torre sul mare: A Marina di Massa la sfida ingegneristica della Colonia Edoardo Agnelli. https://www.giornirubati.it/una-torre-sul-mare-marina-di-massa-la-sfida-ingegneristica-della-colonia-edoardo-agnelli/

La Rovere, L. (2003). 'Rifare gli Italiani': L'esperimento di creazione dell'uomo nuovo nel regime fascista. *Annali di Storia dell'Educazione e delle Istituzioni Scolastiche*, *9*, 51–78.

Labo, M., & Podestà, A. (1942). *Colonie marine, montane, elioterapiche*. Editoriale Domus.

Mira, R. (2019). Pedagogia totalitaria, uomo nuovo e colonie di vacanza: Il fascismo e l'assistenza climatica infantile. In R. Mira, & S. Salustri (Eds.), *Colonie per l'infanzia nel ventennio fascista* (pp. 17–40). Longo Editore.

Mira, R., & Salustri, S. (2019). Le colonie per l'infanzia tra welfare e ideologia. In R. Mira, & S. Salustri (Eds.), *Colonie per l'infanzia nel ventennio fascista* (pp. 9–14). Longo Editore.

Mucelli, E. (2009). *Colonie di vacanza italiane degli anni '30: Architetture per l'educazione del corpo e dello spirito*. Alinea Editrice.

Opera Nazionale Balilla: Tesina. (n.d.). https://doc.studenti.it/appunti/storia/opera-nazionale-balilla.html

Orlandini, L. (2019). Educare al fascismo in colonia. In R. Mira, & S. Salustri (Eds.), *Colonie per l'infanzia nel ventennio fascista* (pp. 149–176). Longo Editore.

Patapan, H. (2014). Patriotic leadership in democracy. In J. Kane, & H. Patapan (Eds.), *Good democratic leadership: On prudence and judgment in modern democracies* (pp. 212–230). Oxford Academic.

Pilat, S., & Sanza, P. (2020). Architectural pragmatism and poetry: Childhood in Fascist era summer camps. *Childhood in the Past*, *13*(2), 109–120. 10.1080/17585716.2020.1791496

Portante, A. (2015, February 15). Fra Razionalismo e Romanità 3: fascismo & architettura. https://www.slideshare.net/pt00400/3fascismoarchitettura

Ricci, G. (1997, November–December). *Profilo di un costruttore che fu anche un capo mio padre Renato*. Italia-RSI. http://www.italia-rsi.it/uomini/riccirenato.htm

Rifugio Scout Vicenza. (n.d.). *Breve storia delle colonie estive GIL*. https://www.rifugioscoutvicenza.com/storia/

Ruinas, S. (1939). Viaggio per le città di Mussolini. Bompiani.

Sanza, P. (2020). Transforming: The rebirth of Bolzano's former GIL. In K.B. Jones, & S. Pilat (Eds.), *The Routledge companion to Italian fascist architecture: Reception and legacy* (pp. 359–369). Routledge.

Vaccaro, G. (1939). La colonia 'Sandro Mussolini' dell'AGIP a Cesenatico. *Architettura*, *18*(1), 1–14.

10

ARCHITECTURE OF HEALTH

Hygiene and schooling in Hong Kong, 1901–1941

Stella Meng Wang

The regulation of school architecture and curriculum for the purposes of improving school health was one of the most defining changes to education in early 20th-century Hong Kong. In the context of a heightened state of anxiety over public health—triggered by a series of plague outbreaks in Hong Kong by the turn of the century—the British colonial government mobilised an army of European sanitary and medical experts to devise a regime of health surveillance in Hong Kong. The imperial preoccupation over the health of youth further drew classroom, dormitory and school playground spaces into the discourse of hygiene, creating a new typology of school architecture on the one hand, and stratifying a class structure in Chinese society on the other. As architectural reform, hygiene education and medical inspection were most rigorously carried out in the state-sponsored English schools (English-medium) that educated a multiracial, but predominantly Chinese middle-class cohort, this strand of schools became the prime site where sanitary innovations and hygiene curriculum materialised. The private vernacular schools (Chinese-medium), however, where the great majority of Chinese children sought schooling, hardly experienced spatial reform due to a lack of funding. In addition to devising architectural reform and sanitary engineering as a means to improve school health, the British colonial government also designed a hygiene curriculum that was enacted differently for middle-class European and Chinese boys and girls. While girls were trained in domestic science, boys were taught in woodcrafts, gardening and more 'outdoor' skills. The discourse of hygiene as it impacted on school architecture and curriculum engaged new class and gender dynamics that resonated with and at times contradicted broader social and cultural changes that were taking place in urban Hong Kong in the early 20th century.

DOI: 10.4324/9781003288671-14

This chapter spotlights how a network of European sanitary, medical and educational experts created a new school typology and health curriculum in Hong Kong schools between 1901 and 1941. To trace how this health infrastructure, enacted through school architecture and curriculum, changed over time, the chapter focusses on one strand of schools where these changes materialised extensively: the state-sponsored English schools. This is not to say that private vernacular schools (Chinese-medium) were left out of the orbit of imperial hygiene and sanitary reform in pre-World War II Hong Kong. Indeed, these schools were criticised heavily by European school inspectors for the period under study, being depicted as in a 'filthy' and 'insanitary' condition that was degenerative to pupils' health (Director of Education, 1912, pp. 4–5; Medical Department, 1938, p. 23). However, paradoxically, in spite of this, vernacular (Chinese-medium) schools hardly received any state financial support to enact sanitary and architectural reform, being ill-situated in shophouse tenements intended for domestic and commercial use. The discourse of hygiene, as it operated in the educational context, thus helped create a stratified class structure within the Chinese community. It should be noted, though, that only a small fraction of school-age children attended state-sponsored English schools, while the vast majority were educated in vernacular (Chinese-medium) schools (including both aided and unaided). By 1934 (this year was chosen because by the late 1930s, the figure of school children in Hong Kong was significantly elevated by the population influx caused by the turbulence in Mainland China):

> of the schools controlled by the Education Department only 20 were 'provided' or government schools, 333 were aided or subsidised by grants from public funds, and 718 were unaided. The number of pupils in attendance at government schools was 5,476; similar figures for the aided and unaided schools were 28,677 and 39,195 respectively, in a total of 73,348.
>
> (Medical Department, 1934, p. 43)

While the aided schools occasionally included vernacular (Chinese-medium) establishments, the unaided schools were predominantly vernacular (Chinese-medium). In 1934, for example, of the 718 unaided schools, 594 were vernacular, and only 123 were English schools (Director of Education, 1934, p. 4). This uneven distribution of state educational funds contributed to a class divide within the schooling context.

The architectural and health curriculum reforms launched in state-sponsored English schools, including both government and grant-in-aid establishments, also resonated with transnational influences that were making their way to Hong Kong in the early 20th century. These included a new planning culture proliferated through the Garden City Movement that brought dramatic changes in urban and suburban landscape, particularly in domestic architecture. Changes in school architecture were thus part of a larger colonial project that served the end of building public health. Putting school health in Hong Kong in its broader British imperial context, concerns over the health of Hong Kong youth echoed with eugenic ideas that gained prominence in the British world by the turn of the century. This imperial concern with the health of Hong Kong youth also drew in the financial support of Chinese elites. Acting as important sponsors for English education (Carroll, 2009), it was through the financial support of Chinese bourgeoisies that architectural reform of Hong Kong schools came into full effect. Against this backdrop, this chapter examines the architectural and curriculum reform in Hong Kong schools.

School architecture and sanitary reform: Background, 1890–1913

The sanitary and hygiene movement that started in Hong Kong in the late 19th century problematised urban shophouse tenements—that accommodated the vast majority of working-class Chinese—as a major public health concern. At the time, the colony was still in recovery from the Bubonic Plague outbreak in 1894 that claimed 2,426 lives just in the first two months of the outbreak. The plague subsequently paralysed the economy of the whole city (The Plague, 1894). In an investigation into the causes of the plague outbreak, medical officer Dr James A. Lowson suggested the structural defects of urban tenements—'the want of ventilation, light and air in them, the inadequate water supply, the want of proper drainage, the overcrowded condition of the houses … the filthy condition of wells'—contributed directly to the rapid spread of the plague in the Chinese quarters (Government Civil Hospital, 1895). While these comments by European medical experts served the primary purpose to discipline the Chinese population on the grounds of health, they ultimately contributed towards a spatial separation of European and Chinese residential quarters. The fact that schools in this period were also housed in shophouse tenements meant that school accommodation was a site for heavy criticism launched in the name of public health. Accelerated by the circulation of both English and Chinese newspapers and journals that published reports on schools, these criticisms reached a wide audience, making school health a site of public debate. For example, in April 1890, an article written by an 'independent reviewer', a Mr C.S. Addis, was published in *The China Review* (an academic journal circulating in Hong Kong between 1872 and 1901) critiquing two defects of the education system in Hong Kong: 'the shortcomings in the matter of school accommodation and the absence of any provision for physical training' (Education Department, 1891, p. 294). The inadequacy of school accommodation critiqued by Addis persisted in different strands of schools. Earlier in 1887, Inspector of Schools Frederick Stewart asserted, 'the question of accommodation seriously affects the results of school teaching in every country, and more particularly so in a tropical climate', however, 'among the 204 schools in the colony there were hardly ten or twelve which were located in suitable premises':

> the vast majority of the schools were accommodated in ordinary semi-Chinese or Chinese dwelling houses, ill-suited for the purpose of classrooms and were in most cases deficient as regards to light and ventilation and especially in respect of lavatories. ... The Aided Schools in the villages were mostly accommodated in window-less cottages ... many of these schools receiving light and ventilation exclusively from the open door-way.
> (Education Department, 1888, p. 403)

In print media and state reports such as these, the educational space in Hong Kong was depicted as architecturally inadequate for the purpose of learning. This image of defects in school accommodation—circulated in public debate—was constructed in the broader context of sanitary reform that highlighted the role European sanitary experts and engineers played in shaping the public health infrastructure in Hong Kong in the early 20th century. In 1882 and 1902, sanitary expert Osbert Chadwick was commissioned to visit Hong Kong and to investigate questions of housing, water supply and sewage as they impacted on the matter of public health. On these two visits, Chadwick pointed out the connection between domestic hygiene and public health and suggested the structural defects of tenement buildings posed myriad urban health concerns (Public Works Office, 1902, p. 590). He subsequently promoted 'public health reforms through better architectural and engineering designs' (Yip et al., 2016, p. 13). Chadwick's advice was incorporated by the British colonial state in Hong Kong in the drafting of the Public Health and Buildings Ordinance of 1903. The Ordinance systematically reshaped urban domestic structure through 'the specific requirements on the provision of skylight, air, and ventilation in rooms used for dwelling'. Also pertinent in this ordinance is the regulation of 'building height, street width, and the inclusion of back-yards and open spaces' (Medical and Sanitary Department, 1932, pp. 12–13).

The emphasis on environmental engineering as a means to improve domestic hygiene reflects the degree to which sanitation and environmental improvements were the main tools of disease control in Hong Kong by the turn of the century (Bu & Yip, 2012, p. 2). Engineers and sanitarians played an important role in public health management (Yip et al., 2016, p. 24). This sanitary approach to public health was also extended to schools. In 1906, for example, the 'unhealthy nature of the surroundings' of the government school Victoria British School (for European children) 'caused some anxiety' for the Education Department. In order to drain the swampy land near the school and clear the grounds of the brushwood, the state sanctioned 'a large sum of money'. Meanwhile, the concrete flooring inside the school caused 'a great deal of trouble', and had made 'it impossible for the school to be kept as clean as it should be'. This defect was also remedied (Education Department, 1907, p. 447).

These earlier sanitary interventions in the schooling site were eventually formalised in the Educational Ordinance of 1913. This ordinance was informed by the Public Health and Buildings Ordinance of 1903 and had specific requirements concerning the spatial arrangement and sanitary condition of schools. As the Director of Education E. Irving explained, the aim of the ordinance was to 'ensure a certain minimum of sanitation and disciplinary and educational attainment in every school in the Colony' (Director of Education, 1913, p. 2). It stipulated:

> in every classroom the windows or other openings to external air shall be situated on at least two sides of the classroom... ... . In addition, no desk shall be placed nearer to the blackboard than three feet, and the blackboard shall be placed in such a position (that is, in the opinion of an Inspector) adequately illuminated and so arranged as to provide every pupil with an easy and unobstructed view thereof... ... . Meanwhile, every classroom shall be swept out daily at least two hours before the opening of the school, and the floors of every classroom shall be washed and treated at least once a week with a dust laying disinfectant.
>
> (Executive Council, 1939, pp. 785–788)

These requirements for the lighting of school buildings and the placement of classroom furniture addressed aspects of school that were viewed as potentially 'damaging' to pupils' health, particularly concerning their spine development and eyesight. The emphasis on ventilation was to compensate for the health effects of overcrowding prevalent in urban schools by the turn of the century; while daily 'sweeping' and 'sanitising' of classrooms were preventative measures against the development and spread of any contagions. These regulations were drafted to address the defects of school accommodation in Hong Kong at the time. The Education Ordinance of 1913 in turn marked the beginning of state intervention in school architecture and a colonial desire to transform schools—state, aided and unaided alike—into conduits for the production of healthy youth. While it may have appeared that the new set of building regulations—specified in the Ordinance—amended the structural defects of private vernacular schools, in practice, the lack of state surveillance and medical inspection, coupled with the lack of funding, limited any significant improvement of the health condition of this type of school. The vast majority continued to be housed in tenement buildings prior to 1941 (Medical Department, 1939, p. 24). In contrast, what contributed to a new era of school health development was the practical teaching of hygiene; the construction of purposefully designed school buildings; and a system of medical examination for European and Chinese children attending government and grant-in-aid schools. These measures also captured the shifting role the educational space played in the management of public health in pre-World War II Hong Kong.

Curriculum of hygiene and school design, 1913–1921

The teaching of hygiene in Hong Kong schools related directly to how the educational space was framed in public health discourse. Informed by the view that 'not only is care of the school child's health of importance in preventing the development and spread of disease but the education of his mind in matters of hygiene and public health is the surest method of spreading the gospel of health among people' (Medical and Sanitary Department, 1936, p. 53), as early as 1905, the Board of Education in Hong Kong issued an outline scheme for teaching hygiene to children attending government elementary schools. The aim of the scheme was to equip children with the necessary knowledge and skills to practice hygiene in their homes and in everyday life. The scheme, drawn up by the Medical Officer of Health Dr W.W. Pearse (Inspector of Schools, 1907, p. 3), covered four principal aspects: 'domestic hygiene; personal hygiene; eating and drinking; and illness'. Therein, pupils were instructed on the cleansing of rooms and furniture on cleanliness, carriage, posture, change of clothing and bedding, quiet speech, and restraint; on food preparation and preservation; and on disease prevention and how to deal with minor illness (Education in Hygiene and Temperance, 1905). By making hygiene a compulsory subject in all government and grant-in-aid English schools (The Teaching of Hygiene, 1906), this new form of hygiene knowledge was first introduced to middle-class European and Chinese children. To stimulate the learning of the subject, the governor Sir Matthew Nathan offered prizes and a shield as a trophy (awarded in the annual hygiene examination, and to be kept for one year) ('Examination in Hygiene', 1906).

The development of hygiene curriculum in Hong Kong schools in the 1900s and 1910s further overlapped with eugenic thought espousing that individuals could learn to take responsibility for healthy conduct through education (Levine & Bashford, 2018). This strand of learning came with the expected outcome that middle-class children would become efficient and responsible professionals and parents. Here hygiene education also had a gendered aspect. Before the subject was made compulsory in all state and grant-in-aid schools, it was taught as part of domestic science (Inspector of Schools, 1907, p. 3). By the late 1910s, hygiene became an integral part of domestic science at English girls' schools. At the government girls' school Belilios Public School for Chinese Girls, for example, 'fresh air in the classrooms, boiled water in the filters, cleanliness of persons and apparel were all matters of the course'. In the upper (senior-grades) school, practical lessons were given with simple equipment in sick-nursing and sick-room matters generally (Director of Education, 1915, p. 12). Additional subjects such as laundry and cookery were all part of this training on domestic hygiene (Director of Education, 1919, p. 7). This teaching of practical homemaking skills for girls connected with eugenic thinking in the training of efficient middle-class mothers.

In addition to equipping Hong Kong children with a toolbox of knowledge to manage the 'tropical' environment that was considered particularly prone to the outbreak of contagions (Pomfret, 2015, p. 22), the colonial state initiated a direct response to change the health function of schools—the design and construction of a type of school architecture that addressed specifically the 'tropical' climate in Hong Kong. While this prototype of colonial school architecture had early precursors in the building design of Queen's College in the 1890s, it was not until the 1910s that the idea to use architecture as a method to combat 'tropicality' became a common practice in the design of government schools. This type of school architecture resembled the 'staple' feature of hospital architecture in the inclusion of a verandah and wide corridors for the perceived health value of fresh air (Bashford, 2004). Furthermore, internal spatial design also took into account of functionality. In 1913, for example, the extension at government school Belilios Public School for Chinese Girls incorporated numerous measures to improve the efficiency and the health function of school buildings. The extension consisted of a two-storey building with 'eight classrooms … four cloak-rooms, four lavatories'. To facilitate the ventilation of the building and to reduce potential clutter, wide corridors were 'provided on both floors throughout the full extent of the building'. Cross-ventilation inside the classrooms was aided by the installation of large windows, a feature that also allowed natural light to penetrate into the building (Director of Public Works, 1913, p. 50). In addition to government schools, the principal grant-in-aid English schools in this period were also designed and built according to modern hygiene principles. At the French Convent, for example, the classrooms of the school were described in local newspapers as 'large, airy and well equipped'; 'the whole building is delightfully cool and commodious' (Anglo-French Convent School, 1916).

The spatial layout and planning of these schools reflects a colonial preoccupation with the health function of school architecture. The emphasis on light, air and cross-ventilation captured how the sanitary approach to public health shaped the spatial design of schools in Hong Kong in the 1900s and 1910s. These building practices also resonated with the modern health movement in Europe during this period. The health feature of these government and grant-in-aid English schools resembled those of open-air schools in their emphasis on 'health amenities, the complexity of their lighting and ventilation systems, and their close links with nature' (Châtelet, 2008). The healthy school architecture that emerged in Hong Kong in the 1910s thus illustrates how ideas on healthy school design in the metropole were reformulated as part of a solution to combat the 'tropical' climate in Hong Kong. By the 1920s, partly resonating with the Garden City movement that gained prominence in Hong Kong (Ho, 2018), small-scale gardening projects were carried out in government and grant-in-aid schools, adding another feature to urban and suburban school architecture. Being generously supported by the Botanical and Forestry Department (1923, p. 7), this experiment again captured the link among colonial agencies for education, urban planning and public health in transforming school architecture and school health.

School gardening, physical education and the School Hygiene Branch, 1921–1931

In the period between 1920 and 1930, woodwork, carpentry, cookery and gardening were among the subjects the Education Department introduced in selected government schools. Rather than training pupils to master these skills, its purpose was to provide middle-class European and Chinese children with hands-on experiments that expanded their previous learning experience. In 1922, for example, at the government district school, the Ellis Kadoorie School for Chinese boys (founded by merchant and philanthropist Mr Ellis Kadoorie in 1901, taken over by the Education Department in 1915), the Inspector of English Schools E. Ralphs observed 'certain classes have taken up basket work'. At the Wantsai School (a government district school for Chinese boys), school gardening was introduced which 'under somewhat trying conditions have produced very creditable results' (Director of Education, 1922, p. 10). As well, at the Ellis Kadoorie School for Indians (founded by Mr Ellis Kadoorie in 1891, relocated to Soo-Kun-Po Valley in 1916), the school ran 'a flourishing garden where flowers, fruit and vegetables are produced in abundance … cotton and coffee were also grown' (Director of Education, 1922, p. 15). Again in 1923, new school gardens had been started at outlying government district schools at Tai Po and Tai Wai (both located in the New Territories) (Director of Education, 1923, p. 10). In fact, the Director of Education E. Irving was the chief advocate for the school gardening movement in Hong Kong in the 1920s. 'Inspired by' what he 'saw of the excellent system of School Garden in the Philippines' on his educational tour, Irving started several school garden projects in government schools with the support of the Botanical and Forestry Department and was instrumental in the introduction of agriculture in outlying district schools (Director of Education, 1923, p. 7).

These school gardens as new additions to school architecture illuminate how ideas that underpinned the management of school health resonated with broader changes in planning practices that took place in Hong Kong over the interwar period. Schooling practices and architectural innovations were combined with landscape and planning experiments that aimed to combat the health problems produced by overcrowded urban living. This, in turn, transformed not only the appearance of schools, but also the function of the educational space in urban health. The 'flourishing garden' with 'flowers, fruit and vegetables' provided a 'remedial' space within the school. It was a response to both the transnational influences such as the school gardening movement and the Garden City movement that were taking place in the educational and urban planning spheres and the changing architectural design practices of schools in Hong Kong.

Physical education was another key practice that underwent dramatic expansion in interwar Hong Kong for its perceived effect on school health. By the mid-1920s, the physical education curriculum at government and grant-in-aid schools had evolved from its earlier focus on gymnastics and drills to include outdoor games and sports. For example at the Ellis Kadoorie School for Chinese boys, a government district school, 'games, drill, excursions by launch, train and motor-bus, swimming and educational walk' were deemed 'an essential part' of the school curriculum. The school headmaster Mr F.J. de Rome suggested that he found:

> time allowed off during the afternoons in which to play volleyball competitions, football at Causeway Bay, to swim at Kennedy Town, to explore the island and the New Territories in connection with geography lesson, to visit the reservoirs, industrial undertakings, etc. does not react unfavourably on the work in school.
>
> (Director of Education, 1927, p. 13)

This expansion of physical education curriculum in schools in the 1920s drew on the same kinds of eugenic ideas that also influenced youth movements such as Boy Scouts (started in Hong Kong in 1913) (Director of Education, 1913, p. 22) and Girl Guides (started in Hong Kong in 1921) (Director of Education 1921, p. 8). Imperial concern with the fitness of Hong Kong youth materialised in a diverse range of settings, instituting a new bodily training regime on the one hand, and transforming urban health architecture on the other.

Curriculum innovations for the purpose of school health moved apace with a gradual institutionalisation of the medical inspection of Hong Kong children. In 1925, in the context of intensified surveillance of school health, a special branch within the Medical Department—the School Hygiene Branch—was established. Hitherto, the medical examination of school children, was performed by government medical officers who also worked at hospitals and therefore could only inspect schools on a limited scope. The founding of the school hygiene branch designated a health officer, Dr (Mrs) Minett, MD (wife of government bacteriologist Dr Edward. P. Minett), who was specially allocated for school medical service (Director of Education, 1925). The purpose of this assignment, as the Medical Department indicated, was 'not only to detect the sick and ailing in their early stages, but also to seek for anomalies of growth and development, so that measures may be taken to prevent not only the progress of ill-health but also its causes' (Medical Department, 1934, p. 44). Upon appointment, Dr (Mrs) Minett conducted a health survey of all children in the 18 government schools and 13 of the grant-in-aid schools, while reports were made on the hygienic aspect of school premises and furniture (Director of Education, 1925, p. 5). These reports served as the basis for the improvement of sanitary infrastructure in schools. In addition, school nurses (mainly Chinese) performed home visits where they advised parents on good habits of health and how to care for their children. Where hospital treatment was necessary, the school nurse often escorted the child and the parent to hospital (Medical and Sanitary Department, 1931, p. 46).

Chaired and staffed by a network of European and Chinese female medical professionals, the founding of the School Hygiene Branch also illuminates the broader changes in the gender dynamics in the professional domain in interwar Hong Kong. Engagement with school health became an important site for European and Chinese female professionals (such as doctors and nurses) to exercise their field of expertise and claim authority to participate in public affairs. By reporting on the efficiency of school and classroom design, daily hygiene and health instruction in schools (Director of Education, 1928, p. 7), this web of medical experts became another group, in addition to sanitarians and engineers, that systematically shaped the architecture of Hong Kong schools. In 1927, Mrs Minett advocated for the inclusion of swimming pool in schools, for example, '[the] swimming-bath in St. Paul's Girls' School has been a great addition to the health equipment of the school' (Director of Education, 1927, p. 7). Again in 1929, Mrs Minett's report on Diocesan Girls' College indicated the function of the school medical officer in safe-guarding school hygiene:

I visited the Diocesan Girls' School, for the purpose of making a half-yearly report, on July 4.

... A physical training mistress has been added to the staff this year, and I saw a number of classes (senior and middle school) at drill. ... The work was excellent, consisting [of] free movement, balancing exercises, good walking and running. The 'special remove' class, of older Chinese girls had obviously taken to the new idea and the improvement in walking, posture, and freedom of movement was well-marked. ... The classrooms and dormitories were all in good order. ... A definite improvement and better use of space has been made in cloakroom provision. (Pupils' Health, 1929)

This inspection of the environmental aspect of school architecture, the health education curriculum and classroom furniture ultimately contributed towards the gradual standardisation of the classroom interior and health instruction at government and grant-in-aid schools. Furthermore, the fact that children were weighed and measured regarding their eyes, hearing, chest, heart, lungs, spine and posture (Director of Education, 1926, p. 8) suggests there was a normalised notion of the child's body and health at play. The medical discourse around child health underlined the routine inspection of schools and functioned as an important factor that shaped the medical surveillance of school children in Hong Kong. The upshot of this medical surveillance on schools is that it not only produced standardised classroom design, but also new engineering of bodily movement in schools, facilitated by the instrument of the timetable.

Timetable and engineering of bodily movement, 1931–1941

While ideas about healthy school architecture had solidified and brought spatial changes to state-sponsored schools well before the interwar period, curricular reform and timetable design were the principal tools that improved the efficient use of school buildings in the interwar years. In the 1930s, bodily movement in schools underwent systematic reform. Short school hours, proper rest and outdoor exercise characterised the timetable of state-sponsored English schools, reflecting the influence of medical discourse around child health and the imperial imperative of hygiene on schooling practice and experience. At the grant-in-aid girls' school, the French Convent, for example, former student Magdalene Fung (b. 1921) recalled:

> every day, we finished at 3pm, I would go to the study room. At about 4.30pm, I would go out and play, first I would have a shower though. At about 6.30pm, it was dinner, and 8.30pm was bed time. In the morning, I got up at 6am to go to the chapel. In the cold days, there would be no water, so I had to save some before I went to bed the day before. … While I was a boarder, we each had a basket, for laundry. About ten of us shared one room, I slept on the upper bunk.
>
> (Oral History Interview with Magdalene Fung, 2001)

What is significant in this recollection is the detailing of how hygiene had been instituted as part of everyday school routine. The shower before dinner, dormitory design and laundry arrangement illuminates how early teaching on personal hygiene materialised into schooling practices as 'a way of school life'. This, in turn, points to the link between personal hygiene conduct and school health. Also prominent is the description of school hours that spotlight the importance of abundant rest and exercise for the perceived benefit of the

development of children. The mechanism of the timetable thus simultaneously enacted the medical debate on proper rest and the hygiene discourse
on personal health conduct for their perceived effect on child health.
Institutional supervision, again, was instrumental in carrying the timetable
into full effect. As the headmistress Miss Sawyer at the Diocesan Girls' School
(a grant-in-aid girls' school) stressed:

> I think that growing girls need plenty of good food and plenty of sleep with
> fresh air, and I try to carry this out in practice with the boarders. All
> dormitory light must be out by 9 pm except Saturday by 9.30 pm. And no
> children are allowed to be downstairs before 7am. It is also forbidden to
> shut a dormitory door or window. We have very little backlash among the
> boarders.
>
> (Diocesan Girls' School, 1930)

Through an army of medical and educational experts, equipped with the
knowledge of modern hygiene, school design and medical inspection, school
health came under intensified scrutiny. Dormitory doors or windows were
'forbidden' to shut, which again reflects how colonial experts translated their
concerns with fresh air and ventilation in the design and daily use of school
buildings. From the inspection of school premises, classroom furniture and
dormitory design to the supervision of timetable and curriculum, it was
through the effort of colonial state officials including doctors and nurses who
worked in the School Hygiene Branch, and the collaboration of headmasters,
headmistresses and teachers that the hygiene discourse materialised into
schooling practice, being instituted as part of the daily school routine.

Conclusion

This chapter has examined how a transnational network of European sanitary,
medical and educational experts helped define the contour of architectural
reform and the hygiene curriculum in Hong Kong between the period 1901
and 1941. Travelling back and forth between Hong Kong and the wider
British imperial world, these colonial experts brought with them new approaches to public health that subsequently shaped the practices in Hong
Kong schools. In the 1900s, the visit of sanitary expert Osbert Chadwick was
instrumental in the drafting of the Public Health and Buildings Ordinance of
1903 that aimed to promote public health in Hong Kong through sanitary
engineering. Translating into the schooling context, this ordinance informed
the Educational Ordinance of 1913, which had specific requirements concerning the spatial arrangement and sanitary condition of Hong Kong
schools. The design and renovation of government schools in this period
(1910s) in part reflected the new building practices stipulated in the

Ordinance. However, more significant regarding the new architectural prototype that proliferated in Hong Kong schools in the 1910s is that it resonated with transnational influences concerning school health, such as the modern health movement in Europe. In the 1920s, the Director of Education E. Irving avidly advocated for the school gardening movement, leading the development of school gardens in urban and suburban areas, as well as in the outlying districts of rural Hong Kong. By then, school architecture had been brought into the fold of landscape and planning experiments that aimed to combat the health problems produced by overcrowded urban living. School gardens were a response to both transnational influences such as the school gardening movement and the Garden City movement that were taking place in the educational and urban planning spheres, and the changing architectural design practices of schools in Hong Kong.

Moving apace with architectural experiments, curriculum innovation was another tool colonial experts used to transform the function of the educational space in public health. Equipped with the knowledge of modern hygiene, Medical Officer of Health Dr W.W. Pearse drafted a scheme for the teaching of hygiene in Hong Kong schools as early as 1905. By the 1910s, hygiene education further engaged with eugenic thought that framed middle-class schoolgirls as the future mothers of the British empire. This then shaped the domestic science curriculum at government schools for middle-class European and Chinese schoolgirls. In addition to hygiene curriculum, eugenic thought also permeated the physical education that blossomed both in the schooling context and through youth movements in interwar Hong Kong. Also significant about the interwar period with regard to school health is the intensified surveillance on classroom furniture and design, daily hygiene and health instruction enacted through the School Hygiene Branch. The upshot of this medical surveillance on schools was that it not only encouraged standardised classroom design, but also a new engineering of bodily movement in schools, facilitated by the instrument of the timetable.

As architectural reform, hygiene education and medical inspection were most rigorously carried out in state-sponsored English schools (English-medium) that educated a multiracial, but predominantly Chinese middle-class cohort, this strand of schools became the prime site where sanitary innovations and hygiene curriculum materialised. The private vernacular schools (Chinese-medium) schools where the great majority of working-class Chinese children sought schooling, however, hardly experienced spatial reform due to the lack of funding. Hygiene discourse, as it operated in the educational context in Hong Kong, thus helped create a stratified class structure within Chinese society. This stratifying effect took place in the context of burgeoning urban middle-class culture that Chinese merchants and professionals contributed to create. Acting as important patrons of English education, it was through the financial support of Chinese bourgeoisies that architectural and hygiene reform came into full effect. School health, as this chapter shows, functioned as an important means to enact new class and gender dynamics in Hong Kong in the early 20th century, entwining with the rise of Chinese bourgeoisies and female professionals, as well as eugenic thought that re-framed the health of Hong Kong youth as directly connected with the future of the British empire.

References

Anglo-French Convent School: New wing at Causeway Bay opened by the governor. (1916, October 7). *Hong Kong Daily Press*, 3.

Bashford, A. (2004). *Imperial hygiene: A critical history of imperialism, nationalism and public health*. Palgrave McMillan.

Botanical and Forestry Department. (1923). Report on the Botanic and Forestry Department for the year 1923. (Appendix N to the *Administrative Reports for the year 1923*). Hong Kong Government.

Bu, L., & Yip, K. (2012). Introduction: Interpreting science and public health in modern Asia. In L. Bu, D.H. Stapleton., & K. Yip (Eds.), *Science, public health and the state in modern Asia* (pp. 1–15). Routledge.

Carroll, J.M. (2009). *Edge of empires: Chinese elites and British colonials in Hong Kong*. Harvard University Press.

Châtelet, A.-M. (2008). A breath of fresh air: Open-air schools in Europe. In M. Gutman, & N. de Coninck-Smith (Eds.), *Designing modern childhoods: History, space, and the material culture of children* (pp. 107–127). Rutgers University Press.

Diocesan Girls' School: Annual distribution of prizes. (1930, February 15). *The China Mail*, 12.

Director of Education. (1912). Report of the Director of Education for the year 1912. (Appendix N to the *Administrative Reports for the year 1912*). Hong Kong Government.

Director of Education. (1913). Report of the Director of Education for the year 1913. (Appendix N to the *Administrative Reports for the year 1913*). Hong Kong Government.

Director of Education. (1915). Report of the Director of Education for the year 1915. (Appendix O to the *Administrative Reports for the year 1915*). Hong Kong Government.

Director of Education. (1919). Report of the Director of Education for the year 1919. (Appendix O to the *Administrative Reports for the year 1919*). Hong Kong Government.

Director of Education. (1921). Report of the Director of Education for the year 1921. (Appendix O to the *Administrative Reports for the year 1921*). Hong Kong Government.

Director of Education. (1922). Report of the Director of Education for the year 1922. (Appendix O to the *Administrative Reports for the year 1922*). Hong Kong Government.

Director of Education. (1923). Report of the Director of Education for the year 1923. (Appendix O to the *Administrative Reports for the year 1923*). Hong Kong Government.

Director of Education. (1925). Report of the Director of Education for the year 1925. (Appendix O to the *Administrative Reports for the year 1925*). Hong Kong Government.

Director of Education. (1926). Report of the Director of Education for the year 1926. (Appendix O to the *Administrative Reports for the year 1926*). Hong Kong Government.

Director of Education. (1927). Report of the Director of Education for the year 1927. (Appendix O to the *Administrative Reports for the year 1927*). Hong Kong Government.

Director of Education. (1928). Report of the Director of Education for the year 1928. (Appendix O to the *Administrative Reports for the year 1928*). Hong Kong Government.

Director of Education. (1934). Report of the Director of Education for the year 1934. (Appendix O to the *Administrative Reports for the year 1934*). Hong Kong Government.

Director of Public Works. (1913). Report of the Director of Public Works for the year 1913. (Appendix P to the *Administrative Reports for the year 1913*). Hong Kong Government.

Education Department. (1888, April 21). Annual report on education in Hongkong for the year 1887. (Government notification no. 171: Supplement to the *Hongkong Government Gazette*). Hong Kong Government.

Education Department. (1891, June 19). The educational report for 1890. (No. 23/91 of the *Papers laid before the Legislative Council of Hongkong 1891*). Hong Kong Government.

Education Department. (1907, July 19). Report of the Inspector of Schools for the year 1906. (Government notification no. 19: Supplement to the *Hongkong Government Gazette*). Hong Kong Government.

Education in Hygiene and Temperance. (1905, September 9). *The Hong Kong Telegraph*, 5.

Examination in Hygiene. (1906, January 13). *The Hong Kong Telegraph*, 4.

Executive Council. (1939, September 1). Hong Kong: Ordinance No. 26 of 1913 (Education). (Government notification no. 711: *Hong Kong Government Gazette*). Hong Kong Government.

Government Civil Hospital. (1895, March 2). Medical report on the epidemic of bubonic plague in 1894. (No. 16/95 of the *Papers laid before the Legislative Council of Hongkong 1895*). Hong Kong Government.

Ho, P.Y. (2018). *Making Hong Kong: A history of its urban development*. Edward Elgar Publishing.

Inspector of Schools. (1907). Report on the study of hygiene in the Hongkong schools, 1906. (No. 7/1907 of the *Papers laid before the Legislative Council of Hongkong 1907*). Hong Kong Government.

Levine, P., & Bashford, A. (2018). Introduction: Eugenics and the modern world. In P. Levine, & A. Bashford (Eds.), *The Oxford handbook of the history of eugenics* (pp. 1–27). Oxford University Press.

Medical Department. (1934). Annual medical report for the year ending 31st December 1934. (Appendix M to the *Administrative Reports for the year 1934*). Hong Kong Government.

Medical Department. (1938). Annual medical report for the year 1938. (Appendix M to the *Administrative Reports for the year 1938*). Hong Kong Government.

Medical Department. (1939). Annual medical report for the year 1939. (Appendix M to the *Administrative Reports for the year 1939*). Hong Kong Government.

Medical and Sanitary Department. (1931). Medical and sanitary report for the year 1931. (Appendix M to the *Administrative Reports for the year 1931*). Hong Kong Government.

Medical and Sanitary Department. (1932). Medical and sanitary report for the year 1932. (Appendix M to the *Administrative Reports for the year 1932*). Hong Kong Government.

Medical and Sanitary Department. (1936). Medical and sanitary report for the year 1936. (Appendix M to the *Administrative Reports for the year 1936*). Hong Kong Government.

Oral History Interview with Magdalene Fung. (2001). *Hong Kong Oral History Archives: Collective Memories.* Hong Kong University Library Special Collections, access no. 32.

Pomfret, D.M. (2015). *Youth and empire: Trans-colonial childhoods in British and French Asia.* Stanford University Press.

Public Works Office. (1902, April 11). Preliminary report on the sanitary condition of Hongkong. (Government notification no. 209: *Hongkong Government Gazette*). Hong Kong Government.

Pupils' Health, Report on Diocesan Girls' School. (1929, July 21). *Hong Kong Sunday Herald*, 8.

The Plague in Hong Kong. (1894, July 31). *The Hong Kong Telegraph*, 2.

The Teaching of Hygiene in Schools. (1906, February 22). *Hong Kong Daily Press*, 2.

Yip, K., Leung, Y.S., & Wong, M.K.T. (2016). *Health policy and disease in colonial and post-colonial Hong Kong, 1841–2003.* Routledge.

11

BETTER TOWNS

Building healthy communities in New Zealand school texts

Frances Kelly

In 1940s Aotearoa New Zealand, town planning promised to provide all members of society access to the *good life,* with opportunities for recreation and community-building fostered by planned neighbourhoods and modern community centres. This was particularly so post-war when New Zealand was at the height of its social democracy, and recreation was regarded as 'every citizen's entitlement', according to Macdonald (2011, p. 71), alongside income protection, good housing and roads, expanded educational opportunities and healthcare. The idea that joining a discussion group or riding a bicycle (safely) was the right of an ordinary citizen shaped postwar urban planning, marking a shift from an earlier predominantly medicalised view of urban life with its preoccupation with sanitation. New Zealand planners, whose powers were extended with the 1948 Town Planning Amendment Act, were influenced by the modern expansive conception of *good health,* which was to do not only with the absence of disease but also active participation in society (Macdonald, 2011).

A particular ideal of citizenship guided governmental involvement in recreation in post-war Aotearoa, framing a citizen's *right* to leisure with the understanding that it carried *responsibility.* According to Caroline Daley, the Labour government promoted certain types of recreation, so that people learned 'to use their increased leisure time in a sensible, worthwhile way' (2003, p. 231). This attitude permeated teacher journals. One article in *National Education* encouraged teachers to spend increased leisure time 'happily and profitably to themselves and to the community'. The wrong kind of leisure, warned the author, 'hours of idleness in which pleasure-seekers try to kill time', was certain to lead down 'the road to ruin' (Caution—Planners at Work, 1946). In *Education,* sixth-former Bobette Clarke (1949) imagined

DOI: 10.4324/9781003288671-15

citizens of post-war New Zealand society as constructively using their leisure whilst taking 'their places in the community' with responsibility, facing 'honestly the problems of living' (pp. 57–58). Town planners also played their part in promoting responsible leisure—the trick was to ensure the public understood their role.

In this chapter, I examine how core precepts of post-war urban design and ideals of active citizenship through leisure were taught to young New Zealanders through school bulletins on town planning, *Towns to Live In* (Town Planning Section, 1948b) and *Better Towns* (Town Planning Section, 1948a), produced by the Town Planning Division of the Ministry of Works and the School Publications Branch (SPB) of the Department of Education. My argument is underpinned by the idea that school texts constitute forms of governance, shaping the behaviours and attitudes of readers, informed by the work of Nikolas Rose (1999). Here, I draw on Rose's analysis with Thomas Osborne of attempts to govern *urban* existence through the spatialisation of virtue, regarding the texts on planning as attempts to 'educate and nurture the urban dweller as a citizen of a democracy in an intrinsically spatial field' (Osborne & Rose, 1999, p. 748). I work with the idea that a particular notion of leisure, conceptualised as virtue within the ideological framework of New Zealand social democracy post-war, is conveyed to readers through spatial representations of mid-century towns. I read these school texts written by 'men who have thought a great deal about how to plan towns' (Town Planning Section, 1948a) as encouraging the generation of children in schools in 1948 to see themselves as citizens of a social democracy—with all attendant rights/responsibilities—in a *spatial field*, reconciling urban dwellers to sanctioned ways of living.

The context

The school bulletins were written during a period of animated discourse on planning and housing during the first Labour government, 1935–1949 (Kelly, in press). Post-war economic recovery and the need to respond to New Zealand's housing shortage and building dilapidation, exacerbated in wartime, focussed attention on the built environment of urban centres framed as a 'blight' on the nation (Cox, 1948). The improvement of towns and cities—the goal to make them *better*—was a focalising agenda for government planners and architects, many of whom were schooled in European modernism (Clark & Walker, 2000) and shared with counterparts in Britain a goal to implement a post-war iteration of the social contract, with its extended citizenship rights and consensus politics underpinned 'by the power of expert knowledge' (Mort, 2012, p. 125). Texts from this era insist that modern planning, carried out by experts from the Ministry of Works, would foster a *good life* and promote opportunities for active, responsible leisure and safe recreation.

Discourse about planning also infiltrates curriculum texts—including school bulletins and pamphlets for adult and returned services discussion groups (Plishke, 1943, 1947)—and teacher journals. The 1946 volume of NZEI's *National Education* alone attests that planning was the *cause de jour*. 'Education must have a plan', headlines one article in the November issue (1946, p. 324). 'What's *your* Post War Plan? You *must* have one', urges another from June (1946, p. 166). However, unlike texts by the Ministry, and in accord with the journal's independent stance on government policy, articles for teachers display scepticism towards the idea that planning might offer a panacea for all societal problems.

The school texts

Children were introduced to basic principles of urban planning in *Towns to Live In* (1948) and *Better Towns* (1948); the third text jointly prepared by Town Planning and School Publications, *Houses to Live In* (1949), is discussed in Kelly (in press). The texts were part of a series of Primary School Bulletins and Post-Primary School Bulletins accompanying the revision of the curriculum post-1945, which introduced social studies as the subject attributed with the task of forming citizens to act 'intelligently in the social interest' (New Zealand Department of Education, 1944, p. 23). Social studies topics in the bulletins focussed on *local* matters, such as housing and planning, whilst staying true to the new education pedagogy that underpinned School Publications from its inception in the 1930s (Beeby, 1957). Thus, while the reader of the school bulletins is addressed as *active*, encouraged to notice, discuss and shape the built fabric of the neighbourhood, architects and town planners are represented as *experts* whose opinions on urban design should be heeded. The expert from the Ministry involved in the bulletins was Helmut Einhorn, who worked in collaboration with Ray Chapman-Taylor and Thelma Maurais of SPB (Kelly, in press).

Not all school publications sang from the same song sheet. 'Our Street' is a serialised story in the *School Journal* (also edited by Chapman-Taylor) written by Brian Sutton-Smith (1949c) and illustrated by Juliet Peter. This story offers a counter-narrative to the school bulletins, revealing the normative improvement agenda that underpins the ideal of the *better* town. 'Our Street' is a run-down street in central Wellington—the zone referred to as a 'blight' by town planners—that fosters community and provides opportunities for mildly destructive fun for a gang of bored boys, whose anti-social leisure activities contrast sharply with the modern recreational ideal-made-virtue of *Towns to Live In* and *Better Towns*.

By analysing these texts in the context of post-war discourse on planning and leisure, this chapter contributes to conversations concerning the relationship between children and the post-war built environment ranging from studies of children's engagement with urban environments (Burke & Jones, 2014) to the urban socialisation of the child (Kozlovsky, 2013). I extend the conversation to *school texts* that confer responsibility for the morphology of towns on a generation of children, presenting ideals of active leisure-as-citizenship through representations of spatial environments. To examine the values shaping the *better towns* in the texts, I begin with an analysis of diagrams in *Towns to Live In*, then consider the unplanned city of 'Our Street', contrasting it with the governmental ideal of a mid-century planned town in *Better Towns*. Thinking with Osborne and Rose (1999), I examine the diagrams, sketches and plans in the school texts for what they reveal about desirable qualities of healthy, active social democratic citizens represented *in* and shaped *through* urban design.

Planning *Towns to Live In*

The first diagram in *Towns to Live In* (Figure 11.1) shows in symbolic form components of *a town* for the junior reader. Diagrammatic sketches explain

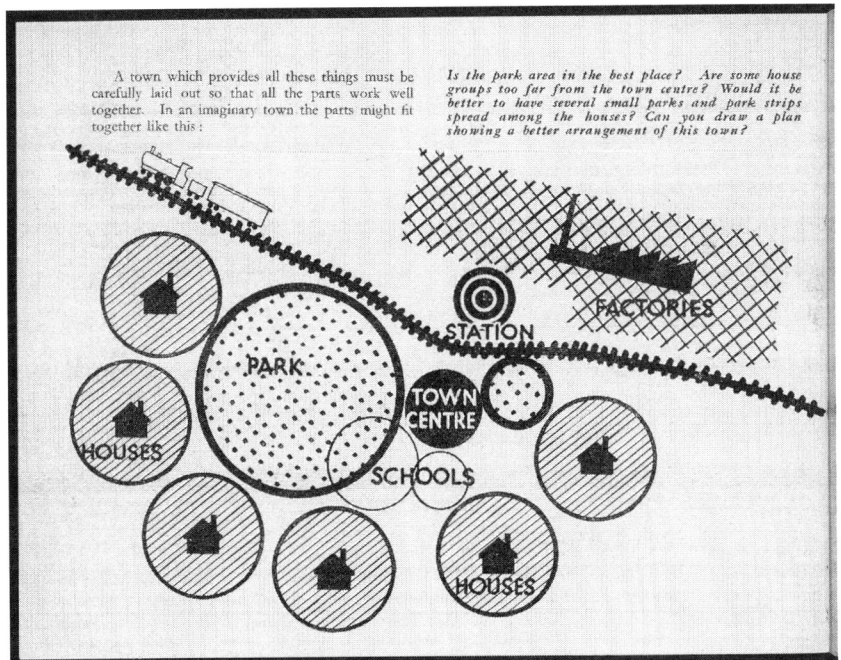

FIGURE 11.1   Diagram, *Towns to Live In*.

Source: Town Planning Section, Ministry of Works and School Publications Branch, Department of Education. (1948b). *Towns to Live In*. R.E. Owen Government Printer. Courtesy of Te Tāhuhu o te Mātauranga / Ministry of Education.

how something works, clarifying a relationship between parts of an entity. Figure 11.1 is not a plan based on a particular town nor a map of a specific location, rather it conveys—in order to promote understanding of—spatial relationships between the *parts* (houses, parks, schools, town centres, stations and factories) that make up the *whole* of a mid-century town. The town model seen here responds to the old model of the industrial town, described by Lewis Mumford (1989) as constituted by the three elements of the factory, the railroad and the slum and underpinned by a laissez-faire ethos. A characteristic of the industrial town was the absence of open spaces for children to play (Mumford, 1989). Note that *this* diagram's basic shapes represent new core elements of a planned town: the *park* constitutes the largest of these and is located beside the town centre, surrounded by houses and intersected by schools. The diagram represents a mid-century aim to reconstruct 'the entire social environment' underpinned by the values of community and co-operation (Mumford, 1989, p. 465).

Diagrams in *Towns to Live In* are representations of simplified urban space which utilise elements of mid-century town plans for public display. According to Frank Mort (2012), simplified town plans appeared in UK booklets for schoolchildren and servicemen, as well as public exhibitions, as part of a *visual strategy* for public education following the publication of *Abercrombie and Forshaw's The County of London Plan* of 1943. New Zealand town planners also took planning to the public in the 1940s, engaging similar strategies for public education. In 1948, the Architectural Centre's public exhibition *Te Aro Replanned* attempted to engage Wellingtonians in actively contributing to the redesign of the built environment of their city's central zone (Cox, 1948). Einhorn, the Ministry planner involved in the school bulletins, was also a member of the Centre (as were other Ministry planners and architects); his collaboration with SPB is indicative of a congruence between the Ministry's and Centre's public education strategy (Kelly, in press). The exhibition used spatial diagrams and models to represent an ideal planned urban environment to the public that, like the diagrams in *Towns to Live In*, reduced essential components to a symbolic form.

The size of the circle representing the park in Figure 11.1 highlights that a key role of mid-century government planners was to ensure the provision and protection of green space near housing areas in towns and cities. Such provision initially arose from concern over poor sanitation (Engels, 1845; Joyce, 2003) and the idea that access to light and clean air promoted good health (de Oliveira, 2015), which was a feature of the 19th-century parks movement (LeGates & Stout, 2005). While nurturing the health of citizens motivated the New Zealand government's intervention in housing and town planning at mid-century—more than a concern with eradicating the threat or burden of an imagined population of unhealthy urban poor, which had characterised earlier interventions—remnants of the earlier goal remained. As Schrader's

(2005) history of state housing in New Zealand has shown, an aim from 1935 on was to 'take out the rotten core' of the dilapidated colonial cities and towns and replace them with clean, planned urban environments that would foster good health (pp. 32–36). In social democratic New Zealand, parks, reframed in line with the more expansive view of good health, became spaces for active participation in social and community activities and leisure (Macdonald, 2011). Labour's Physical Welfare and Recreation Act of 1937 had introduced shorter working weeks which created more time for leisure, as well as physical sites and facilities like community centres, pools and games courts, to encourage sanctioned recreational pursuits. Post-war, Labour reinvigorated this commitment and used its (by this time extensive) modes of dissemination to further encourage the *sensible* use of leisure time (Daley, 2003). Macdonald (2011) has shown that between 1945 and 1949 Labour's *vision for leisure* expanded further, marking a zenith in state involvement in organised sport and demonstrating that recreation was tied to a *societal ideal*. The relative size and positioning of the park in Figure 11.1 point to these concerns.

A governmental conception of leisure is also conveyed in more complex town plans in the school texts—including the cover illustration of *Towns to Live In*. This plan is based on the Ministry's scheme for one of the new Hutt Valley communities—models of 'planned, ideal living' in mid-century Aotearoa (Macdonald, 2011, p. 89). Ministry of Works' plans for Naenae and Upper Hutt town centres were recycled across texts as part of the visual education strategy (Kelly, in press): the repetition of *a* model for a town (the basic elements of which are seen in Figure 11.1) maps out for the public an ideal mid-century-built environment and *how life could be lived* in a social democracy. Diagrams and plans are a matter of discourse, write Osborne and Rose (1999), that intervene in concrete urban space *and* human existence. Each projects an ideal of urban space that intensifies immanent civic *virtues* and pacifies *dangers* according to the dominant mode of governance (Osborne & Rose, 1999). The problem as it is posed in the school bulletins is that most sizeable New Zealand towns were not fit for purpose, having been designed by 'surveyors in England who had no knowledge of this country' on the principle of finding 'the easiest way of cutting up land', limiting rather than enhancing leisure activities. *Better Towns* informs readers that:

> If we want to improve our New Zealand towns, therefore, we must first analyse their purpose and function, to make up our minds how we can make our surroundings help us lead more useful and enjoyable lives. For until we do this, we shall continue to spend unnecessary time in trains and trams and buses, and to lack space for games or the quiet enjoyment of leisure.

(pp. 1–2)

This perspective is echoed in 'Who Wants Community Centres?' in the Architectural Centre's magazine *Design Review*, which identifies 'a growing desire for community life and activity' among New Zealanders. Having achieved material needs (houses, cars and a wireless) the author (echoing arguments in teacher's journals) suggests people seek other ways of achieving happiness. 'We have holidays with pay, but do we know how to use our leisure time? Maybe this is the root of the desire for more "community"'. How will such happiness be achieved? '*This* is the planner's contribution' (1949, pp. 3–4).

A challenge for town planners was to balance the capacity for individuals to live useful and enjoyable lives, whilst enabling operations between different components of a town to run smoothly. In the second diagrammatic sketch in *Towns to Live In*, the positioning of the park adjacent to and surrounding the town centre—now symbolised by a heart—reveals the association of leisure with active citizenship but also the conjunction of commerce with community. The heart is where municipal buildings (town hall and council rooms) sit alongside those for recreation (cinema, library, community centre, hall and bowling green) and shops. That the centre *is* a heart (rather than the circle in Figure 11.1) signifies that one goal is to build a *healthy town* using an analogy with the human body; this is expanded on the following page of the bulletin, with a (male) human form representing the civic body and major arteries signifying roads. The plans reflect the dilemma that roads posed to mid-century planners: they were unsafe, so neighbourhoods and playing children need protection from them, but they were also the veins and arteries vital for keeping the circulation of commerce flowing, the heart pumping. The message in the bulletins is that roads, if planned carefully, can be worked *with* to create better towns—they are an example of an urban danger that requires pacifying (for individual health) but not eradicating (for a healthy town).

While the association in *Towns to Live In* of the urban body with the corporeal is not new, the town-as-body analogy is modified in this mid-century text in line with what Osborne and Rose (1999) term the *good government* of urban space to promote health in its citizens. Promoting health in the 1940s involved modifying urban space to foster the *right kind* of habits and behaviours, amplifying 'virtuous social forces' and reducing those considered destructive or damaging (Osborne & Rose, 1999). *Te Aro Replanned* imagined a place that promised a *full life* (Cox, 1948) but would also *form a better sort of citizen*. As John Cox, head of the Town Planning Division and member of the Centre, asked of the city, 'What kind of people does it tend to produce?' (Te Aro Re-Planned, 1948, p. 4).

Urban play on 'Our Street'

Brian Sutton-Smith's (1949c) 'Our Street' offers a counterpoint to the narrative of planned urban space promoted in the school bulletins although, like these, it too is a SPB text. The protagonists are bored city boys with mildly destructive tendencies—they pick at flaking paint on an old villa porch, use a picket fence as wicket and break a neighbour's property during a cricket game gone awry—which result in a visit from the local policeman. Unusually, the story was pulled from the *School Journal* after its third issue because of complaints about the boys' slang and (what seemed) the glamourisation of their behaviour (O'Brien, 2007). The author was at the time a teacher, researching children's play (Sutton-Smith, 1981, 1990). In *Education*, Sutton-Smith wrote that 'Our Street' represented the real play and vernacular of local children based on his own observations and in keeping with the new education pedagogy of SPB (Sutton-Smith, 1949b). The stories were originally written to introduce vandalism into class discussion after an occurrence at the school, to promote open conversation 'without tension'. According to Sutton-Smith, the 'matter of social discipline' is not easily resolved, as most 'anti-social behaviour of children is perfectly reasonable in the over-organized and restricted environment in which they find themselves'. Destructive acts are framed as *responses to* socialisation forces: 'In imposing a pattern on un-patterned human nature, we inevitably restrict and curb. Just as inevitably, therefore, we must sometimes expect the resulting and apparently irrational outbursts' (Sutton-Smith, 1949b, p. 50).

The setting of 'Our Street' is central Wellington: not the imagined organised environment of *Te Aro Replanned* but a lived-in cityscape known by the 1940s for its dilapidated and overcrowded housing and children playing on the dirty street (Schrader, 2005). This was the zone from which the government aimed to remove families, to be resettled in the Hutt Valley housing schemes and planned suburbs, reflecting what Schrader terms a 'universal belief that safe suburban backyards, not city streets, were the best place for children' (2005, p. 34). However, unlike the bulletins which look forward to *better* towns, 'Our Street' revels in the run-down urban environment, providing a counter-narrative to the improvement agenda; here, the old street provides opportunities for play. Whereas the neat and orderly plans and diagrams of the bulletins represent what Osborne and Rose refer to as a 'governmental dream of a purified, hygenic, moral space' (1999), the dilapidated colonial houses and broken fences in Juliet Peter's illustrations for 'Our Street' (Figure 11.2) represent streets the planners imagined razing in *Te Aro Replanned*—only here they are comfortably ramshackle rather than vice-ridden. All cities have these places, according to Osborne and Rose (1999), where an *unsocial sociability* emerges to counter a governmental ideal. Whilst governments might try to organise and therefore restrict the immanent forces of urban sites, intensifying some and weakening others according to the dominant ideology, cities will continually counter them (Osborne & Rose, 1999). 'Our Street' acknowledges the urban zones which make anti-social forms of play possible, the places that resist the restrictive patterns of

239

Well, one day they had the hard ball and decided to have a real 'test' match with innings and sides. Usually they just played 'Puttings out goes in' and 'tippeny-runs'. This time Alan and Pat, who lived at the top of the street, came down and played. Smitty tried to get Curly to play, too, but he wouldn't play unless they used a soft ball. So Alan and Smitty and Horsey played Pat and Gormie and Brian.

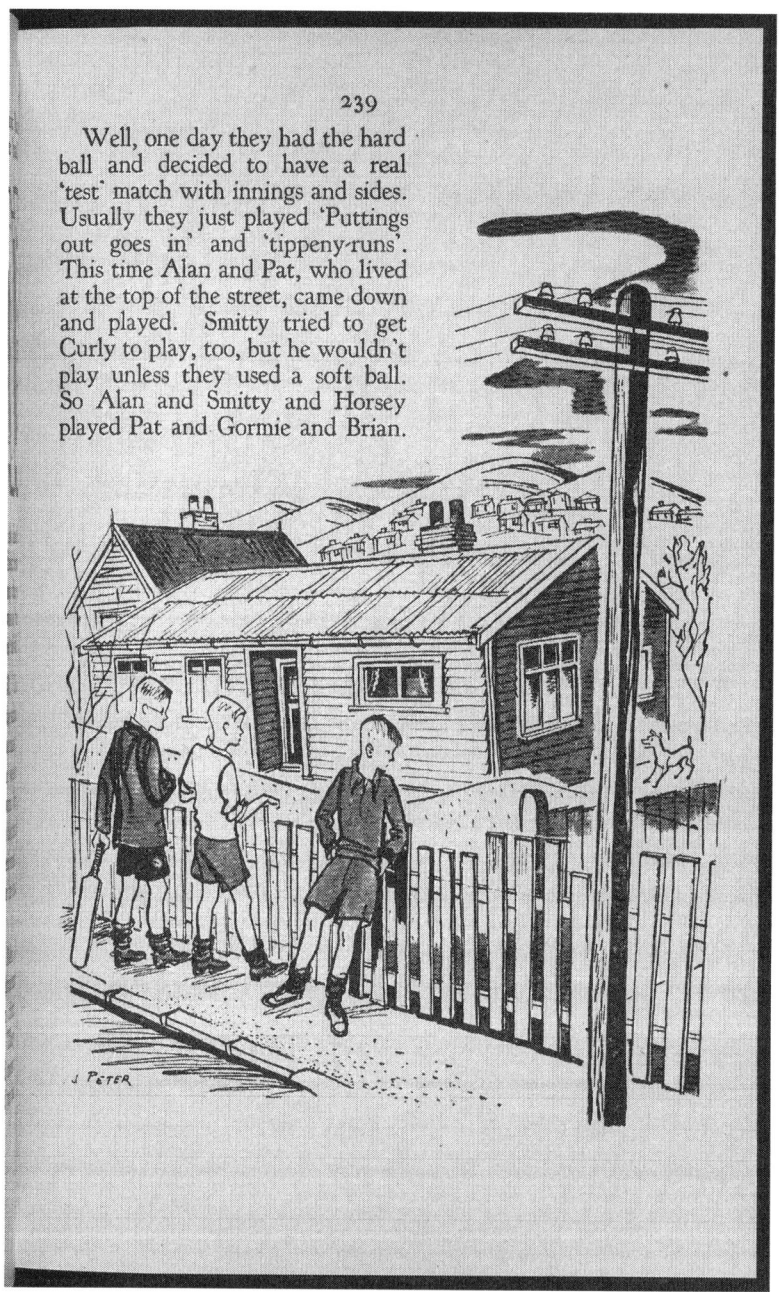

(caption on next page)

FIGURE 11.2 Illustration, 'Our Street'.

Source: Sutton-Smith (1949c). Our street. *School Journal*, *43*(6–8), p. 239. School Publications Branch, Department of Education. Courtesy of Te Tāhuhu o te Mātauranga/Ministry of Education.

organised leisure pursuits and *social sociability* of suburban community centres and games courts.

Sutton-Smith's story for the *School Journal* is not *just* about play or vandalism; rather it contests the ubiquity of modernist planning and the restrictive nature of the built environment promoted by the Ministry of Works and the Architectural Centre. A letter by Sutton-Smith rejecting the universality of modernist values, published in the Architectural Centre's journal *Design Review* (Sutton-Smith, 1949a) supports this claim. His argument in the journal is echoed in 'Our Street' which portrays a homely working-class city street, under threat from planners. Peters' illustrations (Figure 11.2) contribute by utilising the urban vernacular *Design Review* purports to despise—the 'bony telephone poles' (Building Review, 1948, p. 4) evoke the city environment that the empty clean modernist streets in *Better Towns* and *Towns to Live In* replace. Both illustration styles can be traced to *Design and Living* (1947), a curriculum booklet for the Army Education Welfare Service (AEWS) by then-Ministry of Works planner and architect (and muse of the Architectural Centre) Ernst Plishke, whose booklets on planning and housing for the AEWS (Plishke, 1943, 1947) were the inspiration for school texts on planning (Kelly, in press). Plishke's illustrations in these texts convey the problems with the old towns that the new will resolve: 'Typical Result of Uncontrolled Development of Industrial Districts' depicts New Zealand's version of a *slum* with Victorian villas crowded on grid-like roads with obtrusive and unsightly power lines (Plishke, 1947, pp. 72–73).

Sutton-Smith's interest in the changing nature of children's play and its relationship to the physical environment informs 'Our Street'. At the time of writing, he was beginning his lifelong research on the subject; his socio-historical account of play in Aotearoa traces a shift from games defined by the 'physical license of the 19th century', which 'helped produce a child individually autonomous in his management of the physical environment', to games of the mid-20th century reframed by the rapid rise in organised sports (Sutton-Smith, 1981, p. 289). Team sports and community centres, which children attended with adults, radically impacted the nature of play, according to Sutton-Smith: 'The effect of all this organized play can be observed in the playground' (1981, p. 265). According to his piece in *Education*, 'Our Street' represents *actual* games and language of New Zealand children in the late 1940s, in keeping with the new education philosophy of School Publications (Sutton-Smith, 1949b). The dispute over the story which resulted in its removal from the *Journal* highlights a dilemma at the heart of the Branch's pedagogy, shaped simultaneously by a goal to form orderly sociable citizens *and* to show (or even celebrate) the occasional *unsocial* sociability in actual lives of city children.

Contented space of organic sociability or diagram of urban governmentality? *Better Towns*

By introducing children to the principles of town planning, the school bulletins enact the Ministry of Works' goal to educate citizens of a social democracy 'in an intrinsically spatial field' (Osborne & Rose, 1999, p. 748). As social studies texts, the bulletins encourage the new generation to understand themselves as citizens of social democratic communities, reconciling them to the responsibilities associated with that role along with a promise of a good life—which in mid-century Aotearoa was framed in *social* terms. Reading the school bulletins alongside Osborne and Rose (1999), I was struck by their account of the *eudaemonic city* or *spatial projection of social happiness*. According to this argument, the city gets reshaped by an *enlightened administrative imagination* or group of experts that are something like a Town Planning Division within a Ministry of Works: 'men who have thought a great deal about how to plan towns' as *Better Towns* puts it. Various models of eudaemonic cities appear in the school bulletins, including Le Corbusier's Skyscraper city and a diagram of a Reilly town in *Towns to Live In*. The latter is a version of the Garden City, an influential 'diagram of urban governmentality' according to Osborne and Rose (1999) which, as Ben Schrader (2005) outlines, informed the design of suburbs built by the New Zealand Labour government in the 1930s and 1940s. Many state housing suburbs in Aotearoa are based on the model of the repeating cul-de-sac which slows down cars, creating and safely enclosing a shared community space—referred to in *Better Towns* as a *public living room*. It is an imaginary urban space in which immanent energies are tamed and community flourishes. The garden city provided a model for urban space intersected by both capitalism and socialism, according to Osborne and Rose (1999); it certainly held appeal for New Zealand planners juggling productivity, prosperity and economic recovery with moderate socialist agendas.

The town plan on the cover of *Towns to Live In* appears as a double-page spread in *Better Towns*. The plan depicts the Ministry of Works' township for Upper Hutt, versions of which appear in government texts, including Plishke's *Design and Living* (1947), as well as an article in *Design Review* presenting the Ministry's plans for the 'Upper Hutt City Centre' (1949, p. 4). I see this plan as representing the governmental dream of modern urban space within the ideological frame of New Zealand's social democracy of the 1940s. It depicts what Plishke terms 'architectural planning based on the co-ordination of every kind of communal activity' (1947, p. 84). The plan has the essential elements of the original diagrammatic sketch I began with: civic and recreational functions are closely aligned with the town centre flanked by recreation grounds; the cinema, shops and library sit alongside the town hall and municipal offices; major roads are relegated to the perimeter.

Another version of this plan forms the final page of *Better Towns* (Figure 11.3)—the part of a school bulletin reserved for the 'Things to do' and 'Things to discuss' sections written by School Publications' staff, who were well versed in new education pedagogy and aimed to foster active engagement with the texts' key messages. Here, collage is introduced, bringing energy into what is otherwise a static plan and showing cut-out photographs of various sizes of people *doing things*: a runner, cricketer, and golfer; a violinist and pianist; a typist and factory worker. Also pasted into the plan is a group of secondary school students, the intended readers of the bulletin, working collectively around a table. The collage addresses the problem of how

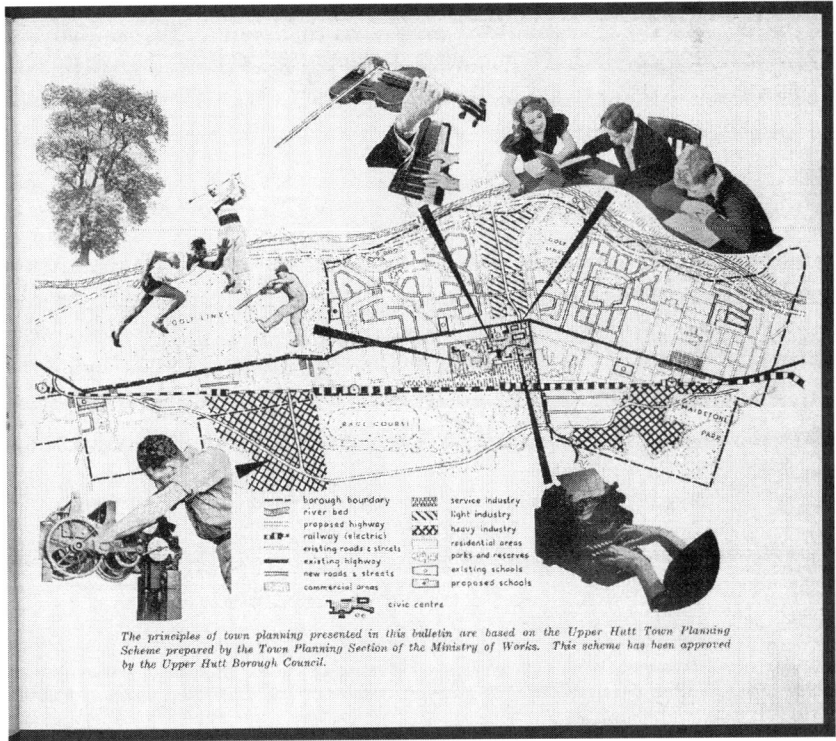

FIGURE 11.3 Collage, *Better Towns*.

Source: Town Planning Section, Ministry of Works and School Publications Branch, Department of Education. (1948a). *Better Towns*. R.E. Owen Government Printer. Courtesy of Te Tāhuhu o te Mātauranga/Ministry of Education.

to manage leisure so that energy is directed in healthy ways and becomes an 'urban virtue' rather than civic disruption: it frames certain types of activities (work, collaboration, sport or music) as desirable and depicts urban spaces that will amplify these and lessen opportunities for other activities, such as picking at paint or playing in dirty streets. It is through these techniques that the texts aim to reconcile the urban dweller to sanctioned and virtuous forms of leisure within a planned spatial environment.

The collage brings *into* The Plan elements of the good life the first Labour government promised to citizens: work and income, housing, leisure and education. Notably, it does not show that other essential—health—at least, not in the form of medical facilities associated with fixing poor health. It does convey *good health* in the form of active participation in leisure, education and work facilitated by the spatial field and contributing to the wellbeing of the individual *and* social body. That is a lesson of *Better Towns*.

Coda: Beyond the plan

To conclude, I draw attention to two subtexts that counter the central normative messages the school bulletins on planning present. The first is to do with the introduction of collage, which also brings other (unintended) associations to the text. Photo-collage was the technique regularly used by town planners to evoke the chaotic nature of the old dilapidated unplanned city: Clark and Walker (2000) show a 1943 collage of bad New Zealand city houses, 'The Case Against Slums', and another from 'Te Aro Re-planned' (p. 75). Collage is used elsewhere in *Better Towns* to illustrate misplaced energy or unchanneled forces with cut-out photographs of oversized cows and cars in incongruous places, clogging up streets and preventing the healthy flow of traffic. Although the collage in Figure 11.3 shows people conducting acceptable activities facilitated by the spatial field, the inclusion of this illustrative technique nonetheless signals the limits of planning, the ways in which *life* exceeds the plan. Whereas the town plan represents a pattern for living that the Ministry hopes will shape New Zealand towns and ways of life, the technique of collage with its out-of-scale interruptions *into* the plan, re-introduces elements (to paraphrase Sutton-Smith (1949b)) that evoke un-patterned human behaviour, in a very School Publications way.

The second subtext is likewise to do with the limits of governmental reach, but also the presence/absence of Māori from these school texts on housing and planning. If the urban street of 'Our Street' contrasts (and counters) the planned communities of *Better Towns* and *Towns to Live In* envisioned by modernist government architects and planners, other spaces fleetingly referred to in Sutton-Smith's story take the reader's attention (momentarily) *further* beyond governmental reach. When one of the boys, Smitty, gets in trouble, he imagines running away to *the bush* and when the boys discuss how to escape punishment, after accidentally breaking someone's property during cricket, they consider absconding to Māori Bush. Both references evoke a place imagined by the boys to be less subject to the conventions of mid-century governmental Pākehā society than modern towns, or even city streets visited regularly by policemen. These references draw attention to the absence of Māori from the town planning bulletins (Kelly, in press), which is indicative of the government's neglect of Māori housing in the 1940s (Harris, 2008). Whereas urban dwellers were targets of housing reform in the 1940s and were relocated to the suburbs, rural Māori became so in the 1960s, when the state aggressively pursued its policy of integration (Harris, 2008). The boys' remarks are also a reminder that Te Aro was once a pā site for Taranaki and Ngāti Ruanui, before there were British surveyors with their grids or Ministry/Centre planners with modernist diagrams imposing western norms of *how to live* through reshaping the built environment.

Acknowledgements

All images are printed with permission from Te Tāhuhu o te Mātauranga/ Ministry of Education.

References

Beeby, C. (1957). Introduction. In P. Wells (Ed.), *The New Zealand School Publications Branch* (pp. 5–7). UNESCO Educational Studies and Documents 25. UNESCO.

Building Review: A group of four shops at Naenae, Lower Hutt. (1948). *Design Review, 1*(1), 4.

Burke, C., & Jones, K. (Eds.). (2014). *Education, childhood and anarchism: Talking Colin Ward.* Routledge.

Caution—Planners at Work. (1946, June 4) *National Education, 28,* 166.

Clark, J., & Walker, P. (2000). *Looking for the local: Architecture and the New Zealand modern.* Victoria University Press.

Clarke, B. (1949). What a sixth form thinks. *Education, 2*(4), 56–59.

Cox, J. (1948). A town planning exhibition. *Landfall, 2*(2), 132–136.

Daley, C. 2003. *Leisure and pleasure: Reshaping and revealing the New Zealand body, 1900–1960.* Auckland University Press.

de Oliveira, F.L. (2015). Abercrombie's green-wedge vision for London: The County of London Plan 1943 and the Greater London Plan 1944. *Town Planning Review, 86*(5), 495–518.

Education must have a plan. (1946, November 1). *National Education, 28,* 324.

Engels, F. (1845/2003). The great towns. In R.T. LeGates, & F. Stout (Eds.), *The city reader* (pp. 58–66). Routledge.

Harris, A. (2008). Concurrent narratives of Māori and integration in the 1950s and 60s. *Journal of New Zealand Studies, 6–7,* 139–155.

Kelly, F. (in press). *Houses to Live In*: Planning social democracy in New Zealand school texts. *History of Education.*

Kozlovsky, R. (2013). *Architectures of childhood: Children, modern architecture and reconstruction in postwar England*. Ashgate.

LeGates, R., & Stout, F. (Eds.). (2005). *The city reader*. Routledge.

Macdonald, C. (2011). *Strong, beautiful and modern: National fitness in Britain, New Zealand, Australia and Canada, 1935–1960*. Bridget Williams Books.

Mort, F. (2012). Fantasies of metropolitan life: Planning London in the 1940s. *Journal of British Studies, 43*(1), 120–151.

Mumford, L. (1961/1989). *The city in history: Its origins, its transformations and its prospects*. Harcourt Brace Jovanovich.

New Zealand Department of Education. (1944). *The post-primary curriculum: Report of the Committee appointed by the Minister of Education in November, 1942*. Government Printer.

O'Brien, G. (2007). *A nest of singing birds: 100 years of the New Zealand School Journal*. Learning Media.

Osborne, T., & Rose, N. (1999). Governing cities: Notes on the spatialisation of virtue. *Environment and planning: Society and space, 17*(6), 737–760.

Plishke, E. (1943). About houses. *New Zealand Services Current Affairs Bulletin 1*(20). Department of Internal Affairs.

Plishke, E. (1947). *Design and living*. Army Education Welfare Service, Department of Internal Affairs.

Rose, N. (1999). *Governing the soul: The shaping of the private self*. Free Association Books.

Schrader, B. (2005). *We call it home: A history of state housing in New Zealand*. Reed Publishing.

Sutton-Smith, B. (1949a). A matter for agreement. *Design Review, 2*(2), 23–24.

Sutton-Smith, B. (1949b). Our street. *Education, 2*(2), 49–51.

Sutton-Smith, B. (1949c). Our street. *School Journal, 43*(6–8). School Publications Branch, Department of Education.

Sutton-Smith, B. (1981). *A history of children's play: The New Zealand playground, 1840–1950*. New Zealand Council of Educational Research.

Te Aro Re-planned: A Study in Teamwork. (1948). *Design Review, 1*(2), 1–4.

Town Planning Section, Ministry of Works and School Publications Branch, Department of Education. (1948a). *Better towns*. R.E. Owen Government Printer.

Town Planning Section, Ministry of Works and School Publications Branch, Department of Education. (1948b). *Towns to live in*. R.E. Owen Government Printer.

Upper Hutt Community Centre. (1949). *Design Review, 1*(5): 4.

Who wants community centres? (1949). *Design Review, 1*(5): 3–4.

PART 4

Routines and disciplinary practices

12

GLIMPSES INTO THE BLACK BOX OF SCHOOLING

Continuities and discontinuities in 'gymnastics between the desks', the 1880s–1970s

Marta Brunelli

The school desk, as a real 'icon of the pedagogical materiality and the school culture' (Depaepe et al., 2012, p. 50), has over the past two decades given rise to many studies demonstrating how it has been given multiple functions in parallel with the evolution of pedagogical theories and school practices. Historians of education, architecture, school hygiene and school industries have increasingly explored the history and functions performed by this piece of school furniture: as a device aimed at rationalising school spaces for modern schooling (De Giorgi, 2014; Hnilica, 2003, 2010, 2020; Schoning, 1998); as an educational-hygienic apparatus for disciplining bodies and minds (Herman, et al., 2011; Hnilica, 2003; Moreno Martinez, 2005, 2006; Nakayama, 2012; Peyranne, 1999); and as the product of emerging school industry (Depaepe et al., 2012; Meda, 2016, 2018; Müller, 1998; Müller & Schneider, 1998).

There is however a further dimension that should be explored—which would give concrete and visible shape to what Burns et al. (2020) have defined as the 'curriculum of the body', the range of teaching/learning activities 'organized around the bodies of children'—and that is the gymnastic function of the school desk. In the 19th century, in fact, this object was drawn upon to serve as gymnastic equipment in schools, especially in Italy where the advent of mass schooling highlighted the importance of providing students with gymnastics that was easy to perform in the classroom from the early stages of elementary education, and without using a gym (Brunelli & Meda, 2017). Such activity was primarily intended as a necessary break after long hours of mental work and motionless sitting posture: two conditions that characterised the modern school years as the 'sitting years'—an expression the Austrian orthopaedist Adolf Lorenz coined in 1888 when analysing hygiene issues linked to school desks (Hnilica, 2020, p. 151).

DOI: 10.4324/9781003288671-17

However, this practice of gymnastics has remained relatively marginalised in the official history of school practices, and somehow forgotten both in collective and individual school memories, hidden inside the so-called 'black box of schooling' (Braster et al., 2011). In Italy, such gymnastics has rarely been the object of a systematic literature, except for the research by Gaetano Bonetta on the history of bodily education (1990), by Mirella D'Ascenzo (1997, 2010, 2018) on the gymnastics teacher Emilio Bauman, and by Paolo Alfieri (2013, 2017) on the introduction of gymnastics in Italian schools. Usually explored as a 19th-century practice, and 'an Italian speciality' responding to the aims of nationalisation as well as the physical and moral regeneration of young Italians (Bonetta, 1990, 2009), recent studies have not only revealed that this gymnastics persisted after the Second World War (Scaglia, 2011) and even up to 1970 (Brunelli & Meda, 2017), but also that it had connections with similar practices carried out abroad and related to Swedish and German gymnastic traditions (Brunelli & Meda, 2017, pp. 185–186). The current aim is to analyse how an Italian 'curriculum of the body' was constructed around the gymnastic use of school desks, and how it evolved (or did not) in a country that has always been characterised by slow modernisation in social, economic and cultural ambits (school included). Finally, we examine which pedagogical ideas led this practice to extend past the 19th century and reach the threshold of the 1970s.

The birth of gymnastics between school desks in Italy

Following the Unification of Italy, the young nation brought together populations that were diverse in terms of literacy rates, socio-economic conditions and perception of the new state. The task of 'making Italian citizens' required in school an educational action able to combine alphabetisation with the construction of a solid ethical conscience imbued with bourgeois virtues as a basis for the national identity (Ascenzi, 2009; Ascenzi & Sani, 2016; Chiosso, 2011; Fiorelli, 2012; Morandini, 2003; Soldani & Turi, 1993; Scotto di Luzio, 2007).

The school, however, would have to take on another task: that of relieving the miserable health conditions of young Italians. The high percentage of frail and sick young people emerging from the responses to the first military drafts from 1862 to 1877, combined with the results of the parliamentary *Inquiry on the Italian agriculture and the conditions of the agricultural class* carried out between 1877 and 1887, revealed situations of poverty and malnutrition across Italy. Therefore, a universal education system aimed at physically and morally regenerating the Italian people (Bonetta, 1990) became the prime concern of a political class that needed a population able to physically cope with the civil and military commitments required by the nation (Mosse, 1996). In schools, health experts focussed on how to provide healthy school environments (including hygienic school desks) designed to facilitate class-room work, in order to support the healthy development of children's bodies and prevent school disease.

Despite this, explicit attention towards gymnastics emerged slowly among Italian educational policymakers. The first school law (the 1859 *Casati Law* of the Sardinia Kingdom) was in fact primarily concerned with language and moral education and no compulsory physical activity was envisaged in ele-mentary schools. It was only in 1878 that the *De Sanctis Law* (n. 4442, 7 July 1878), with the attached *Regulation, Programs, and Instructions for Gymnastic Teaching in Schools* (Royal Decree n. 4677, 16 December 1878), introduced gymnastics in the elementary school as an obligatory activity for boys and girls alike. On this occasion, *gymnastics between school desks* was specifically imposed for the first two elementary classes (the so-called 'lower order') to be carried out 'daily, repeatedly and for a few minutes at a time, to obtain the double advantage of recreating the minds of children..., and sat-isfying the need for movement, so natural at that tender age' (Ferrari & Morandi, 2015, p. 98). The 1878 Programs for the lower classes specified, in fact, that gymnastics between school desks should be performed (Ferrari & Morandi, 2015, p. 99):

a at the beginning of each lesson;
b after writing exercises;
c whenever considered useful to allow a little rest;
d at the end of each lesson as preparation for going out.

This commitment to gymnastics was achieved thanks to the experimental work carried out by some Italian gymnastics teachers and especially by Emilio Baumann, who, after testing the first exercises in Bologna schools, spread the practice through his seminal books: *Gymnastic Handbook for Primary Teachers* (1867), *Physical Education in Schools, Especially Elementary* (1873) and *Programs of Gymnastics Between School Desks for the Three Male and Female Popular Classes for Bologna Schools* (1877). Despite being initially at variance with the Turinese movement (inspired by Rudolf Obermann, the founder in Italy of a military-style educational gymnastics), gymnastics between school desks was accredited at the Fifth Congress of Gymnastics held in Florence in 1874, which paved the way for its introduction in schools in 1878 (Alfieri, 2013, 2017; D'Ascenzo, 1997, pp. 147–150; D'Ascenzo, 2010; Ferrara, 1992, pp. 55–69).

From that time on, an increasing number of dedicated manuals was pub-lished in coincidence with the main steps of this acknowledgement process. Felice Valletti, a representative of the Turinese school, not only began dedi-cating sections of his manuals to exercises in the classroom but also together with Baumann wrote the 1886 *Gymnastics School Programs* which consecrated such gymnastics in elementary schools. In addition to dedicated booklets, a large production of more general gymnastics handbooks containing sections on gymnastics between desks equally attests to the spread of this practice after 1878, such as the *Gymnastic Manual for Elementary Teachers* (1879) by the teacher and advocate for a hygienic approach to motor exercises Francesco Ravano; or Giuseppe A. Silvestri's *Manual of Educational Gymnastics for Girls' Elementary Schools of the Kingdom* (1881).

From 1874 to 1886, the traditional ethical-militarist gymnastic approach—characterised by military exercises, collective choreographies and 'regulatory exercises' aimed at forming a disciplined and strong citizen-soldier—was gradually joined by a more rationalist attitude. Especially in the early years of elementary school, gymnastics had to meet the physiological needs of youth, offer recreation from intellectual work by counteracting school se-dentariness and educate the pupils' soul and will by providing for better knowl-edge of the self and one's own body (Alfieri, 2017, pp. 117–179; D'Ascenzo, 2010; Morandi, 2015a). In an emerging curriculum of the body, such a mild recreational activity to carry out at school desks seemed to be the perfect com-promise between the traditional aims and a new focus on children and their needs. In addition, it was easy to perform in all schools, even the poorest ones: this exact reason would influence the history and persistence of this practice.

No wonder, then, that it continued to spread despite criticisms raised by gymnasiarchs, teachers and hygienists. This practice was in fact denounced as insalubrious by the promoters of open-air games and sports such as the physi-cian Angelo Mosso who, from the journal *Nuova Antologia* of 16 March 1892, accused gymnastics in the classroom of being a real 'crime' due to the 'dark and unhealthy environments where it is practised' (Mosso, 1892); or the positivist teacher Costantino Melzi who, in his 1899 treatise, *Antropologia Pedagogica*, condemned the damages caused by lifting 'microbes and bacilli from the floor and from the bench into the air, which is then breathed' (p. 137). All Italian teachers, however, had to come to terms with the reality of poorly ventilated school spaces and a lack of gyms, so they made the best of a difficult situation. This was the case with Michelangelo Rustia who, although disagreeing with the ministerial imposition, published his booklet *Short Guide to Regulative Exercise and Gymnastics Between Desks* (1876), which only contained selected exercises that he considered the least harmful. Similarly, in the teachers' magazine *L'Osservatore Scolastico*, the female gymnastics teacher Salvadorita Dasara declared in a teacher training conference that any 'zealous teacher' would manage to find 'a small entrance hall, a corridor, a waiting room' where little girls could perform at least some movement 'while waiting for schools to expand and municipalities to provide needed spaces' (1882, p. 693). Unfortunately, such underdeveloped conditions of gymnastics in Italian schools would persist for a long time, being the result of a combination of causes: scarce government funds, economic inability of municipalities to build schools and gyms, a lack of trained teachers, and finally the low regard in which gymnastics and gym teachers were generally held by families (Elia, 2018; Scotto di Luzio, 2004).

Gymnastics between school desks in the new century

The Royal Decree n. 914 of 26 November 1893 promulgated new *Instructions and Programs for Gymnastic Teaching*, in which the expression 'educational gymnastics' was replaced with 'physical education', to highlight a new curriculum of the body built around the concept of outdoor games and activities and aimed at promoting health, strength and dexterity from the earliest age. The programs seemed to scale down the role of gymnastics between the desks, replacing the practice in infant schools with various games (gardening, games with toys and suchlike) to be played in the open air 'when the weather permits'. For elementary schools, it was clearly stated that:

> Exercises between school desks should be limited to those that, are either indispensable preparation for outdoor movements, or serve to accustom the ear to rhythm, or loosen the limbs and reorder circulation, or warm up the hands and feet, with movements that do not imply lifting the whole foot off the floor: therefore, hopping or marching in place in the schoolroom is not allowed.
>
> (Ferrari & Morandi, 2015, p. 115)

The most innovative indications were not effectively implemented because many teachers were not adequately prepared (Bonetta, 1990, pp. 123–137; Morandi, 2015a; Ragazzini, 2001) and, consequently, the traditional manuals on gymnastics between desks kept on being published. Dalla Dea's *Between School Desks*, first published in 1893, was reprinted in 1895 in a 'third revised and expanded edition' alongside a new manual by the same author: *Inside and Outside the Desks: Small Theoretical-Practical Guide of Exercises and Gymnastic Games to be Performed in the Classroom and in the Gym, Prescribed by the Programs …of 26 November 1893*; Valletti's 1886 *Manual of Gymnastics for Schools, for Girls' Schools and Kindergarten*, presenting exercises at school desks as particularly suitable for girls and boys, was reprinted in 1894 and 1896.

A similar situation occurred in the years following the 1909 *Law on Physical Education and Teachers* (Law n. 805, 26 December 1909) and the 1914 *Instructions, Programs and Hours for Infant Schools and Kindergartens* (Royal Decree n. 27, 4 January 1914), where we find an explicit call to female educators 'not to turn the young into soldiers', 'to usually perform open air gymnastics' and, only whenever forced to perform indoor gymnastics, 'to avoid practicing real gymnastics between school desks' (Ferrari & Morandi, 2015, pp. 138–139).

Once again, the reality was different, and the usefulness of this gymnastics continued to be praised, as seen in contemporary magazines like *La Lettura* of November 1908, which included an anonymous report (translated from the Berliner journal *Die Woche* n. 10, 1908) on gymnastic exercises performed in the classroom by a Prussian teacher (i.e. Fritz Schmale) as winter workouts or as an interlude between lessons. Based on the Swedish gymnastic system combined with the German tradition, this practice was perceived as an aid to combat tuberculosis, musculoskeletal disorders and school diseases.

The enduring interest of Italian teachers in the gymnastic use of the school desk is demonstrated by the continuous flourishing of manuals: old ones (such as Valletti's *Manual of Gymnastics for Schools, for Girls' Schools and Kindergarten*, reissued in 1902 and 1914) alongside new ones by Ettore Patini (*Compensatory or Balancing Gymnastics and Gymnastics Between School Desks*, 1909), Luisa Grisolia (*The Elementary Gymnastic Exercises in the Gym and Between the Benches*, 1913) and Camillo Viganò (*Gymnastics Between School Desks, for Voice and Piano*, 1914). The continuing promotion of such old-style gymnastics can be attributed not only to the infrastructural deficiencies, but—as explained in 1916 by the young gymnastic teacher Maria Susanna Giavelli—also to educators who believed in the superiority of traditional methodical gymnastics over free exercises, games or sport: 'because here in Italy, besides achieving the hygienic goal, we still tend to educate the spirit and especially the will, i.e. to form the character' (Giavelli, 1916, p. 958). Therefore, when the fascist regime began redesigning a new curriculum of the body, gymnastics between desks was still a strongly rooted real.

Fascism and gymnastics between school desks: A conflicting curriculum of the body

Fascism marked the return to an ethical-militaristic approach to gymnastics, considered crucial in raising healthy Italians, educated in military values of obedience and sacrifice for the fatherland. The fascist myth of the body (Barbanera, 2016; Gori, 2000, 2004; Giorio, 2019) led to the exaltation of physical and sports education (Canella & Giuntini, 2009; Dogliani, 2000; Fabrizio, 1976) which had to be supported by a network of places and opportunities for the training and indoctrination of the young. For this purpose, the regime entrusted the management of physical and sports education to entities outside the school—first, the ENEF -*National Agency for Physical Education*, then the fascist youth organisations ONB-*Opera Nazionale Balilla*, and finally the GIL-*Italian Youth of the Lictor*—and boosted the modernisation of dedicated infrastructures by implementing three strategic actions: (a) to build sports facilities and schools with gyms, courtyards and open spaces as prescribed by the *New Regulations for Designing School Buildings*, issued in 1939 by the Ministry of Education, Giuseppe Bottai (Viola, 2019, p. 18); (b) to modernise schools and gyms with updated equipment produced by national school industries 'to support the State in the healthy battle for the physical education of the Breed', as we read in the *Catalogue of gymnastic equipment* published by the Turinese company Paravia in 1931 (*Catalogo Degli Attrezzi e dei Giuochi Ginnastici*, 1931, p. 3); and (c) to build open-air schools (D'Ascenzo, 2018) as well as marine and mountain colonies (Mira & Salustri, 2019; Nucelli, 2009), which were expressly designed for educating and preventing disease among children from the poorer classes.

Architecture, pedagogy, physical education and medicine collaborated in arranging infrastructures designed to foster the correct physical development of the Italian race while instilling fascist ideology. In the light of such an effort of modernisation, it is jarring that the regime accepted and even promoted gymnastics between school desks, in open contradiction with the new, ideal fascist curriculum of the body promoted by the 1923 Gentile Reform. The 1923 *Programs and Teaching Prescriptions for Elementary Schools* (issued with Ministerial Order 11 November 1923), in fact, basically confirmed the innovative 1893 *Programs*, declaring the superiority of 'collective gym games' to be performed 'in school yards or playgrounds' over class teaching, 'since [games] allow to know the soul of single children and to modify it' (Ferrari & Morandi, 2015, p. 140). In addition, the importance of competition was stressed 'which so closely resembles, in its beneficial effects, the "esprit de corps" of military departments', and brought moral benefits such as:

1 Individual and hierarchical discipline.
2 Care for cleanliness, health and elasticity of the body.
3 Gradual, severe and continuous preparation for exertion.
4 Readiness to help the weaker; spirit of sacrifice in letting the smaller and clumsy ones play; appreciation without envy of others' worth or spirit of emulation.
5 Aptitude for leadership and moral ability to resume the cordial tone of comrade as soon as the office of leader held during play has ceased. (Ferrari & Morandi, 2015, p. 141)

The fascist curriculum of the body combined new hygiene aims with moral and patriotic-militaristic education, meant as a legacy of the 19th-century tradition more than an expression of fascist ideology (Alfieri, P., 2021, p. 74). Contrary to claims and expectations, gymnastics in the classroom—although never mentioned in the programs—continued playing a central role in the daily school practice, as testified by contemporary manuals. In 1933 Serafino Mazzarocchi (Director of the National Academy of Physical Education) published the popular *Physical Education: Handbook Following the Programs for Elementary Teaching*, whose reprints contained, in 1937, eight pages dedicated to gymnastics between desks, which became 27 pages in the 1939 edition. In the same years, workouts at school desks appeared also in other manuals, but the final confirmation of the continued existence of this practice came from two handbooks issued by the aforementioned youth fascist association GIL, directly controlled by the Fascist Party. The first book (PNF-GIL, 1942) published the winning papers by gymnastics teachers who had created workouts 'between desks' (to be executed while sitting) and 'in the classroom', i.e. performed alternately by each half of the class group standing in the aisles between the desks. The second (PNF-GIL, 1943) was a manual openly addressed to teachers, to whom the manifold benefits of the *gymnastics in the classroom* were illustrated (pp. 8–9):

1 It can be done at any time, at the teacher's discretion.
2 It is a useful and restful break for the body and spirit.
3 It avoids restlessness due to enclosure and immobility: therefore, it has a high disciplinary value.
4 It allows for air exchange in the classroom because, during exercises, windows can be opened even in the colder seasons.
5 It is an effective introduction to gymnastics in the gym, as it facilitates the study of small elementary exercises.
6 It allows the study of the nomenclature of the parts of the body and gymnastic terminology.
7 It prevents deformations, correcting bad posture assumed by pupils seated at school desks.
8 It brings balance back to the body parts most sacrificed by immobility.

Authors were conscious of the contradiction with the regime's policies on outdoor education, therefore, the Preface, after mentioning the 'narrowness of many poor classrooms, with no aisles and with irrational desks', highlighted how the handbook would illustrate 'the importance, value and even necessity of gymnastics in the classroom' (PNF-GIL, 1943, p. 3). Indeed, a bitter realisation shines through the manuals mentioned: teachers were aware that—contrary to the loudly proclaimed modernisation—gymnastics between school desks would be the only gymnastics that Italian children could perform in many rural and mountain schools for a long time yet.

The second post-war period in fact saw a revival of gymnastics in the classroom. This practice had initially been cancelled by the 1945 *Teaching Programs for Elementary and Infant Schools* (Ministerial Decree 9 February 1945; Legislative Decree n. 549 24 May 1945), inspired by the Deweyan pedagogist Carleton Washburne, member of the Commission in charge. These programs introduced a modern vision of 'the body as a tool of the soul', and of physical education that—finally associated with moral and civic education—was meant to educate sociality and instil autonomy by 'abandoning the *caporalismo* [vulgar authoritarianism] which had deadened the spirit of youth' (Ferrari & Morandi, 2015, p. 142).

An unexpected turnaround arrived with the *Programs for Teaching Physical Education in Elementary and Secondary Schools* (Decree of the Provisional Head of State n. 383 8 November 1946). Although refusing any militaristic approach to physical education (i.e. public parades, choreographic exercises, etc.) and reasserting the educational value of sport games, the *Programs* were presented in three parts: (a) methodical and preventive-corrective gymnastics; (b) games; and, once again (c) *gymnastics between school desks*. The first two parts were to be implemented for at least one hour per week (increased to two hours for the fourth and fifth classes) and, possibly, outdoors. Regarding the third part, the legislator prescribed 'to perform it several times daily in all classes and more frequently in the lower ones, in order to intercalate study lessons and to reduce the burden of sedentariness and the damage it does to children' (Ferrari & Morandi, 2015, p. 143).

The gymnastic function of school desks was thus reaffirmed, and, in the same year, Mazzarocchi published the first post-war manual dedicated to this practice: *Gymnastics in the Classroom* (Mazzarocchi, 1946), designed as an appendix to complement his main gymnastics handbook for teacher training schools (Mazzarocchi, 1937). After establishing that 'the best gymnastics is that which we do outdoors', Mazzarocchi stated that gymnastics between desks was nonetheless 'a didactic necessity and a practice with considerable merits' (Mazzarocchi, 1946, p. 14). Just a year later the female gymnastics teacher Costantina D'Amato in her *A, B, C of Physical Education* (1947) presented gymnastics in the classroom as integral to activities 'in the gym', and a healthy daily practice necessary for 'allowing children to move and recreate their mental work' and preventing other problems such as 'cold hands and feet in winter' (D'Amato, 1952, p. 81).

The subsequent 1955 *Programs for the Primary School* (Presidential Decree n. 503 4 June 1955) generically indicated, for the first and second grades, 'games and exercises' to be performed in the open air 'if possible': which indirectly confirms the persistence of indoor practices, as corroborated by the reissue of the mentioned manuals (Mazzarocchi, reprinted through 1962; and D'Amato, released in a second edition in 1954). Classroom gymnastics was mentioned, again, by Giorgio Zampori who, in his 1956 manual, *Educational Gymnastics: Practical Guide for Elementary Teachers According to Current Programs*, claimed that it was 'especially appreciable in those schools where the deficiency of suitable rooms impedes normal [gymnastic] practice' (Zampori, 1956, p. 117; see also Lovera, 1958). This situation is confirmed by oral sources: among the interviews collected by Macerata University, there is that of Marialaura Capuzzi, born in 1952, who recalls that during elementary school (i.e. from 1958 to 1963) 'we very often did gymnastics in classroom or in the corridor, we didn't do it in the gym, there weren't many spaces' (Museo della Scuola, 2020, min. 5:52–5:58).

Just as significant is the case of the renowned educationalist Giovanni Calò. Always attentive to the improvement of physical education in schools (Petronelli, 2015; Scaglia, 2011), Calò recommended performing gymnastics between school desks in schools lacking gyms in his widely used *Course of Pedagogy*, written for future teachers. These manuals—especially those by Mazzarocchi and Calò, reprinted until the mid-1960s—formed future generations of teachers who would be called in the years to come to face the most difficult challenge: that of reconciling an evolving curriculum of the body with, on the one hand, still backward school infrastructures, and on the other, the hidden curriculum and related implicit pedagogy that had been instilled in them.

From the 1960s to the 1970s: Towards a new curriculum for the body?

Between the 1960s and 1970s, the Italian school experienced a succession of political, social and cultural innovations. Contrary to the traditional, classist and authoritarian school models, new active, democratic and libertarian experiences were implemented by innovative educators such as Mario Lodi, Fiorenzo Alfieri and Bruno Ciari from the MCE-Movimento di Cooperazione Educativa (Educational Cooperation Movement); Ernesto Codignola, founder in 1945 of Pestalozzi School-City; or Don Lorenzo Milani who, over the years 1954–1967, carried out his experimental Barbiana School in a poor mountain village north of Florence. On a normative level, a real revolution was the establishment of the Unified Middle School in 1962, which cancelled the separation between vocational schools (for the working classes) and high-school education (for the ruling classes), replacing them with a unique school equal for all. In this scenario, however, gymnastics continued to maintain the role of a minor discipline, being entrapped between the fear of evoking the memory of the propagandistic value attributed to it by Fascism, and the need for new epistemological and institutional recognition (Morandi, 2015b, 2018).

Nevertheless, in the cultural climate of 1968, a new vision of the body emerged, combining the cultural stimuli of the time, such as the fight against authoritative models and the implementation of active educational experiences, with what Ivano Gamelli (2011, 2019) calls the 'psychomotor revolution' of the 1970s. Following Psychomotor Education, which was introduced in the 1960s as a form of rehabilitative practice, this approach moulded a new concept of the body, no longer to be regarded as a passive object but as a subject capable of—through the pivotal activity of playing—interacting with the world, building social relations and discovering the self by developing motor mastery.

This new approach merged with the experimentations implemented in the early 1970s by the Group of Bodily Education of the MCE (Alfieri, 1974), as well as the recreational gymnastics in primary schools described by the teachers Imeroni and Margaira (1976). All these educators agreed in reporting the persistence among Italian teachers of an obsolete perception of gymnastics and bodily dimension. This clash between an old and a new curriculum of the body was denounced by Mario Lodi in his article 'How School Beheads Children', which appeared in the newspaper *Paese Sera* on 18 September 1973:

> In classrooms, the 'breaking of the unity of the physical person' takes place. … The aggression happens by 'decapitating' children, whose heads are removed from their bodies and filled with notions. The body, considered a useless tool, is buried in a bench, wrapped in aprons equal for all, on which tradition in many schools hangs a huge ridiculous bow as a garland. And even when the child is called to do gymnastics, with gestures the same for all, commanded from outside as movements for the resuscitation of the paralyzed, his will be a lifeless body. The living body does not make imposed gestures: it sets in motion every faculty of the person to express and communicate ideas, to work, to invent, to sing, to dance, according to his/her inner rhythm that will become collective not by order of an organizer but by vital need. To get an idea of the traditional school's respect for the body, just look at how it is represented in textbooks and on wall posters: it is even sexless. School should no longer mortify the person, no longer reject the body but accept it as an integral part of a whole, as a language and means of relationship with others.
>
> (Lodi 1973/2022, pp. 87–88)

The request for a new vision of the body and a new physical education based on children's free creativity and expression collided both with the prevailing teaching culture and—once again—with the reality of school infrastructure. Iconographic sources from the 1960s and 1970s, such as photographs portraying pupils still performing old-style exercises between school desks, open a real window on the 'black box of schooling'.

Audio–visual sources also offer a precious contribution, for example, the documentary series *Abbasso Evviva l'Educazione Sportiva* (Down with, Hooray for, Sports Education) on sports education in Italy, shot and broadcast by the national television company RAI in 1973. In the first episode of 20 February 1973—emblematically entitled *Il moto in scatola* (Exercises in a Box)—the authors attributed the Italian underdevelopment in sports education to economic and socio-cultural causes such as: 'unsafe or absent gyms' in schools; the shortage of public sports facilities and/or green areas for children; and finally, a 'traditionally hostile to sports' family and social education (Avallone, 1973, min. 2:30–4:46). The voices of educators claiming the importance of playing outdoors or doing sport in schools, clash with video footage representing a classroom where schoolgirls in tracksuit do exercises poised over their wooden school desks (Avallone, 1973, min. 47:15–49:30). A time when the young are no longer considered (to use Mario Lodi's words) 'a head detached from the body' but a 'unitary physical person who needs, and has the right, to use his body as a language to fulfil himself, both at individual and social level', is still to come.

Conclusion

The research confirms how many educational practices have long remained hidden in the 'black box of schooling', such as gymnastics between school desks, which—although considered a 19th-century practice—persisted over the second half of the 1900s. All the various sources analysed—school regulations, gymnastics manuals, teachers' magazines, teacher training manuals, educational essays, oral testimonies and audio–visual sources—converge in attesting to what has been the daily use of the school desk for many generations, finally depicting a dynamic and no longer static 'portrait of the class next to or at their desks', as required by Depaepe et al. (2014, p. 23).

From its experimental introduction in Italian schools in the 1860s, and for more than a century, gymnastics between desks was the subject of judgements fluctuating between condemnation (as a practice considered unhygienic and harmful) and resigned acceptance (as the only gymnastics practicable without gyms or other suitable spaces). In such a scenario, school environments really worked as 'containers' which, far from being 'neutral or passive' (Burke, 2005, p. 490), shaped the school experience of generations of pupils and teachers alike. The latter, in fact, continued for a long time to implement an educational practice deeply rooted in the 'hidden curriculum of the body' that they had assimilated for years: (a) first in their role as pupils; (b) then as pre-service teachers trained in traditional methods and on gymnastic manuals used for a long time; (c) and, finally, as professionals working in still inadequate school spaces. Such reciprocal conditioning between spaces, bodies and pedagogies was at the heart of the persistence of this educational gymnastic practice. Equally persistent was the pedagogical vision which considered, on the one hand, the pupils' body an object of disciplining, and gymnastics as compensatory to sedentary schooling, on the other. However, the reflection carried out during the 1970s sowed a seed that was destined to grow in the following decades, when a debate arose around a 'pedagogy of the body' (Gamelli, 2011), able to overcome an obsolete conception of physical education and make room for a more modern vision of the child's body and the school environment.

References

Alfieri, F. (Ed.). (1974). *A scuola con il corpo*. La Nuova Italia.

Alfieri, P. (2013). 'A quale fine vero e proprio debba rispondere la ginnastica nelle scuole': Emilio Baumann e la manualistica ad uso dei maestri elementari all'indomani della legge De Sanctis. *History of Education & Children's Literature*, 7(2), 195–220.

Alfieri, P. (2017). *Le origini della ginnastica nella scuola elementare italiana: Normativa e didattica di una nuova disciplina*. PensaMultimedia.

Alfieri, P. (2021). Physical education for Italian school children during the totalitarian Fascist regime. *Historia Scholastica*, 7(1), 71–84. 10.15240/tul/006/2021-1-004

Ascenzi, A. (2009). *Education and the metamorphoses of citizenship in contemporary Italy*. Eum-Edizioni Università di Macerata.

Ascenzi, A., & Sani, R. (2016). *Tra disciplinamento sociale ed educazione alla cittadinanza: L'insegnamento dei Diritti e Doveri nella scuola dell'Italia unita (1861–1900)*. Eum-Edizioni Università di Macerata.

Avallone, M. (Director). (1973, February 22). Il moto in scatola (Episode 1) [Documentary series episode]. In *Abbasso evviva l'educazione sportiva*. RAI-Radio Televisione Italiana. Historical Archive Teche RAI, C16890.

Barbanera, M. (2016). *Il corpo fascista: Idea del virile fra arte, architettura e disciplina*. Aguaplano.

Bonetta, G. (1990). *Corpo e nazione: L'educazione ginnastica, igienica e sessuale nell'Italia liberale*. Franco Angeli.

Bonetta, G. (2009). Nelle palestre del Regno: Le vicende della ginnastica educativa nei primi 50 anni dalla legge Casati. *Lancillotto e Nausica*, 39(1), 16–25.

Braster, S., Grosvenor, I., & Pozo Andrés, M.M. (Eds.). (2011). *The black box of schooling: A cultural history of the classroom*. Peter Lang.

Brunelli, M., & Meda, J. (2017). Gymnastics between school desks: An educational practice between hygiene requirements, healthcare, and logistic inadequacies in Italian primary schools (1870–1970). *History of Education Review*, 46(2), 178–193. 10.1108/HER-01-2016-0008

Burke, C. (2005). Containing the school child: Architectures and pedagogies. *Paedagogica Historica*, 41(4–5), 489–494. 10.1080/00309230500165635

Burns, K., Proctor, H., & Weaver, H. (2020). Modern schooling and the curriculum of the body. In T. Fitzgerald (Ed.), *Handbook of historical studies in education* (pp. 1–21). Springer. 10.1007/978-981-10-0942-6_34-1

Canella, M., & Giuntini, S. (Eds.). (2009). *Sport e fascismo*. Franco Angeli.

Catalogo degli attrezzi e dei giuochi ginnastici. (1931). G.B. Paravia & C.

Chiosso, G. (2011). *Alfabeti d'Italia: La lotta all'ignoranza nell'Italia unita*. Sei.

D'Amato, C. (1952). *L'a, b, c. dell'educazione fisica: Guida per gli insegnanti delle scuole elementari*. (2nd reprint of the 1st ed.). G.B. Paravia & C.

Dasara, S. (1882, September 5). L'associazione pedagogica in Sassari. *L'Osservatore Scolastico*, 17(44), 690–694.

D'Ascenzo, M. (1997). *La scuola elementare nell'età liberale: Il caso Bologna, 1859–1911*. Clueb.

D'Ascenzo, M. (2010). Alle origini delle attività sportive nella scuola italiana: La ginnastica 'razionale' di Emilio Baumann (1860–1884). In R. Farné (Ed.), *Sport e infanzia: Un'esperienza formativa tra gioco e impegno* (pp. 194–215). Franco Angeli.

D'Ascenzo, M. (2018). *Per una storia delle scuole all'aperto in Italia*. Edizioni ETS.

De Giorgi, F. (2014). Appunti sulla storia del banco scolastico. *Rivista di Storia dell'Educazione*, *1*(1), 85–98.

Depaepe, M., Simon, F., Herman, F., & Van Gorp, A. (2012). Brodskys hygienische Klappschulbank: Zu leicht für die schulische Mentalität? *Zeitschrift für Pädagogik*, *58*, 50–65. http://hdl.handle.net/10993/7910

Depaepe, M., Simon, F., & Verstraete, P. (2014). Valorising the cultural heritage of the school desk through historical research. In P. Smeyers, & M. Depaepe (Eds.), *Educational research: Material culture and its representation* (pp. 13–30). Springer.

Dogliani, P. (2000). Sport and Fascism. *Journal of Modern Italian Studies*, *5*(3), 326–348.

Elia, D.A. (2018). La formazione dei docenti di ginnastica nell'Ottocento: Nascita di una professione in Italia. *Studi sulla Formazione*, *21*(2), 175–190.

Fabrizio, F. (1976). *Sport e Fascismo: La politica sportiva del regime 1924-1936*. Guaraldi.

Ferrara, P. (1992). *L'Italia in palestra: Storia, documenti e immagini della ginnastica dal 1833 al 1973*. La meridiana.

Ferrari M., & Morandi, M. (Eds.). (2015). *I programmi Scolastici di 'educazione fisica' in Italia: Una lettura storico-pedagogica*. Franco Angeli.

Fiorelli, V. (2012). (Ed.). *La nazione tra I banchi: Il contributo della scuola alla formazione degli italiani tra Otto e Novecento*. Rubbettino.

Gamelli, I. (2011). *Pedagogia del corpo*. Raffaello Cortina.

Gamelli, I. (2019). Bisogna innanzitutto essere corpo: La proposta della Pedagogia del corpo per la formazione dell'educatore. *Giornale Italiano di Educazione alla Salute, Sport e Didattica Inclusiva*, *3*(4), 27–34. 10.32043/gsd.v3i4.148

Giavelli, M.S. (1916, June 30). Dei locali per la educazione fisica. *Rivista di Ingegneria Sanitaria e di Edilizia Moderna*, *12*(12), 135–140.

Giorio, M.B. (2019). La scultura fascista di soggetto sportivo tra bellezza e propaganda ideologica. *Italies*, *23*, 65–80. 10.4000/italies.6979

Gori, G. (2000). Model of masculinity: Mussolini, the 'New Italian' of the Fascist Era. In J.A. Mangan (Ed.), *Superman supreme: Fascist body as political icon—Global fascism* (pp. 27–61). Frank Cass.

Gori, G. (2004). *Italian fascism and the female body: Sport, submissive women and strong mothers*. Routledge.

Herman, F., Van Gorp, A., Simon, F., & Depaepe, M. (2011). The school desk: From concept to object. *History of Education*, *40*(1), 97–117.

Hnilica, S. (2003). *Disziplinierte Körper: Die Schulbank als Erziehungsapparat*. Edition Selene.

Hnilica, S. (2010). Schulbank und Klassenzimmer—Disziplinierung durch Architektur. In R. Egger, & B. Hackl (Eds.), *Sinnliche Bildung? Pädagogische Prozesse zwischen vorprädikativer Situierung und reflexivem Anspruch* (pp. 141–162). VS Verlag für Sozialwissenschaften. 10.1007/978-3-531-92383-3_9

Hnilica, S. (2020). The school bench as a disciplinary apparatus. In G. Griffith, & D. Kuhlmann (Eds.), *What, if anything, is a rabbit? Kari Jormakka, architecture theorist / Gedenkschrift* (pp. 151–170). (Datutop 39). Tampere University.

Imeroni, A., & Margaira, R. (1976). *C'era una volta la ginnastica: Un'esperienza di attività ludico-motoria nella scuola elementare*. Emme Edizioni.

Lodi, M. (1973/2022). Come la scuola 'decapita' i bambini. *Paese Sera*. 1973, September 18. Reprinted in: Lodi, M. (2022). *Cominciare dal bambino: Scritti didattici pedagogici e teorici* (pp. 87–89). Mondadori Libri (ebook).

Lovera, T. (1958). *Educazione fisica: Teoria e didattica per l'istituto magistrale.* Principato Editore.

Mazzarocchi, S. (1937). *Educazione fisica: Manuale redatto sulla traccia dei programmi ufficiali per l'insegnamento elementare* (2nd rev. and enl. ed.). Tipografia Mareggiani.

Mazzarocchi, S. (1946). *Ginnastica in aula per l'insegnamento elementare.* Tipografia Mareggiani.

Meda, J. (2016). *Mezzi di educazione di massa: Saggi di storia della cultura materiale della scuola tra XIX e XX secolo.* Franco Angeli.

Meda, J. (2018). L'évolution du banc d'écolier en Italie de la fin du XIXe siècle à la première moitié du XXe siècle. In M. Figeac-Monthus (Ed.), *Éducation et culture matérielle en France et en Europe du XVIe siècle à nos jours* (pp. 89–108). Honoré Champion.

Melzi, C. (1899). *Antropologia pedagogica.* Tipografia economica.

Mira, R., & Salustri, S. (Eds.). (2019). *Colonie per l'infanzia nel ventennio fascista: Un progetto di pedagogia del regime.* Longo editore.

Morandi, M. (2015a). Corpo e carattere: 'L'educazione fisica' scolastica dall'Unità al secondo dopoguerra. In M. Ferrari, & M. Morandi (Eds.), *I programmi scolastici di 'educazione fisica' in Italia: Una lettura storico-pedagogica* (pp. 20–40). Franco Angeli.

Morandi, M. (2015b). Introduzione: Le burrascose sorti di una disciplina 'speciale'. In M. Ferrari, & M. Morandi (Eds.), *I programmi scolastici di «educazione fisica» in Italia: Una lettura storico-pedagogica* (pp. 11–19). Franco Angeli.

Morandi, M. (2018). Storia di una straniera: L'educazione fisica in Italia. *La Ricerca*, 6(14), 6–11. [Monographic issue: *Corpi intelligenti: La ginnastica a scuola: Pedagogia, ricerca e cultura*]. https://laricerca.loescher.it/storia-di-una-straniera-l-educazione-fisica-in-italia/

Morandini, M.C. (2003). *Scuola e Nazione: Maestri e istruzione popolare nella costruzione dello Stato unitario (1848–1861).* Vita & Pensiero.

Moreno Martínez, P.L. (2005). History of school desk development in terms of hygiene and pedagogy in Spain (1838–1936). In M. Lawn, & I. Grosvenor (Eds.), *Materialities of schooling: Design, technology, objects, routines* (pp. 71–95). Symposium Books.

Moreno Martínez, P.L. (2006). The hygienist movement and the modernization of education in Spain. *Paedagogica Historica*, 42(6), 793–815.

Mosse, G.L. (1996). *The image of man: The creation of modern masculinity.* Oxford University Press.

Mosso, A. (1892, March 16). La riforma della ginnastica. *Nuova Antologia*, 27(2), 237–267.

Müller, T. (1998). Die Entwicklung des schulmöbels als Industrieprodukt. In T. Müller, & R. Schneider (Eds.), *Das Klassenzimmer: Schulmöbel im 20. Jahrhundert* (pp. 9–27). Prestel.

Müller, T., & Schneider, R. (Eds.). (1998). *Das Klassenzimmer: Schulmöbel im 20. Jahrhundert.* Prestel.

Museo della Scuola: Paolo e Ornella Ricca. (2020, October 1). *School memories: Interview with Marialaura Capuzzi.* [Video]. YouTube. https://www.youtube.com/watch?v=5KyvcX4vZGc

Nakayama, I. (2012). Posturing for modernity: Mishima Michiyoshi and school hygiene in Meiji Japan. *East Asian Science, Technology and Society: An International Journal, 6*(3), 355–378. 10.1215/18752160-1727678

Nucelli, E. (2009). *Colonie di vacanza italiane degli anni '30: Architetture per l'educazione del corpo e dello spirito.* Alinea.

Petronelli, G. (2015). *Etica ed educazione fisica in Giovanni Calò.* Il Pozzo di Micene.

Peyranne, J. (1999). *Le mobilier scolaire du XIXe siècle à nos jours: Contribution à l'étude des pratiques corporelles et de la pédagogie à travers l'évolution du mobilier scolaire.* (Publication No. CB05125). [Doctoral dissertation, Université de René Descartes (Paris V)]. Proquest Dissertations & Theses Global.

PNF-GIL (1942). *Concorso per progressione di esercizi ginnastici con attrezzi e per ginnastica fra i banchi: Atti del concorso e lavori premiati.* A. Vallecchi.

PNF-GIL (1943). *Ginnastica nell'aula scolastica.* Società anonima tipografica operaia romana.

Ragazzini, D. (2001). Dalla ginnastica educativa all'educazione fisica nella scuola elementare. In A. Semeraro (Ed.), *L'educazione dell'uomo completo: Scritti in onore di Mario Alighiero Manacorda* (pp. 29–40). La Nuova Italia-RCS libri.

Scaglia, E. (2011). L'educazione fisica nella riflessione pedagogica di Giovanni Calò. *Cqia, 2*(3), 10–24.

Schoning, B. (1998). Die unbewegliche Schulbank und das bewegliche Kind: zu den Auswirkungen der Lebensreformbewegung auf Möblierung und pädagogisches Leben im Klassenzimmer. *Mitteilungen & Materialien, 50,* 37–52.

Scotto di Luzio, A. (2004). Corpo politico e politiche del corpo nella storia dell'Italia unita. Le vicissitudini della 'ginnastica' a scuola. In G. Bertagna (Ed.), *Scuola in movimento: La pedagogia e la didattica delle scienze motorie e sportive tra riforma della scuola e dell'università* (pp. 51–54). Franco Angeli.

Scotto di Luzio, A. (2007). *La scuola degli italiani.* Il Mulino.

Soldani, S., & Turi, G. (1993). (Eds.). *Fare gli italiani: Scuola e cultura nell'Italia contemporanea. Vol. 1: La nascita dello Stato nazionale.* Il Mulino.

Viola, V. (2019). L'edilizia scolastica in Italia ai tempi del Fascismo. *Revista História da Educação, 23,* e82787. 10.1590/2236-3459/82782

Zampori, G. (1956). *Ginnastica educativa: Guida pratica per gli insegnanti elementari e gli allievi degli Istituti Magistrali.* La Scuola.

13

WHO OWNS THE BODY OF THE CHILD?

Human rights and corporal punishment in 1980s Australia

Helen Proctor, Kellie Burns, and David Magro

Corporal punishment in schools—the permissible physical striking or 'caning' by a teacher of the body of a child or young person as punishment for aberrant behaviour—was a hot political topic in Australia during the 1980s. This chapter focuses on how this one specific and very dramatic bodily practice, unusually amongst the myriad impositions on bodies within schools—keeping quiet, staying inside a classroom, lining up, sitting straight, dress rules and so on—broke through the walls of the classroom to become a focus of politicised public contestation about teacher violence and who had rights over the body of the schoolchild. In this chapter, we focus on two elements of the public debate about whether corporal punishment should continue to be allowed inside Australian schools. One is the activity of a grassroots advocacy organisation formed in the 1970s with the aim of achieving a legislative ban and the second is a report on 'Corporal punishment in schools and the Rights of the Child' compiled by the national Human Rights Commission with the aim of 'generating public discussion and comment' (Human Rights Commission, 1983a, p. 1). In previous work, two of this chapter's authors have argued for the utility of focussing on the 'curriculum of the body' in the history of schooling (Burns et al., 2020; also Proctor & Burns, 2017). In this chapter, we describe some of the tactics and strategies of the cane's activist opponents and examine the expression of an array of competing claims over expertise and authority on the matter—from parents and others. We note that the location of this form of discipline inside the school and away from family is a key distinction, and even so it was unclear in the 1980s just how much appetite there was for a state-wide ban (e.g. see Seymour, 1992). Proposals to legislate against corporal punishment of children by family members have little traction in Australia (e.g. see Saunders & Cashmore, 2011).

DOI: 10.4324/9781003288671-18

We situate our account in three main fields of inquiry. First, there is a historical literature of schooling that has, particularly since the translation of Michel Foucault's works into English, thematised discipline, bodily regulation and governmentality (e.g. Gleason, 2018; Hunter, 1994; Kirk, 1998; Norlin, 2018; Rousmaniere et al., 1997). Second, we are interested in the question of schools of this period as a site for community organising (e.g. see Proctor et al., 2023; Yeatman, 1998). In the case of the advocacy group described in the chapter, this organising manifested in a set of activities that were underpinned by an evident confidence that citizens had both the responsibility and the means to influence the policymaking process in a modern democratic state, especially about the nurture of children. Third, public debate about children during the 1980s occurred in the context of historical developments in international commitments to children's human and legal rights, including discussion of the implications of Australia becoming a signatory to and then ratifying the United Nations Convention on the Rights of the Child in 1990 (e.g. Barrett Meyering, 2022; Funder, 1996; Kilkelly & Lundy, 2017).

By the 1980s, corporal punishment was a practice that education people internationally had expressed reservations about for decades and more, abhorring the violence of it and/or preferring the inculcation of what was often called 'self-discipline' (e.g. Dewey, 1916). The hitting of the child's body was a form of punishment that had its own specialist equipment and language, part of yet also distinct from other forms of coercion. The 'cane' was both a commonly used name for the practice of teachers striking children and the long thin stick used as a tool for the purpose. Depending on context the term, 'the cane' can be seen as euphemistic, in that elides what it is used for; the term also makes concrete the literal separation between wielder and recipient that was intended to render the practice of beating children more rational and acceptable than it really ever was. Other terms for the equipment and practice included, in the Australian state of Victoria, 'the strap' (made of leather) (Slee, 1992); in the United Kingdom, 'birching' and 'six of the best' (Human Rights Commission, 1983a), or in Canada, the 'rod' and the 'strap' (Axelrod, 2010). Apparently in the United States, where the equivalent of the cane might be a 'switch' or a 'paddle', one US school jurisdiction distinguished in the 1980s between 'hand spanking', which was permissible, and the use of 'instruments', which was not (Human Rights Commission, 1983a, p. 11).

The real life of the cane is challenging to track. In a history of the banning of corporal punishment in Toronto, Canada, Paul Axelrod (2010) makes use of punishment statistics generated by the bureaucratic reporting requirements of public schools to document the declining use of the cane over the middle decades of the 20th century, the rarity of caning girls, and the substantial variation in numbers of instances between schools. As Scribner and Warnick (2021) point out in a recent historical and philosophical study of punishment in US schools, factual data is elusive for many reasons, not least because of a division between approved practices and the rage and anger that might erupt behind the classroom door. In Australia as elsewhere historical archives sometimes include accounts of punishments that were formally contested by parents or students. These almost by definition were not routine cases but do offer instances where school people and interested others recorded rationales and explanations that were more often tacit. Proctor (2000), for example, describes how a case against one high school teacher in the late 1910s turned on such questions as whether he lost his temper rather than meting out punishment in a planned and rational way, and whether he struck with a fist or an open hand. Holbrook (1997) proposes that most cases of classroom violence were neither reported nor recorded in official documents. In analysing a large collection of oral histories of people who had attended Australian primary schools from the 1910s to the 1950s, she found schools to be violent places with interviewees recalling beatings being delivered for such offences as singing out of tune and misspelling. In a number of accounts, the public shaming and showy performance of caning in front of a class group was integral to the punishment.

Much work criticising or condemning the practice of caning came from the field of child psychology (e.g. Holden et al., 2018; Miller, 1983; Slee, 1995), and by the 1980s the voices of opponents were dominant in the public domain, despite the persistence of the practice they condemned. Even the cane's many supporters, as we outline below, were not so much recommending its use as objecting to its prohibition on various grounds, including teacher and parent rights. Internationally, full legislative abolition gained pace after the United Nations General Assembly adopted the UN Convention on the Rights of the Child, in 1989 (Global Partnership to End Violence Against Children, n.d.-b). According to the UN-affiliated organisation the Global Partnership to End Violence Against Children, by 2022 a total of 136 nation-states offered legislative protection for children and young people against corporal punishment of children in schools (Global Partnership to End Violence Against Children, n.d.-a). This does not include Australia where the outlier is the northern state of Queensland. In Queensland, the use of corporal punishment is proscribed (by policy rather than law) only in government schools while (technically at least) still permitted in private schools (Australian Institute of Family Studies, 2021; Corporal Punishment of Children in Australia, 2023).

The 1980s was the last decade during which corporal punishment was a legal practice in all Australian states. Public debate was animated by the prospect of the introduction of comprehensive prohibitions in several of the school systems administered by state governments, with the first state-wide public-school ban implemented in the state of Victoria during the early to mid-1980s (see Slee, 1992; Slee & Knight, 1992). In New South Wales during the 1980s and 1990s, the cane went from being a routinised disciplinary practice that was institutionalised and inflicted onto thousands of student bodies to something that was legally impermissible, although an initial ban in the mid-1980s implemented by Labor education minister Rodney Cavalier was overturned by his newly elected conservative party counterpart Terry Metherell before being reinstated and extended to all schools during the 1990s (e.g. Seymour, 1992; Slee & Knight, 1992). The next section of the paper introduces and outlines the campaign against corporal punishment in schools by the purposely formed community group, Parents and Teachers Against Violence in Education (PTAVE). After that we attend to the Human Rights Commission (1983a, 1983b) discussion paper, 'Corporal Punishment in Schools and the Rights of the Child', which was apparently drafted in response to an approach by PTAVE (Human Rights Commission, 1983a, p. 2.)

Parents and Teachers Against Violence in Education

Sometime in the late 1970s, the father of a Sydney school student handed himself over to a local suburban police station with a confession. He had 'stolen' the cane used by his son's primary school and buried it in his garden. A faded, undated newspaper clipping shows a grainy photograph of father, son and garden spade as if caught in the act (Power, n.d.). The man, Jordan Riak, was a US academic, employed in Australia for a few years, who apparently became politicised by his discovery that the cane was not only legal in the state of New South Wales, but also in regular use in local public schools. Riak moved back to the United States in the late 1980s and expanded his anti-corporal punishment advocacy. Thirty years later, the Australian origins of his public campaigning were rendered as a well-polished anecdote in an interview he gave to a Californian newspaper (Kurhi, 2008):

> Riak went to the school and asked to see the switch that was used. He then refused to return it.
>
> 'I told the headmaster, "This is a weapon. It has no business in schools, and no business being used on children"'. Riak said. 'Then I called all the media outlets and told them I'm turning myself in to the Paddington Police Station for the theft of government property'.
>
> Riak took the publicity stunt and ran with it, often posing for photographers in his yard, burying the headmaster's switch.
>
> 'Then I'd dig it up again and rebury it when another photographer came by', he said. 'I did it several times and probably still have (the switch) around here somewhere'.

Grassroots community organisers do not always leave many traces in the public record. Our brief account in this chapter of the early years of the group, PTAVE partly relies on the group's own commitment to posterity and partly on its ability to make news that has survived. A detailed although now inert website, 'Project NoSpank', includes a memorial page for co-founder Jordan Riak, who died in 2016, and a historical clippings file. There are traces of PTAVE activity in online media repositories such as the *Sydney Morning Herald* archives and the Australian National Library's 'Trove', and collections of papers deposited in the National Library and New South Wales state libraries. While various historical archives show school parents contesting the treatment of their own children, Riak's story is one of the transformations of the personal into the political via the school—which as an institution is, in this case, a bridging space between the private domain of the family and the public domain of collective policymaking. Part of this process can be seen in his 'first move against corporal punishment', constituting an open letter he wrote in 1975 to the parents of his local public high school in Sydney:

> Two months ago at a meeting of the Dover Heights Parents and Citizens Association a resolution was introduced endorsing the continued use of corporal punishment. There were only eight or nine parents present at the meeting and, except for my dissenting vote, the resolution would have passed unanimously. ... The association's majority decision was primarily influenced by the assumption that [the school Principal's] experience and professionalism would preclude the unfair use of the punishment. ... The cane at Dover Heights Boys' High School is dispensed like aspirin: a cure for everything. It is prescribed at whim and administered with a vengeance.
>
> (Riak, 1975)

In the letter, Riak is frustrated by what he sees as the credulousness of his fellow Parent and Citizens members, and much of PTAVE's work after it was founded in 1978 or 1979 (dates vary) was collecting evidence for the purposes of raising public consciousness and lobbying governments.

PTAVE let it be known via various media outlets that they were collecting data. A 1979 letter to the editor of the NSW Teachers Federation journal signed by Federal Labor Senators Ken Wriedt and Mal Colston, for example, encourages parents to contact PTAVE with their concerns (Wriedt & Colston, 1979). PTAVE also designed and distributed a pro forma 'Child abuse in schools incident report' for the recording of cases (see Human Rights Commission, 1983a; Seymour, 1992). Three such forms were published as an appendix to the 1983 Human Rights Discussion Draft. They make for tough reading. In one case, a Vietnamese migrant student reports being caned for 'playfully' 'flicking water' and for 'misunderstandings' caused by language and cultural differences. The assaults cause emotional injury—especially shame—rather than just fleeting pain: 'It was obvious to the PTAVE informant that Van found his interview a catharsis, a chance to rationally and sympathetically discuss what had happened to him at school'. The second informant is a student teacher who powerlessly witnesses an assault on two disabled children ('slow learners', to use the terminology of the report's authors), who according to 'Julie N.' as a result 'became more hostile' and were 'sent into a "shell"'. She tells a PTAVE interviewer, 'caning was routine' and that she 'believes that some teachers enjoyed doing it'. The third report includes the information that a child's concerned mother was told by a school principal that she was 'overzealous', that he 'doesn't believe in psychology' and that her son was 'playing up to get attention'.

It is likely that PTAVE's activism contributed to both a 1984 public school teacher union (NSW Teachers Federation) resolution calling for the abolition of corporal punishment and the subsequent (1987–1988) state-wide ban (Seymour, 1992). Yet as Brenda Seymour argues in her account of the initial short-lived ban, 'Still, despite the teachers' union pronouncements and PTAVE's thunderings, the community (of parents and educators) was still strongly divided on abolishing the cane' (Seymour, 1992, p. 47).

Corporal Punishment in Schools and the Rights of the Child

This section of the chapter briefly examines a piece of grey literature entitled 'Corporal Punishment in Schools and the Rights of the Child' published in 1983 under the auspices of Australia's nascent human rights bureaucracy (Human Rights Commission, 1983a). A Human Rights Commission had been established in December 1981—which would be succeeded by the Human Rights and Equal Opportunity Commission in 1986—and amongst its earliest projects was the assembling of 'Discussion Draft papers' on various issues. Prepared by project director Dr Helen Ware, the main part of the corporal punishment paper is 17 pages long, with another 12 pages of appendices. It opens with an explanatory introduction informing that it was drafted in response to a request by PTAVE to 'draw the attention of State Ministers for Education to Australia's obligations as a signatory of the International Covenant on Civil and Political Rights' (Human Rights Commission, 1983a, p. 2). This strategy by PTAVE of appealing to the peak national human rights organisation was a long way from the kinds of local disputes over school violence documented in school or department correspondence files. Instead, it declared corporal punishment to be the domain of international rights principles and practices, far removed from the lone teacher wielding a stick in the closed-door classroom or principal's office.

Reading the discussion paper from a poststructural policy analysis perspective (Bacchi & Goodwin, 2016) we ask not only what its conclusions were about the substantive issue, but how the question of corporal punishment in schools was framed as a problem to be addressed by the Commission. It is important that the paper explicitly framed corporal punishment as a currently open question, to be argued for or against, a matter that public opinion could legitimately weigh in on. In 1983, the matter of the abolition of caning discursively permitted an opposing voice. People who rejected bans on corporal punishment in school, or teachers who wielded the cane in the 1980s, were not placed out of bounds—unlike in some of the PTAVE material. At the same time, the paper found that 'it is very hard to find a reasoned argument in favour of the imposition of corporal punishment in schools' and this finding was picked up by the news media (Corporal-Punishment Paper, 1983). The inclusion of an appendix of the PTAVE cases outlined above also weights the argument in favour of a ban.

A question implicitly asked and answered by the paper is the question of what information or evidence might be brought to bear, which kinds of authorities might provide direction. As had been a long tradition in Australia, precedents were sought from overseas—from Britain, Western Europe and the United States. The first authority invoked, other than PTAVE's 'committee of advisers drawn from the Senate, the church and the legal procession' (Human Rights Commission 1983a, p. 2), is the European Court of Human Rights. The paper identifies two cases concerning school students from the United Kingdom in which, essentially, corporal punishment (in each specific context) was found to be either 'degrading' or that parents had the right to object to the practice on philosophical grounds on behalf of their own children. In each case, a lone dissenting voice came from a British judge—a detail salient for settler colonial Australia. Sweden is advanced as an example of the banning of physical punishment at home as well as school. The United States is offered as a place with a mix of practices including some state-level bans. The main part of the paper ends with a 'for and against' summary and a brief interpretation of the *UN Declaration of the Rights of the Child*, the 1959 set of principles which preceded the 1989 Convention on the Rights of the Child in which it proposes that corporal punishment is against the spirit of the Declaration even if not yet enshrined in so many words.

A significant gap in the Human Rights Commission paper is the voice of young people. Except for their appearance in the PTAVE case reports there is no seeking of advice from current or former school students. Their absence is neither noticed nor are they addressed directly within the pages of the document. The authorities are institutional, with certain kinds of formal representative standing. While it would have been surprising to find young people consulted at this time for this kind of document, it is interesting to note that the Human Rights Commission had plans to do exactly that (Human Rights Commission, 1983b, p. 26) although we have not yet been able to find evidence of this further step having been taken.

An emerging tension is whether corporal punishment—unacceptable or not—was a routine sanction that was applied to everyone more or less equally or could be understood politically and sociologically as something that structurally divides and discriminates. PTAVE had queried 'what action the Commission considers should be taken with respect to the A.C.T. Education Authority's regulations on physical punishment' which they maintained discriminated between 'males and females' (Human Rights Commission, 1983a, p. 2). PTAVE's mobilisation of gender as an example of how discipline practices discriminate was likely partly a tactic of using workable angles to achieve a ban but does raise the question of other ways in which discipline was unevenly administered in terms of race and class. Was corporal punishment in schools merely an aberrant, albeit widespread, detail or did it shore up an inequitable institutional structure? Even more than the arguments advocating a ban, the arguments opposing prohibition were framed around the idea that all young people were in the same boat—with a few easily understood exceptions, such as older girls. Glimpses of the implication of corporal punishment in the pro-duction or reinforcement of educational inequality are few, and somewhat buried, but present nevertheless, as in the example mentioned above in the PTAVE data that was appended to the Human Rights Commission paper—the kids flicking water. In the paper itself, it is briefly observed that corporal pun-ishment has become a 'civil rights' issue in the United States (pp. 11–12). In the summary of arguments for a ban, it is argued, 'Whilst middle class boys may accept such punishment as part of the ethics of the school, working class boys may regard it as evidence of the bankruptcy of the school which preaches against violence but also practises it' (p. 15).

At the time of the report's writing, the publication of the *Little Red Schoolbook* (Hansen & Jensen, 1972) in Australia was within recent living memory (see Barrett Meyering, 2022, pp. 103–105), and it offers an inter-esting comparison with both the PTAVE campaigns and the Human Rights Commission paper in terms of what was thinkable and sayable in the time period. This book, the original version of which was published in Denmark in 1969, was best known not only for offering frank advice to school students about sex, but also included many details about students' rights in relation to schools and other authority structures. Its tone and mode were one of direct address to students, encouraging them to become informed and take control of their own lives. A section of several pages describes the continued use of corporal punishment in Australian schools and its popularity with parents despite its ineffectiveness and despite the damage it causes (Hansen & Jensen, 1972, pp. 63–71). The section concludes with this advice: 'You shouldn't put up with continued bad treatment. You're told often enough about your duties. Remember that you have rights too' (Hansen & Jensen, 1972, p. 71). Furthermore, the book argued that the corporal punishment was 'used most frequently on precisely… … the unfortunate kids [who] often show their distress in "abnormal" or "delinquent" behaviour' (Hansen & Jensen, 1972, p. 66) and implied that it was also used disproportionately on working class, immigrant and Aboriginal students (Hansen & Jensen, 1972, p. 67). The authors recommended that school students educate themselves on the topic by reading Jonathan Kozol's 1967 book *Death at an Early Age*, a classic sociological text of the Civil Rights Era in the United States which offered an excoriating account of racialised violence and alienation in an inner-city Boston school (Hansen & Jensen, 1972, p. 68; also Johns, 1997).

Conclusion

In this chapter, we draw attention to ways in which the 1980s history of debates about corporal punishment illuminates the curriculum of the body in modern mass schooling. While individual parents had protested against school violence in the past, the activist group PTAVE claimed expertise over, rather than personal opposition to, this aspect of the professional domain of the school teacher and the school principal. Rather than claiming their authority as parents personally invested in or protecting the interests of their own children, PTAVE sought to frame corporal punishment as an issue of good education in the broadest sense, and of collective, even international, human rights. Among the many campaigns of PTAVE was a request to the recently founded national Human Rights Commission. The Draft Discussion paper that was prepared as a result constitutes the basis for the second main part of this chapter, in which we look at how the legitimacy of corporal punishment was framed as a debate in relation to human rights law and international administrative or legal precedent, and in relation to the 1959 UN Declaration of the Right of the Child. The debate was framed in the Human Rights Commission paper ostensibly as one between two allowable sides, even though the scales were weighted in favour of abolition. In considering the overarching question, 'who owns the body of the child?', we turn to the 1972 *Little Red Schoolbook*, which proposed in very direct language that young people have rights over their own bodies, and suggested that they inform themselves, and act accordingly. Finally, considering the curriculum of the body, the proposed banning of corporal punishment in Australian schools in the 1980s shows how this longstanding, violent practice could animate public interest in how schools operated and challenge the idea that schools were little worlds, sealed off from the outside. Classrooms of the 1980s were both closed off, secretive places and leaky sites that some were working to prise open to public scrutiny and voice.

References

Australian Institute of Family Studies. (2021, August). *Physical punishment legislation*. https://aifs.gov.au/sites/default/files/publication-documents/2107_physical_punish-ment_resource_sheet_0.pdf

Axelrod, P. (2010). No longer a 'last resort': The end of corporal punishment in the schools of Toronto. *The Canadian Historical Review, 91*(2), 261–285.

Bacchi, C., & Goodwin, S. (2016). *Poststructural policy analysis: A guide to practice.* Palgrave Macmillan.

Barrett Meyering, I. (2022). *Feminism and the making of a child rights revolution: 1969–1979.* Melbourne University Publishing. 10.2307/jj.1176767

Burns, K., Proctor, H., & Weaver, H. (2020). Modern schooling and the curriculum of the body. In T. Fitzgerald (Ed.), *Handbook of historical studies in education* (pp. 1–21). Springer. 10.1007/978-981-10-0942-6_34-1

Corporal Punishment of Children in Australia. (2023). https://www. endcorporalpunishment.org/wp-content/uploads/country-reports/Australia.pdf

Corporal-Punishment Paper. (1983, March 27). *Canberra Times,* 3.

Dewey, J. (1916). *Democracy and education.* Free Press.

Funder, K. (Ed.). (1996). *Citizen child: Australian law and children's rights.* Australian Institute of Family Studies.

Gleason, M. (2018). Metaphor, materiality and method: The central role of embodiment in the history of education. *Paedagogica Historica, 54*(1–2), 4–19. 10.1 080/00309230.2017.1355328

Global Partnership to End Violence Against Children. (n.d.-a). *Corporal punishment in schools.* https://endcorporalpunishment.org/schools/

Global Partnership to End Violence Against Children. (n.d.-b). *End corporal punishment.* https://endcorporalpunishment.org/

Hansen, S., & Jensen, J. (1972). *The little red schoolbook* (B. Thornberry, Trans.). Alister Taylor and Brolga Books. (Original work published 1969)

Holbrook, A. (1997). Rewards and punishments in New South Wales classrooms in the early twentieth century. *Critical Studies in Education, 38*(1), 1–30. 10.1080/1 7508489709556289

Holden, G.W., Wright, K.L., & Sendek, D.D. (2018). History of and progress in the movement to end corporal punishment in the United States. In B. Saunders, P. Leviner, & B. Naylor (Eds.), *Corporal punishment of children: Comparative legal and social developments towards prohibition and beyond* (pp. 293–320). Brill Nijhoff.

Human Rights Commission (1983a). *Corporal punishment in schools and the rights of the child.* (Discussion Draft Paper No. 1). https://humanrights.gov.au/sites/ default/files/HRC_DP1.pdf

Human Rights Commission (1983b). *Human Rights Commission Annual Report 1982–83* (Parliamentary paper No. 244, 1983). Commonwealth of Australia.

Hunter, I. (1994). *Rethinking the school: Subjectivity, bureaucracy, criticism.* Routledge.

Johns, R.W. (1997). [Reconsideration of the book *Death at an early age: The destruction of the hearts and minds of Negro children in the Boston Public Schools,* by J. Kozol]. *Educational Studies, 28*(1), 3–14. 10.1207/s15326993es2801_1

Kilkelly, U., & Lundy, L. (Eds.). (2017). *Children's rights.* Routledge. 10.4324/ 9781315095769

Kirk, D. (1998). *Schooling bodies: School practice and public discourse, 1880–1950.* Leicester University Press.

Kurhi, E. (2008, January 7). Hands off those kids—A 30-year crusade. *San Ramon Valley Times.* http://nospank.net/riak130.htm

Miller, A. (1983). *For your own good: Hidden cruelty in child-rearing and the roots of violence.* Farrar, Straus & Giroux.

Norlin, B. (2018). Exploring violence(s) in the history of education. *Nordic Journal of Educational History*, 5(2), 1–15. 10.36368/njedh.v5i2.115

Power, M. (n.d.). Father steals cane as a protest. https://www.nospank.net/riak80.htm

Proctor, H. (2000). Gender, grievance and bad behaviour at a NSW state high school, 1913–22. *Change: Transformations in Education*, Monograph *1*, 53–65.

Proctor, H., & Burns, K. (2017). The connected histories of mass schooling and public health. *History of Education Review*, 46(2), 118–124.

Proctor, H., Gerrard, J., & Goodwin, S. (2023). Working with and against the bureaucratic state: Histories of grassroots organising for public education reform, 1970s–1980s. *Journal of Educational Administration and History*. 10.1080/0022 0620.2023.2211911

Riak, J. (1975, June 23). An open letter of protest to the parents of the students of Dover Heights Boys' High School. https://www.nospank.net/dover.htm

Rousmaniere, K., Dehli, K., & de Coninck-Smith, N. (Eds.). (1997). *Discipline, moral regulation, and schooling: A social history*. Routledge.

Saunders, B., & Cashmore, J. (2011). Australia: The ongoing debate about ending physical punishment. In J.E. Durrant, & A.B. Smith (Eds.), *Global pathways to abolishing physical punishment: Realizing children's rights* (pp. 83–97). Routledge.

Scribner, C.F., & Warnick, B.R. (2021). *Spare the rod: Punishment and the moral community of schools*. University of Chicago Press.

Seymour, B. (1992). A sparse sparing of the rod: The changing status of student welfare and discipline in New South Wales schools. In R. Slee (Ed.), *Discipline in Australian public education: Changing policy and practice* (pp. 45–60). Australian Council for Educational Research.

Slee, R. (1992). Changing disciplinary policy in Victorian schools: A critique of the policy process. In R. Slee (Ed.), *Discipline in Australian public education: Changing policy and practice* (pp. 13–44). Australian Council for Educational Research.

Slee, R. (1995). *Changing theories and practices of discipline*. Falmer Press.

Slee, R., & Knight, T. (1992). Recent changes in discipline policies and implications for the future. In R. Slee (Ed.), *Discipline in Australian public education: Changing policy and practice* (pp. 1–12). Australian Council for Educational Research.

Wriedt, K., & Colston, M. (1979, November 19). Against violence. *Education: Journal of the N.S.W. Public School Teachers Federation*, 60(19), 450.

Yeatman, A. (1998). Activism and the policy process. In Yeatman, A. (Ed.), *Activism and the policy process* (pp. 16–35). Allen & Unwin.

14

HISTORICAL AND CONTEMPORARY PERSPECTIVES ON GENDERED SCHOOL UNIFORMS IN AUSTRALIA

Heather Weaver

The history of school uniforms in Australia is a history of ideas about the gender binary: the earliest iterations, modelled on forms of dress worn in exclusive single-sex British schools, first appeared around 1900 in Australian private schools and prestigious public secondary schools. This chapter looks at those gendered dress codes and takes them as a springboard for examining subsequent changes to school uniforms in Australia in the latter half of the 20th century—when uniform dress became ubiquitous in the nation's public schools—through to the present, with a focus on how Australian culture has represented and interpreted those changes.

Uniformity is about sameness in the face of difference. Codes of uniform dress render individual bodies of a piece. Sartorial uniformity can be seen as an 'embodied social practice' (Tynan & Godson, 2019, p. 2). The uniform serves as a vehicle for sociality, with sociality understood as the process of relating to others by action (Sillander, 2021). But in the case of school uniforms, this 'relating' is mandated rather than voluntary and can be very specific and targeted, with not only institutional affiliation, but also, often, gender, social class and internal rank designated in the fabric (Meadmore & Symes, 1997, p. 174).

School uniforms impose order on the student body—they set standards of sameness that pupils are required or at the very least expected to embody. To take an example of a longstanding boys' school in Sydney, the uniform can be a 'mould' that students are meant to fit, or a 'role' that students are meant to fulfil (Proctor, 2011). Such a regime of order can seem to work in opposition to expressions of individuality and personal creativity (Synott & Symes, 1995, pp. 140–141; also Park, 2013). An item like a school blazer can symbolise a structure that seems to allow entry into paths for some and not others.

DOI: 10.4324/9781003288671-19

Writing of boys who grew up in Sydney and Adelaide during the latter 20th century, Lovett argues that 'one's cultural, social and economic survival ... was mediated through [one's] preference in school clothing' (2013). A school blazer can present a fate that some recognise and some embrace. Others can find themselves confounded or repelled.

Symes and Meadmore construe school dress codes in Australia and beyond in terms of a cultural syntax: they see school uniforms as 'a key tactic in the production of a grammatical body' (1996, p. 190). This builds on Tyack and Cuban's assertion that 'grammar' in schooling goes beyond a regularised set of linguistic rules taught in schools: just as there is grammar that dictates the composition of words on a chalkboard, so too is there a conservative 'grammar' that dictates the look and function of schooling (1995). Schooling teaches 'grammar' not only in its lessons, but also in its rules and practices. The bodies of students, hemmed in by requirements regarding conduct and appearance, become vehicles for the popular understanding of schooling. Bidwell observes that 'the school system is responsible for a uniform product of a certain quality' (1965, p. 974). This chapter seeks to explore how schools in Australia have come to render the bodies of students themselves as a sartorially uniform and comprehensible product.

School uniforms as failed copies of gendered ideals

When a school requires that its students don, for example, a blue school blazer, the school is tying itself to a sartorial practice that goes back to longstanding institutions in 19th-century Britain such as Harrow School (Meadmore & Symes, 1996). In this way, the school is aligning itself, at least to some degree, with cultural stasis and a resistance to change. Details on the blazer can reinforce this position: Synott and Symes (1995) show how a school crest on the breast of a blazer can serve as a symbol of stability, an expression not only of the school's image of its own standing, but also of the school's connection to a larger tradition.

Butler theorises that gender identity is produced over time by a 'stylized repetition of acts' that eventuates in a 'corporeal style' (1988, pp. 519, 521). A person's 'style' can be seen as equivalent to personal taste, however, Butler notes that the embodiment of gender is 'never fully self-styled, for living styles have a history, and that history conditions and limits possibilities'. The embodiment of gender involves strategizing within and through such limits (1988, pp. 521–522). 'Style' conjures up changing fashions and fads, but it also functions as a space for the 'classic': that which is understood as perennial, transcending the latest trend or whimsy. The uniform, with its putatively static appearance, deposits itself over time into the classic sartorial space. The uniform wearer is obliged to don the same clothing day after day: repetition is the intended result of a mandatory uniform. The uniform wearer is compelled to engage in a 'stylized repetition of acts', and in this way is compelled to wear and wear again a set of garments that contributes to a particular gender identity.

And yet inherent in Butler's theory of repetition is their idea of the failed copy (1990, p. 186), which holds that a repeated act fails to perfectly emulate the act or acts that came before it. But, crucially, just as the repeated act serves as a failed copy, so too did the 'original' act. Gendered ideals always fail to be produced and reproduced (Warren, 2008, p. 299), which is to say fail to be ideally embodied, even as gendered identities are formed. Meaning and change are created in the compromise between the imagined ideal and the failed copy.

Therefore although a school uniform may seem to stand as a bulwark against individuality and change, there is more to it. If uniforms are about sameness in the face of difference, the repeated attempts at sameness also create opportunities for difference. Craik (2003, pp. 128–129) puts it this way:

> The uniform … is not as obvious as commonly thought. Uniforms have overt and covert lives. … There is a constant play between the intended symbolism of uniforms (sameness, unity, regulation, hierarchy, status, and roles) and the informal codes of wearing and denoting uniforms (subversion, individual interpretation, and difference).

The interplay between sameness and difference in uniforms hides and reveals much about gender. Uniforms have long iterated gendered ideals, with masculinity often the default (Craik, 2005; Tynan & Godson, 2019, p. 9), as seen in the history of naval attire (Geczy & Karaminas, 2017, pp. 67–84; Miller, 2015). School uniforms are no exception—they generally require the making of 'gender binary choices' (Bragg et. al., 2018; also Connell, 1996; Stephenson, 2019) because schools with dress requirements have historically tended to articulate the rules of dress in gendered terms. This is an explicit manifestation of the 'curriculum of the body' (Burns et al., 2020). Uniforms have taught students that boys and girls are to don their clothes of learning differently. Yet the gendered norms of uniform wearing can open up space for difference and change. Students may 'appear to conform' while at the same time trying to 'customize' their school dress 'in defiance' of regulations (Spencer, 2007, p. 228; also Dussel, 2005, p. 118; Swain, 2002). And the uniforms themselves diverge over time. The regulations change, both in direct response to students' wishes, and, arguably more commonly, in general response to changes in prevailing fashions and attitudes.

The rest of this chapter seeks to shed light on examples of the uniform-wearing student—the embodied young scholar—in the history and present of Australia. This exploration is a cultural history, drawing upon personal and institutional records as well as mass-marketed texts and images (found in sources such as popular fiction, magazines, newspapers and advertising campaigns) in order to further understanding of how Australian society has used school uniforms to posit statements and questions about gendered bodies.

'Well cut in regulation style': The 1900s–1930s

Regulated school attire began to appear in Australia around 1900 in schools seeking to convey superior status by emulating the clothing styles found in British Public Schools and grammar schools. Key pieces included the blazers and ties that had emerged in England on the playing fields and waterways of elite boys' schools beginning around 1860, which in turn had antecedents in men's boating and naval wear (Meadmore & Symes, 1996, pp. 212–213). It is important to note that the majority of early 20th-century Australian schools did not require a blazer or a tie, nor any specific complement of particular items: only certain expensive and/or more rigorous schools (as well as some wishing to seem so) stipulated any such attire. This led to the popular conception that the 'successful' student was uniform-clad and attended a uniform school (Meadmore & Symes, 1997, p. 177).

At first, school uniform styles in Australia were quite varied, with highly distinctive looks in girls' and boys' schools. In 1906, for example, the prestigious boys' Geelong Church of England Grammar School in the Australian state of Victoria opened an affiliated girls' school called the Hermitage. Geelong Grammar students wore a uniform drawn exactly from their counterparts at elite boys' British schools, including a blazer with school crest, collared shirt and tie (Wilmot, 1915) (Figure 14.1). The students at their new girls' school dressed quite differently. The *Australian Women's Weekly*, a remarkably widely read magazine for much of the 20th century, featured decades later a photograph of the Hermitage's 1906 opening day ('Uniform Revolution', 1958). The image shows a group of students in long white dresses: many are in high collars, punctuated by the occasional one in turned-down collar and tie; the majority seem to be wearing school-crested straw boaters, however, some wear hats

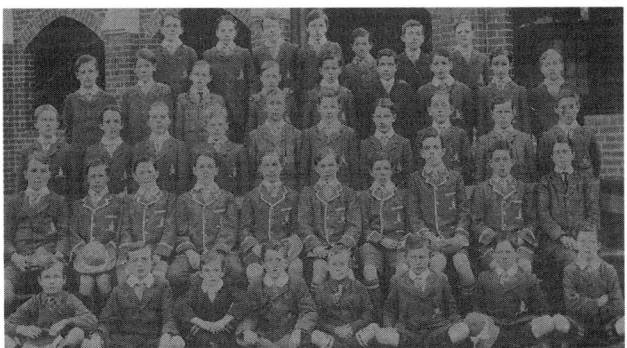

FIGURE 14.1   Group photograph of students at the boys' Geelong Grammar School in 1915.

Source: Wilmot (1915), *Junior House, Manifold House, Geelong Grammar* [Photograph], Pictures Collection, State Library Victoria.

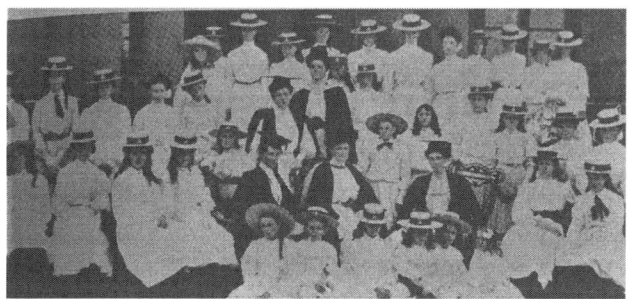

FIGURE 14.2 Group photograph of students at the girls' Hermitage School in 1906.

Source: Uniform Revolution (1958, January 22), *Australian Women's Weekly*, 29. Courtesy of Are Media Pty Limited.

without the crest, and several wear no hat at all (Figure 14.2). The sartorial variations, as subtle as they are, hint at meaningful differences, perhaps about personal circumstances, status or inclination. When compared with their boy counterparts, however, the schoolgirls come together in their sameness, so unlike are their outfits to those at Geelong. For the *Weekly*, from the vantage of a half-century later, the girls in the photograph were all of a piece, in 'high-necked, buttoned-all-down-the-front, long-sleeved' garb with 'ruched, frilled hems' and 'leg-o'-mutton sleeves' (Uniform Revolution, 1958). The main lesson the magazine offered was that such outfits would have required great domestic care: 'Garments that … had to be pressed with a flatiron represented hours of hard work' ('Uniform Revolution', 1958).

Joan Lindsay, writing from a similar mid-20th-century perspective about a girls' school in 1900 in her classic Australian novel, *Picnic at Hanging Rock*, also highlights the work involved in such clothing, but for her the effort was in the wearing of the garments rather than their maintenance: she describes schoolgirls as bodily encumbered by 'corsets pressing on the solar plexus' and 'voluminous petticoats' (1967/2012, p. 23). The school in Lindsay's novel—Appleyard College—was fictional, but as a 'select and suitably ex-pensive boarding school … for Young Ladies' (1967/2012, pp. 3–4), it was not unlike the Hermitage. (Lindsay in fact modelled Appleyard on her alma mater, Clyde Girls' Grammar School, which in the 1970s joined with the Hermitage in amalgamating with Geelong Grammar to form a co-educational school.) Like the girls of Appleyard (Gorman, 2015), the girls at the Hermitage were preserved for memory in their white muslin dresses.

But in both worlds—fiction and fact—turn-of-the-century schoolgirls donned other outfits, notably during their gymnastics lessons. Lindsay calls the gymnasium a 'Chamber of Horrors' and characterises the 'black serge bloomers' worn by the girls during gym lessons as 'mad' 'instruments of torture' (1967/2012, pp. 192–193, 197). Bloomers had originated in America in 1851 as long, loose trousers gathered at the ankle and layered underneath a long skirt, identified with the movement for women's 'rational dress' (Fischer, 2001). By the turn of the 20th century, some girls' schools had incorporated knee-length bloomers as a functional item suitable for the gymnasium. There is of course an irony in the fact that Lindsay chose to characterise as torturous a garment meant for freedom of movement, but in the novel's gymnastics scene, the use of the word 'torture' is not hyperbolic. The gymnasium, arrayed with 'various instruments for the promotion of female health and beauty', features a 'horizontal board fitted with leather straps, on which the child Sara, continually in trouble for stooping, was to pass the … hour' (Lindsay, 1967/2012, pp. 192–193). The gymnastics lesson descends into chaos when most of the girls attack one of their peers, pressing her for details about the disappearances on Hanging Rock. Sometime after the lesson, it becomes apparent that something is still very wrong for Sara, the 'youngest boarder' (Lindsay, 1967/2012, p. 203):

> From the far corner of the room now almost in darkness came a single rasping cry. Miss Lumley, under the stress of a most unpleasant afternoon, had forgotten to unfasten the leather straps that held the child Sara rigid on the horizontal board.

The space meant to promote movement, health and beauty had here turned into a space of restriction, neglect and misery. 'Rational dress' could be quite irrational.

The trend in favour of 'freedom of movement' for schoolgirls expanded beyond bloomers to the box-pleated tunic. The tunic, a garment going from the shoulders to the knees, dated back to various ancient styles. By the late 19th century starting in England, a sleeveless, pleated, woollen version was gaining acceptance in women's sporting contexts as being appropriate for competition wear. Seen as 'sexless'—pleated for mobility, but at the same time 'modest'—this tunic was worn in private spaces out of the public gaze (Atkinson, 1978). Within a few decades, the tunic had gone public as standard girls' school-uniform wear. This is seen in a 1926 advertisement in the *Australian Woman's Mirror* for a 'girls' well-made fine navy serge regulation school tunic, cut on generous lines, with three Box Pleats back and front' (Big Savings on Winter School Clothes, 1926). The advertisement was by the Sydney retail giant Anthony Hordern & Sons. (Known as Hordern's, it was around this time the largest department store in the world). Typical of this era in Australian culture, Hordern's aimed this 1926 advertisement at schoolgirls' mothers: 'Well cut in regulation style, from superior hard-wearing materials. Mothers can depend on their serviceability' (Big Savings on Winter School Clothes, 1926). Just as the clothing in the advertisement was gendered, so was the physical and emotional labour behind it (Proctor & Weaver, 2017).

The advertisement also listed navy flannel blazers together with navy serge skirts, coats and frocks, and collared blouses. When Hordern's referred to the 'regulation' aspect of the items, this was not aimed at a particular set of schools or rules. Their 'regulation' status was aspirational. Hordern's used the word at a time when the majority of Australian schools lacked uniform codes, to suggest their school garments were suited to the world of exclusive schools and required uniforms.

By about 1930, codes of mandatory school dress had coalesced in Australia into standard forms centred around key pieces such as the blazer, collared shirt and tie. As noted above, these items were not worn by the majority of Australian students, but they were now worn by enough students in many of the country's private schools and some selective public secondary schools that they had become a very recognisable and emulated look. 1930s advertisements for popular sewing patterns, aimed at Australian housewives, featured light-skinned, fair-haired children, ready for school in their blazers and ties (Figures 14.3 and 14.4). The children

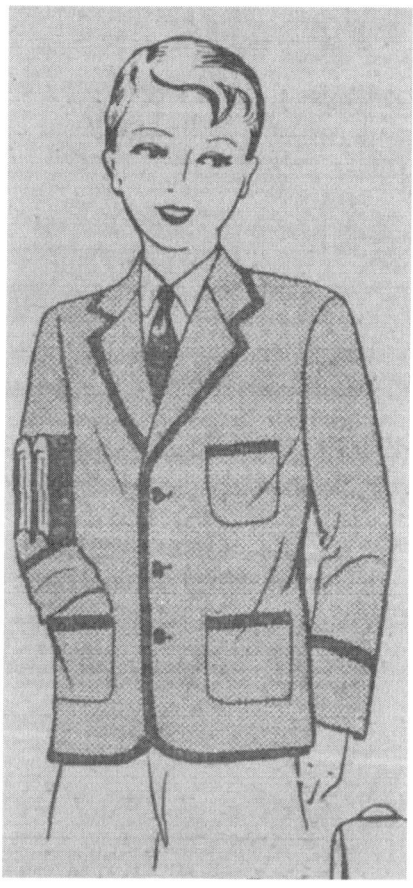

FIGURE 14.3 Idealised 1930s Australian schoolboy.

Source: Our Fashion Service and Free Pattern (1934, July 7), *Australian Women's Weekly*, 27.

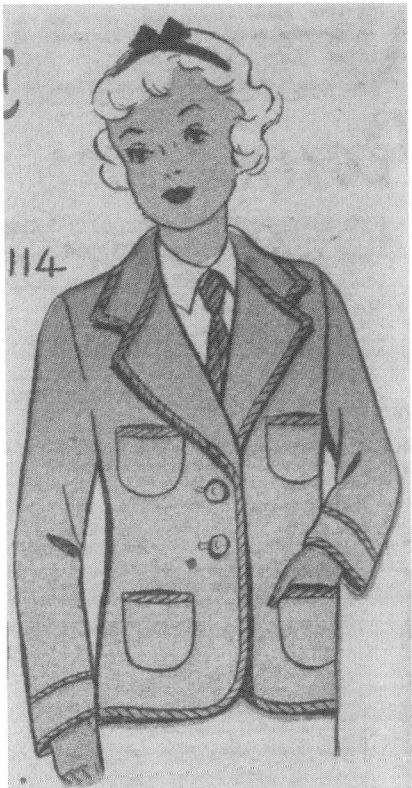

FIGURE 14.4   Idealised 1930s Australian schoolgirl.

Source: Our Fashion Service and Free Pattern (1936, March 14), *Australian Women's Weekly*, 58.

look like they could be siblings, which was not a coincidence or a particular artist's convention so much as it was a reflection of and a move to replicate Australia's dominant Anglo culture (Carey, 2006). In the case of boys, the blazer and tie drew upon well-established tropes from military and sport traditions. But in the case of girls, these pieces reflected rapidly evolving norms that sought to reconcile traditional docile femininity with new views about the modern active girl (e.g. Collins, 2010). The shift in idealised girls' school wear over these several decades must be noted. The turn-of-the-century paradigm of the schoolgirl in a long white muslin dress had been erased, replaced by a model schoolgirl in tailored blazer and tie, dressed effectively, from the waist up, as an oppositely buttoned counter-point of the model schoolboy.

Renewal and resistance: The 1940s–1970s

The blazer, shirt and tie ideal for both boys and girls appeared and reappeared in representations of Australian school wear in the decades that followed, but it underwent contestations and reinterpretations. In the 1940s, there was concern in Australia about avoiding the trend of American schoolgirls wearing oversized garments: either girls' clothing 'made several sizes too large, fit any old way round the chest and waist' or 'tweed jackets discarded by boys on war service' (Clinch, 1944; see also Cahill, 1936). This was partly an objection to the lack of school uniform codes in the United States, but it also relayed a fear that uniform codes would not necessarily prevent this sort of dressing. Here again, it was the tailoring, or lack thereof, that was perceived as making crucial statements about gender.

Throughout this period, there were objections to the ways in which traditionally British uniform styles were not appropriate for the warmer Australian climate—these too could come from a gendered perspective, as in this lead letter to the editor from an *Australian Women's Weekly* reader:

> In most Australian cities high school and college boys are often dressed up like little men to go to school; but most mothers would welcome a more free-and-easy style. There would be a great saving in money ... if the boys wore shorts and sports shirts, and it would be much healthier. To see a schoolboy in collar and tie when the temperature is round the hundred mark is pathetic. ... [B]oys ... in shorts and shirts ... look just as smart as the more dressed-up boys, and what's more they really do look like boys.
> (Fletcher, 1946)

This reader framed health in terms of avoiding heat stress, but she went on to imply a connection between gender conformity and healthiness. In saying boys 'in shorts and sports shirts' really did, as compared with their peers in collars and ties, 'look like boys', she was suggesting that being less 'dressed up' was more consonant with the true nature of boyhood (Fletcher, 1946).

Somewhat the opposite anxiety was growing about girls in school uniform. By the mid-century, there was the idea that girls, like boys, would appreciate wearing 'sports clothing' (lightweight nylon and cotton separates) to school rather than 'clumsy lace-up shoes, and a heavy, drab uniform' (Bruckell, 1965). On both girls and boys, the blazer, collar and tie no longer communicated athleticism and modernity as much as they did fustiness and impracticality. But in the case of girls, there was the added worry that old-fashioned uniforms would stand in the way of learning how to be fashionable. This dated back to the consolidation of uniform codes in the 1930s, when the question arose, 'Should not each girl have an opportunity of developing her individuality even during her school years?' (Bard, 1934). A generation later, such complaints were joined to observations about staid designs: 'The ones that students wear now are almost identical to those our parents wore. Surely a collar and tie is not necessary in a girl's uniform' (Mills, 1962). Popular concerns about 'individuality' versus uniformity tended to be about girls and their development into women: there was no similar level of concern about boys. It was girls who were expected to develop a sense of individual style.

In the 1960s, some girls' schools responded to such concerns by updating their required attire. The *Australian Women's Weekly* profiled an array of 'new-look uniforms' from across the country over two consecutive issues (Bright New Look in School Uniforms, 1963; also More New-Look School Uniforms, 1963):

> Throughout Australia students in public, private, and church schools are being given a new look, with the introduction of glamorous and practical uniforms. The days of thick serge tunics, heavy stockings, and unflattering velour hats are numbered, and in their place are uniforms with style and color.

The pages featured teenage girls happily modelling their schools' new uniforms and showing old uniforms for contrast. Fabrics included 'bright and cool gingham' and 'light, drip-dry cotton', and colours included sky blue, butter yellow, lilac, spearmint, turquoise and candy pink. Apart from the light blue, the pastel colours represented a departure from tradition. Standard colours for school dress had long been restricted to more subdued shades such as navy, grey, tan, and dark red and green. Blue had a particularly long history in school wear, dating back to British charity schools as well as exclusive institutions like Harrow, Oxford and Cambridge (Ewing, 1977, pp. 32–35; Meadmore & Symes, 1996, pp. 212–213). The modern rainbow made school seem new and fun. Indeed, at a time when the majority of students neither were required to nor did, remain in high school until the final year, some high-schoolgirls were quoted as saying that fashionably updated uniforms would motivate them to stay in school longer than if they were dressed in their old garb: 'This would encourage many girls to go on to sixth year'; and 'our new uniform … has encouraged many of us to stay at school' (Smarter School Uniforms, 1965).

Updating the old uniform was one thing, but rejecting it entirely was another. The late 1960s and 1970s proved to be a time of resistance to the school uniform (Meadmore & Symes, 1996, pp. 217–218). This was less of an option in private schools with substantial authority when it came to setting rules and, importantly, expelling students if the rules were not followed. But public schools gave students more space for opting out of sartorial conventions. This was not necessarily the intention of school administrators, but rather more often the product of ambivalence or aversion on the part of students and parents (e.g. Government Secondary Schools Discipline Committee, 1972, p. 116) coming up against a lack of enforceable policy (e.g. Morris, 1975). The wearing of school uniforms had ebbed previously: during the depression and war years of the 1930s and 1940s, many students who attended schools with uniform mandates could not meet the requirements due to financial constraints and/or material scarcity. Yet even though the 1970s were also a time of economic challenge, there was more to the retreat from uniform at this time, including the popularisation of denim and the ubiquity of casual collar-less tops, which made traditional school uniforms, with their collars and ties, their wool serge and tailoring, seem all the more outdated. But this new resistance also involved a growing sense of personal autonomy. As a *Canberra Times* reporter observed, with dismay and shock, 'It is quite clear that in some schools, the official attitude to the wearing of uniform goes quite beyond normal bounds, and almost constitutes an assault on the person and privacy of pupils. One Sydney school actually asks all girls to wear Cottontails [a brand of women's briefs]!' (Connors, 1975; also Weaver & Proctor, 2018, p. 250). The line between 'normal bounds' and the 'person and privacy of pupils' had never been fixed, but there was a growing emphasis on 'person and privacy'. Bounds that would have previously been considered 'normal' were now being questioned.

Conclusion: 'Unisex' and beyond, 1980s–present

Although uniforms had begun to emerge in Australian schools by the turn of the 20th century, it was only towards the end of the century that the overwhelming majority of schools in Australia had mandated uniform dress. The first school uniforms in Australia emerged in a handful of elite institutions around the turn of the 20th century, with highly gendered looks for boys (blazers and ties) and girls (flowing muslin dresses). By the 1930s, uniforms had become somewhat more widespread, but by no means ubiquitous: they were mandated only in certain private schools and selective public secondary schools. At this point, girls' uniforms were typically 'feminine' versions of boys': 'modern' skirts or tunics worn with blazers, collared shirts and/or ties. It was only in the last decades of the 20th century that uniforms became a standard requirement across all school sectors in Australia—public as well as private, comprehensive as well as selective, and primary as well as secondary. By the 1980s and 1990s, many public schools, not only secondary schools but also primary schools, had instituted garments such as jumpers, polo shirts, sport shorts and sunhats meant to be worn interchangeably by boys and girls. These items were categorised as 'unisex', a word coined in the late 1960s to describe clothing and hairstyles that were aimed at both men and women, boys and girls (Antonelli & Fisher, 2017, pp. 261–262; Hines, 2015). This was in line with new official frameworks in the 1980s, for example, the Gender

Equity Education Policy instituted by the Australian Capital Territory Schools Authority in 1987, which insisted on the importance in the context of schooling of 'the treatment of members of both sex groups as human beings of equal value and with equal rights and the potential to undertake the full range of human activities'. The phenomenon of boy and girl classmates donning the same school jumper could now be understood as a visual representation of the egalitarianism inherent in Australia's self-concept.

Yet the movement could 'feel like an uphill battle at times'—this was the description given by primary-school teacher and gender-equity consultant Kate Rosewarn, who said she would 'like to see a unisex school uniform' (Kennedy, 1990). The problem when it came to school dress lay in negotiating the difference between traditional gendered norms and new ideals. Such negotiations, even with modernising intentions, could easily go in the direction of conservatism. A South Australian public high school in the 1990s touted its 'fresh new look', in which 'students have a wide choice of unisex clothing for everyday wear'. In actuality, this meant the choice of 'unisex navy or grey ... style shorts' and 'long grey trousers for boys and the traditional skirts for girls', combined with 'navy or white polo shirts' (Fresh New Look at Victor High, 1995). Even in an encouraging 'unisex' school environment—a public school seemingly unencumbered by old-fashioned private school styles—many girls in Australia could still by the end of the century be expected to wear 'traditional skirts'.

Enter the recent 'push for pants'. It was only in 2017 and 2018 that several Australian states announced uniform policies mandating shorts and pants options for all government school students (Osbich, 2018). The conservative 'grammatical body' holds sway in the Australian imagination—many private schools in Australia still mandate skirts or dresses for girls (Kleyn, 2019). The shift towards 'trousers for girls ... unisex shirts, and hoodies now often for both sexes' (Williams, 2017) is in many respects newly underway (Heath, 2016; Mergler, 2017).

A school uniform that today demands skirt- or dress-wearing forces a stark differentiation of girl from boy (Happel, 2013). This differentiation, however, is arguably just as enforced by the schools that mandate the wearing of shorts or trousers. The idea of a boy in a dress can elicit a degree of fear and apprehension in Australia (Gerrard, 2020). A schoolboy in a skirt or pinafore would have long been accepted only in the context of a passing joke or prank, or as theatre, as was the case when UK schoolboys wearing skirts appeared in Australian media coverage employing elements of prank and theatre to protest requirements that they wear trousers in warm weather (UK Schoolboys, 2017). There is a growing space in the culture, however—opened up by 'gender benders' such as Little Richard, David Bowie, Billy Porter and Harry Styles—for the serious fact that some people who were assigned male at birth may occasionally or regularly prefer to wear traditionally 'female' clothing. In the context of schooling, this space is allowing for the idea that all students deserve the same sartorial freedoms and options: a few schools in Australia are now letting all of their students have all of the clothing options that were once limited to a particular gender, including allowing boys to wear dresses or skirts (Fitzsimmons, 2021).

When a school requires that its students wear a uniform, it is often teaching them to embody a set of gendered values. These values may be particular to an institution, but whatever a school's motto, whatever its traditions, the donning of a uniform teaches students that they are literally of a piece, cut from the same cloth. The irony inherent in this curriculum of sameness is that it has also long been a curriculum of twoness, an embodiment of the gender binary. To what extent school uniforms can continue to go beyond both sameness and twoness to instead sanction individuality remains to be seen.

References

Antonelli, P., & Fisher, M.M. (2017). *Items: Is fashion modern?* The Museum of Modern Art.

Atkinson, P. (1978). Fitness, feminism and schooling. In S. Delamont, & L. Duffin (Eds.), *The nineteenth-century woman: Her cultural and physical world* (pp. 92–133). Croom Helm.

Bard, F. (1934, December 15). School uniforms. *Australian Women's Weekly*, 21.

Bidwell, C.E. (1965). The school as a formal organization. In J. March (Ed.), *Handbook of organizations* (pp. 972–1022). Routledge.

Big Savings on Winter School Clothes at Anthony Hordern's. (1926, April 6). *Australian Woman's Mirror*, 41.

Bragg, S., Renold, E., Ringrose, J., & Jackson, C. (2018). 'More than boy, girl, male, female': Exploring young people's views on gender diversity within and beyond school contexts. *Sex Education, 18*(4), 420–434.

The Bright New Look in School Uniforms. (1963, June 12). 'Teenagers' weekly' supplement to the *Australian Women's Weekly*, 4–5.

Bruckell, N. (1965, August 11). Suggestions for the Wyndham Scheme. *Australian Women's Weekly*, 64.

Burns, K., Proctor, H., & Weaver, H. (2020). Modern schooling and the curriculum of the body. In T. Fitzgerald (Ed.), *Handbook of historical studies in education* (pp. 1–21). Springer. 10.1007/978-981-10-0942-6_34-1

Butler, J. (1988). Performative acts and gender constitution: An essay in phenomenology and feminist theory. *Theatre Journal, 40*(4), 519–531.

Butler, J. (1990). *Gender trouble: Feminism and the subversion of identity.* Routledge.

Cahill, F. (1936, November 21). School uniforms. *Australian Women's Weekly*, 19.

Carey, J. (2006). White anxieties and the articulation of race: The women's movement and the making of White Australia, 1910s–1930s. In J. Carey, & C. McLisky (Eds.), *Creating white Australia* (pp. 195–213). Sydney University Press.

Clinch, L. (1944, October 28). U.S. dress designers fight 'Sloppy Sue' craze. *Australian Women's Weekly*, 9.

Collins, T.J.R. (2010). Athletic fashion, *Punch*, and the creation of the new woman. *Victorian Periodicals Review, 43*(3), 309–335.

Connell, R.W. (1996). Teaching the boys: New research on masculinity, and gender strategies for schools. *Teachers College Record, 98*(2), 206–235.

Connors, L. (1975, May 26). Education '75: Voices from the world of roll-calls and chalk dust. *Canberra Times*, 2.

Craik, J. (2003). The cultural politics of the uniform. *Fashion Theory, 7*(2), 127–147.

Craik, J. (2005). *Uniforms exposed: From conformity to transgression*. Berg.

Dussel, I. (2005). The shaping of a citizenship with style: A history of uniforms and vestimentary codes in Argentinean public schools. In M. Lawn, & I. Grosvenor (Eds.), *Materialities of schooling: Design, technology, objects, routines* (pp. 97–124). Symposium Books.

Ewing, E. (1977). *History of children's costume*. Scribner.

Fischer, G.V. (2001). *Pantaloons & power: A nineteenth-century dress reform in the United States*. Kent State University Press.

Fitzsimmons, C. (2021, May 2). Kids can be comfortable without judgement: The schools adopting gender-neutral uniforms. *Sydney Morning Herald*. https://www.smh.com.au/national/nsw/kids-can-be-comfortable-without-judgement-the-schools-adopting-gender-neutral-uniforms-20210427-p57msv.html

Fletcher, C. (1946, August 10). Australian schoolboys overdressed. *Australian Women's Weekly*, 28.

Fresh New Look at Victor High. (1995, January 24). *Victor Harbor Times*, 8.

Geczy, A., & Karaminas, V. (2017). *Fashion and masculinities in popular culture*. Routledge.

Gerrard, J. (2020). Boys in dresses: Same-sex marriage, children and the politics of equivalence. *Australian Feminist Studies, 35*(103), 70–80.

Gorman, A. (2015, August 6). Oz stylewatch: Still haunted by Picnic at Hanging Rock, 40 years on. *The Guardian*. https://www.theguardian.com/fashion/2015/aug/06/oz-stylewatch-still-haunted-by-picnic-at-hanging-rock-40-years-on

Government Secondary Schools Discipline Committee. (1972). *Discipline in secondary schools in Western Australia*. Education Department of Western Australia.

Happel, A. (2013). Ritualized girling: School uniforms and the compulsory performance of gender. *Journal of Gender Studies, 22*(1), 92–96.

Heath, N. (2016, April 22). It's 2016. Why are school uniforms gender-specific? Special Broadcasting Service.

Hines, A. (2015, May 13). How his'n'her ponchos became a thing: A history of unisex fashion. *Smithsonian Magazine*. https://www.smithsonianmag.com/arts-culture/his-her-ponchoes-became-thing-history-unisex-fashion-180955240/

Kennedy, J. (1990, June 25). All men (and women) are created equal. *Canberra Times*, 9.

Kleyn, B. (2019, January 21). Many private schools resist push for pants, shorts options for girls' uniforms. ABC News. https://www.abc.net.au/news/2019-01-21/girls-school-uniforms-rules-shorts-pants-qld/10640388

Lindsay, J. (1967/2012). *Picnic at hanging rock*. Viking.

Lovett, T. (2013). 'What the blazers?' The effect of cultural symbols on class identity and learning outcomes. *Journal of Educational Enquiry, 12*(1), 1–14.

Meadmore, D., & Symes, C. (1996). Of uniform appearance: A symbol of school discipline and governmentality. *Discourse: Studies in the Cultural Politics of Education, 17*(2), 209–225.

Meadmore, D., & Symes, C. (1997). Keeping up appearances: Uniform policy for school diversity? *British Journal of Education Studies*, *45*(2), 174–186.

Mergler, A. (2017, January 9). Why do we still make girls wear skirts and dresses as school uniform? The Conversation. https://theconversation.com/why-do-we-still-make-girls-wear-skirts-and-dresses-as-school-uniform-69280

Miller, A. (2015). Clothes make the man: Naval uniform and masculinity in the early nineteenth century. *Journal for Maritime Research*, *17*(2), 147–154.

Mills, H. (1962, August 1). A uniform uniform for girls? 'Teenagers' weekly' supplement to the *Australian Women's Weekly*, 2.

More new-look school uniforms. (1963, June 19). 'Teenagers' weekly' supplement to the *Australian Women's Weekly*, 4–5.

Morris, A. (1975, April 16). Are school uniforms really necessary? *Australian Women's Weekly*, 7.

Osbich, L. (2018, August 1). Gender-neutral school uniforms: Queensland and New South Wales join the push for pants. School Governance. https://www.schoolgovernance.net.au/news/2018/08/02/gender-neutral-school-uniforms-queensland-and-new-south-wales-join-the-push-for-pants

Our fashion service and free pattern. (1934, July 7). *Australian Women's Weekly*, 27.

Our fashion service and free pattern. (1936, March 14). *Australian Women's Weekly*, 58.

Park, J. (2013). Do school uniforms lead to uniform minds? School uniforms and appearance restrictions in Korean middle schools and high schools, *Fashion Theory*, *17*(2), 159–177.

Proctor, H. (2011). Masculinity and social class, tradition and change: The production of 'young Christian gentlemen' at an elite Australian boys' school. *Gender and Education*, *23*(7), 843–856.

Proctor, H., & Weaver. H. (2017). Creating an educational home: Mothering for schooling in the *Australian Women's Weekly*, 1943–1960. *Paedagogica Historica*, *53*(1–2), 49–70.

Sillander, K. (2021). Introduction: Qualifying sociality through values. *Anthropological Forum*, *31*(1), 1–18.

Smarter school uniforms. (1965, October 13). 'Teenagers' weekly' supplement to the *Australian Women's Weekly*, 84.

Spencer, S. (2007). A uniform identity: Schoolgirl snapshots and the spoken visual. *History of Education*, *36*(2), 227–246.

Stephenson, K. (2019). Uniform adoption in English Public Schools, 1830–1930. In J. Tynan, & L. Godson (Eds.), *Uniform: Clothing and discipline in the modern world* (pp. 67–86). Bloomsbury Visual Arts.

Swain, J. (2002). The right stuff: Fashioning an identity through clothing in a junior school. *Gender and Education*, *14*(1), 53–69.

Symes, C., & Meadmore. D. (1996). Force of habit: The school uniform as a body of knowledge. *Counterpoints*, *29*, 171–191.

Synott, J., & Symes, C. (1995). The genealogy of the school: An iconography of badges and mottoes. *British Journal of Sociology of Education*, *16*(2), 139–152.

Tyack, D., & Cuban, L. (1995). *Tinkering toward utopia: A century of public school reform*. Harvard University Press.

Tynan, J., & Godson, L. (2019). Understanding uniform: An introduction. In J. Tynan, & L. Godson (Eds.), *Uniform: Clothing and discipline in the modern world* (pp. 1–22). Bloomsbury Visual Arts.

UK schoolboys wear skirts to protest against shorts ban, cope with summer heat. (2017, June 23). ABC News. https://www.abc.net.au/news/2017-06-23/uk-schools-boys-wear-skirts-protest-shorts-ban-cope-with-heat/8645352

Uniform revolution. (1958, January 22). *Australian Women's Weekly*, 29.

Warren, J.T. (2008). Performing difference: Repetition in context. *Journal of International and Intercultural Communication*, *1*(4), 290–308.

Weaver, H., & Proctor, H. (2018). The question of the spotted muumuu: How the *Australian Women's Weekly* manufactured a vision of the normative school mother and child, 1930s–1980s. *History of Education Quarterly*, *58*(2), 229–260.

Wilmot, G.C. (1915). *Junior House, Manifold House, Geelong Grammar* [Photograph]. Pictures Collection, State Library Victoria.

Williams, S. (2017, March 3). Nothing uniform about school uniforms now. *Sydney Morning Herald*. https://www.smh.com.au/national/nsw/nothing-uniform-about-school-uniforms-now-20170302-gup7ll.html

INDEX